FUNCTIONAL NEUROLOGY

# CONSIDERING CONSCIOUSNESS CLINICALLY

# FUNCTIONAL NEUROLOGY

## *GERRY LEISMAN AND JOAV MERRICK – SERIES EDITORS –*

ISRAEL

**Neuroimmunity and the Brain-Gut Connection**
*Aristo Vojdani (Editor)*
2015 - 4th Quarter. ISBN: 978-1-63483-969-3
(Hardcover)

**Considering Consciousness Clinically**
*Gerry Leisman and Joav Merrick (Editors)*
2016 - 1st Quarter. ISBN: 978-1-63484-260-0
(Hardcover)

**Neuroplasticity in Learning and Rehabilitation**
*Gerry Leisman and Joav Merrick (Editors)*
2016 - 1st Quarter. ISBN: 978-1-63484-305-8
(Hardcover)

FUNCTIONAL NEUROLOGY

# CONSIDERING CONSCIOUSNESS CLINICALLY

GERRY LEISMAN
AND
JOAV MERRICK
EDITORS

NOVA BIOMEDICAL

*New York*

**Library of Congress Cataloging-in-Publication Data**

ISBN: 978-1-63484-260-0

Library of Congress Control Number: 2015956837

*Published by Nova Science Publishers, Inc. † New York*

# CONTENTS

# INTRODUCTION

In: Considering Consciousness Clinically
Editors: Gerry Leisman and Joav Merrick

ISBN: 978-1-63484-260-0


*Chapter 1*

# CONSIDERING CONSCIOUSNESS CLINICALLY

***Gerry Leisman, MD, PhD[1-3,*], Calixto Machado, MD, PhD, FAAN[3] and Joav Merrick, MD, MMedSc, DMSc[4-8]***

[1]The National Institute for Brain and Rehabilitation Sciences, Nazareth, Israel
[2]Biomechanics Laboraatory, ORT-Braude College of Engineering, Karmiel, Israel
[3]Institute for Neurology and Neurosurgery, Universidad de Ciencias Médicas de la Habana, Facultad Manuel Fajardo, Havana, Cuba
[4]National Institute of Child Health and Human Development, Jerusalem
[5]Office of the Medical Director, Health Services, Division for Intellectual and Developmental Disabilities, Ministry of Social Affairs and Social Services, Jerusalem
[6]Division of Pediatrics, Hadassah Hebrew University Medical Center, Mt Scopus Campus, Jerusalem, Israel
[7]Kentucky Children's Hospital, University of Kentucky College of Medicine, Lexington, Kentucky, United States
[8]Center for Healthy Development, School of Public Health, Georgia State University, Atlanta, United States of America

## ABSTRACT

Intensive care has led to an increase in the number of patients who survive after severe acute brain damage. Most comatose patients who survive begin to awaken and recover gradually within 2–4 weeks. Although some of these individuals lastingly lose all brain function leading to brain death (BD), oftentimes this state is treated as synonymous with the death of the individual. Nonetheless, other individuals progress to "wakeful unawareness" defined as vegetative state (VS). Disorders of consciousness (DOC)

* Correspondence: Professor Gerry Leisman, Director, The National Institute for Brain and Rehabilitation Sciences, Biomechanics Laboratory, Department of Mechanical Engineering, ORT-Braude College of Engineering, Snunit 51 Street, POBox 78, IL-21982 Karmiel, Israel. E-mail: gerry.leisman@staff.nazareth.ac.il

terminology may be useful clinically, but does little to explain the nature of consciousness.

## Introduction

Disorders of consciousness (DOC) represent one of the most complex and crucial challenges for neuroscientists. A precise and reliable assessment of the arousal and awareness of consciousness in patients with severe brain damage would allow for a comprehensible classification of DOC. Intensive care has led to an increase in the number of patients who survive after severe acute brain damage. Most comatose patients who survive begin to awaken and recover gradually within 2–4 weeks. Although some of these individuals lastingly lose all brain function leading to brain death (BD), oftentimes this state is treated as synonymous with the death of the individual. Nonetheless, other individuals progress to "wakeful unawareness" defined as vegetative state (VS). DOC terminology may be useful clinically but does little to explain the nature of consciousness.

The clinical diagnostic nomenclature includes five abnormal states of consciousness that can result from a brain injury: stupor, coma, persistent vegetative state, locked-in syndrome, and brain death.

Stupor is a state in which the patient is unresponsive but can be aroused briefly by a strong stimulus, such as sharp pain. Coma is a state in which the patient is totally unconscious, unresponsive, unaware, and non-arousable. Patients in a coma do not respond to external stimuli, such as pain or light, and do not have sleep-wake cycles. Coma results from widespread and diffuse trauma to the brain, including the cerebral hemispheres of the upper brain and the lower brain or brainstem. Coma generally is of short duration, lasting a few days to a few weeks. After this time, some patients gradually come out of the coma, some progress to a vegetative state, and others die.

## Vegetative state

Patients in a vegetative state are unconscious and unaware of their surroundings, but they continue to have a sleep-wake cycle and can have periods of alertness. Unlike coma, where the patients eyes are closed, patients in a vegetative state often open their eyes and may move, groan, or show reflex responses. A vegetative state can result from three main neuropathological patterns: widespread and bilateral lesions of the cerebral cortex, diffuse damage of intra- and subcortical connections in the cerebral hemispheres white matter, and necrosis of the thalamus (1).

Anoxia, or lack of oxygen to the brain, which is a common complication of cardiac arrest, can also bring about a vegetative state, although severe brain injury of different etiologies may also lead to this state.

Many patients emerge from a vegetative state within a few weeks, but those who do not recover within 30 days are said to be in a persistent vegetative state (PVS). The chances of recovery depend on the extent of injury to the brain and the patient's age, with younger patients having a better chance of recovery than older patients. Generally adults have a 50 percent chance and children a 60 percent chance of recovering consciousness from a PVS within the first 6 months. The Multi-Society Task Force on PVS has defined the precise use of the terms persistent and permanent. "Persistent refers only to a condition of past and continuing disability with an uncertain future, whereas permanent implies irreversibility." This Task Force likewise wrote that "a patient in a persistent vegetative state becomes permanently vegetative when the diagnosis of irreversibility can be established with a high degree of clinical certainty." According to the etiology, a period of observation has been proposed to define when a persistent vegetative state, has become a permanent vegetative state:" three months for postanoxic encephalopathy and one year for traumatic injury (2, 3).

Nonetheless, after a year, the chances that a PVS patient will regain consciousness are very low and most patients who do recover consciousness experience significant disability. The longer a patient is in a PVS, the more severe the resulting disabilities will be. Rehabilitation can contribute to recovery, but many patients never progress to the point of being able to take care of themselves.

## LOCKED-IN SYNDROME

Locked-in syndrome is a condition in which a patient is aware and awake, but cannot move or communicate due to complete paralysis of the body. Unlike PVS, in which the upper portions of the brain are damaged and the lower portions are spared, locked-in syndrome is caused by damage to specific portions of the lower brain and brainstem with no damage to the upper brain. Most locked-in syndrome patients can communicate through movements and blinking of their eyes, which are not affected by the paralysis. Some patients may have the ability to move certain facial muscles as well. The majority of locked-in syndrome patients do not regain motor control, but several devices are available to help patients communicate.

DOC nomenclature cannot be used as terms in which to understand and explain conscious experience. While consciousness has been variously defined in the literature, its operational definition in the neurosciences is largely problematic for a variety of reasons. Convention portrays consciousness as an emergent property of classical computer-like activities in brain's neural networks. The prevailing views in this camp are that patterns of neural networks correlate with mental states that synchronous network oscillations in the thalamus and cortex temporally bind information, and that consciousness emerges as novel property of computational complexity among neurons (4).

## DEATH

What we mean by "death" that includes the absence of consciousness in a physiological sense is puzzling. While we know a dead body when we see one and death appears to us as a real event; being dead as an indisputable condition. Yet it turns out that even the dead body retains, for a while, some residual processes of life. Some individual cells still live; some "nests of cells" still communicate. But no one would argue that the human being is still alive just because every isolated process that might be called life has not yet ceased.

Much more complicated are those cases when a crucial part of the body-the brain-has died, yet the rest of the body, including the heart, is maintained by our technological interventions. In the past, whole-brain death led imminently and irreversibly to the death of the whole person; the entire body shut down. In the age of modern medicine, this process of shutting down is potentially suspended, making it difficult to know when or whether death has occurred.

The brain can lose function or be irreversibly damaged in a variety of ways. Certain insults will destroy the actual brain tissue anatomy, while others will lead to loss of function due to anoxic "starvation" of cells in the brain. While we can generate rules based on the interaction between environmental and anatomical circumstances, exceptions to those rules make the development of universals and therefore a definition of death difficult.

Anoxic conditions typically result from lack of oxygenated blood flow, which is often a direct result of cardiac arrest (asystole), severe brain swelling, drug intoxication and strokes. Under ischemic or anoxic conditions, the different parts of the brain succumb at different rates. After only a few minutes (~ 2-4), the cerebrum and cerebellum may suffer irreparable damage. The brainstem is much more resilient, however, and may be revived after many minutes (~ 15-20) of anoxia. It is this resilience that enables the condition known as the "persistent vegetative state," in which a person's brainstem continues to function after the upper brain has been destroyed or rendered non-functional. Such an individual entirely lacks cerebral functions of self-awareness or purposeful communication. "Awake but unaware," he exhibits brainstem functions of spontaneous breathing, reflexes to light and pain stimulus, and sleep-wake cycles. This is in contrast to wholly "brain dead" patients who have no functional brainstem and exhibit none of these traits. If anoxia persists, the brainstem too will eventually become damaged beyond the possibility of revival, in many instances. While this is not the only neuropathological scenario explaining this state, it is one example of our being able to state that the entire brain has died, and lacking medical intervention the body will undergo rigor mortis and putrefaction. However, if a mechanical ventilator is instituted quickly enough to a victim who has suffered death of the whole brain, the heart may be resuscitated and circulation and other bodily functions may be restored, including brain function. This individual, sustained on a respirator and exhibiting total and irreversible lack of all functions of the entire brain, is considered by clinicians to be "brain-dead."

## BRAIN DEATH

Clinicians generally employ the term "brain death" to refer to a person whose whole brain has died and who is thus declared dead within standard medical practice. This usage has been criticized widely including by the Institute of Medicine (IOM), since it seems to present an ambiguity between a "dead organism," i.e., a person who is declared dead due to brain injury, and a "dead organ," i.e., the brain itself. When discussing donation from those who have normally been called "brain dead," the IOM recommends the modified term "donation after neurological determination of death," or DNDD (5). The question in dispute is precisely whether those who are brain dead should in fact be declared dead.

As thinkers began to wrestle with the new problems of death that confront us in the age of ventilators, a salient distinction was made between death of the organism as a whole and death of the whole organism. The latter term would imply that all processes that could be called "life" have ceased in an individual for whom they once were operative. It is that absolute lifelessness that happens sometime after the human person has died. The death of the "organism as a whole," by comparison, is a much more difficult concept to grasp. To say that there is an organism as a whole implies that there is something (someone) that (who) exists over and above the organism's individual material parts. This entity that exists "over and above its parts" is mortal in a way that the parts of which it is composed are not. Put differently, the death of the organism as a whole can leave behind living components that contributed, perhaps crucially, to the organism's "alive-ness" while it was still living, but those components taken separately are not "a" living organism.

Once this notion of a mortal organism as "a whole" is accepted, the task is set to determine what life-like activities of its component parts can persist without being absolute indicators of continuing organismal life. No one has trouble with positing the co-existence of life in isolated cells with death of the organism as a whole. Yet the advent of the ventilator introduces a much more difficult case: continued function in some of the living parts of an organism after the organism, itself, may already have died.

## WHAT IS DEATH?

This leaves us with a series of rather difficult questions: Is the death of the person equivalent to the death of the integrated organism functioning as a whole? Is the wholly brain dead person still functioning as a whole organism? Are there other physiological failures besides that of the whole brain that might signal that death has occurred? What functions of the body are necessary for the human person to continue living? Can we really ever know? And if not, is death better defined "the old-fashioned way," as the permanent and irreversible cessation of breathing and heartbeat, when the individual is indisputably dead as seen through the prism of ordinary human experience? While these are not physiological questions alone, we cannot address them philosophically without a more detailed understanding of modern physiology-that is, of how the parts of the body relate to the human whole.

The "brainstem" formulation and the "higher brain" formulation of the definition of death both challenge the standard paradigm by suggesting that it has not adequately articulated the basic concept of death. The practical consequence of a successful challenge from either of these camps would be an expansion-either small or large-of the class of patients considered to be dead by neurological criteria, i.e., dead despite the continuation of ventilator-supported somatic functioning. A third challenge to the standard paradigm is of a much different sort. Shewmon (3-5) reports an understanding that has thrown the standard paradigm of the physiological and philosophical understanding of death into uncertainty. Shewmon (6) argues that that if we accept the definition of death as the loss of integrative function of the organism as a whole, then we cannot consider brain dead patients to be dead. And, conversely, if we maintain that brain dead patients are indeed dead, then we must abandon the loss of integrative functioning as the underlying definition.

Shewmon has shown that neither bodily disintegration nor asystole necessarily follow imminently after brain death (6). Over one hundred documented cases demonstrate chronic survival past a week's time, with one extreme case surviving over 14 years. Furthermore, he demonstrates that factors such as age, aetiology, and underlying somatic integrity variably affect the survival probability of brain dead patients. Thus, not only is asystole not necessarily imminent upon brain death, but also it is the integrity of the rest of the body (the underlying somatic plasticity) and not the condition of the brain that most strongly influences survival.

## Spinal shock

Shewmon also argues against the consensus that the somatic disintegration that is observed in brain dead patients has as its cause the loss of neural regulatory centres; instead, he presents clinical evidence that dis-integration may be explained by the condition known as "spinal shock." Spinal shock is a transient condition that occurs following a sudden acute spinal cord injury, resulting in the temporary loss of function of the spinal region below the lesion. Such functions may be regained after 2 to 6 weeks, and include autonomic reflexes, sympathetic and parasympathetic tone, and thermoregulation. In several brain dead patients in whom life-support is sustained long enough, this loss and subsequent recovery of spinal cord regulation has been observed (7, 8).

Shewmon (8) build on these arguments in a 2001 paper that looks directly at the issue of integration and integrative unity. His philosophical exploration of these notions leads him to the following conclude that the body has no integrator but rather the holistic property of integration. In support of this idea, Shewmon discusses the various functions of the organism that qualify as integrative. Some of these seem to warrant the designation "brain-mediated," but many others do not. Among those that do not are, for example, wound-healing, immunological defence of "self" against "non-self," proportional growth, and even successful gestation of a foetus. These functions, and many others he names, have been exhibited by at least some brain dead bodies. Shewmon is careful to point out that calling these functions "non-brain-mediated" does not mean that the brain has nothing to do with them in an intact organism.

## Consciousness

While the content of consciousness is mainly a function of the higher brain, arousal or the capacity for consciousness resides mostly in the brainstem. The brainstem and the higher brain play an important role in directing the integrative functions of an organism. Integrative functions are those complex processes and spontaneous innate activities that involve communication, coordination, and regulation of several subsystems within the body. Examples include respiration, heartbeat, blood pressure, temperature regulation, coordinated muscle movement, neuroendocrine control, and response to light and sound. Yet while some of these integrated functions directly correspond to a function in the brain (such as the ability to moderate the depth and pace of breathing), others (such as blood-pressure and body temperature regulation) are less clearly dependent on the brain's regulation. The extent to which brainstem regulation is necessary for somatically integrative functioning is a central matter of controversy. Clearly, however, the ability to behave in an integrative way is the some and substance of consciousness. That is while there may well be profound anatomical compromises to the nervous system, if the individual's nervous system can behave in an integrative fashion, then there is no functional compromise and there is a possibility of recovery through plasticity.

We can easily measure and quantify stages of the continuum of consciousness, at least from coma to states of elation exemplified in Figure 1.

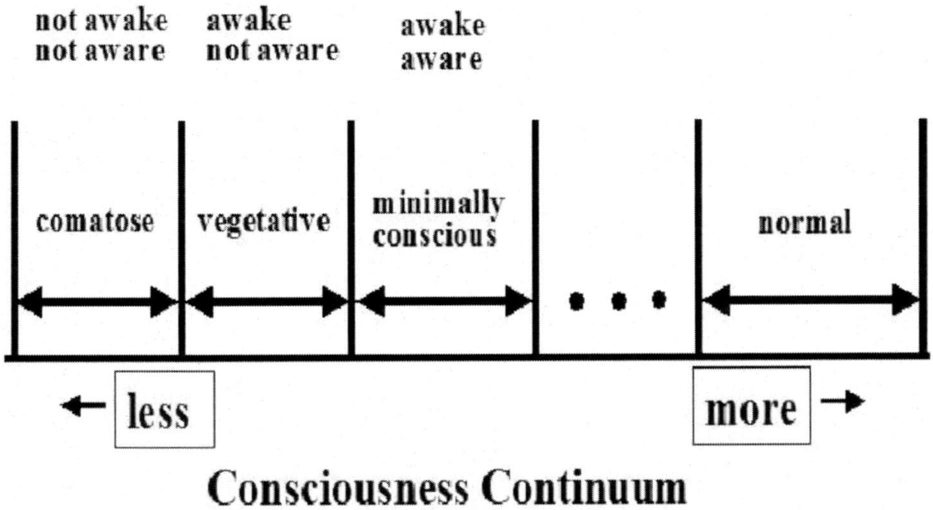


Figure 1. Clinically compromised states of consciousness.

We can actually see these functional disconnectivities in sleep (9). In sleep, brain areas loose ability to communicate with each other as compared to awake subjects who create responses in different destinations unlike sleep subjects who are more likely to create responses to single or fewer destinations. Reduced brain consciousness is associated with breakdown into non-coherent activity. Consciousness then could be considered to be the ability of the brain to integrate information with consciousness being the coherent communication between brain areas. Clinically altered states seem to be a compromise in that integration process. The result is in some cases that these altered states of consciousness can be seen as a dysfunction resulting in primitive awareness of self and the environment.

## CONCLUSION

The unity of consciousness is based on a "centrencephalic system" that includes the reticular formation and thalamus. While it is not known which portions of the brain are responsible for cognition and consciousness; what little is known points to substantial interconnections among the brainstem, subcortical structures and the neocortex. Thus, the 'higher brain' may well exist only as a metaphorical concept, and not in reality. The role of cortex allows for the interface between world, the individual's body and the conscious self as well as well as in the integration of sensory input and motor output. Functional disconnectivities represent the behavioural traits observed and reconnection may be engineered. Nonetheless, it is important to emphasize that we cannot simply differentiate and locate arousal as a function of the

ARAS, and awareness as a function of the cerebral cortex. Substantial interconnections among the brainstem, subcortical structures and the neocortex, are essential for subserving and integrating both components of human consciousness (10).

## REFERENCES


[1] Kinney HC, Korein J, Panigrahy A, Dikkes P, Goode R. Neuropathological findings in the brain of Karen Ann Quinlan. The role of the thalamus in the persistent vegetative state. N Engl J Med 1994;330:1469-75.

[2] The Multi-Society Task Force on PVS. Medical aspects of the persistent vegetative state (1). N Engl J Med 1994;330:1499-1508.

[3] The Multi-Society Task Force on PVS. Medical aspects of the persistent vegetative state. N Engl J Med. 1994;330:1572-9.

[4] Leisman G, Koch P. Continuum model of mnemonic and amnesic phenomena. J Int Neuropsychol Soc 2000;6:589-603

[5] Institute of Medicine. Organ donation: Opportunities for action. Washington, DC: National Academies Press, 2006.

[6] Shewmon DA. Chronic "brain death": Meta-analysis and conceptual consequences. Neurology 1998;51(6):1538-45.

[7] Shewmon DA. Spinal shock and "brain death": Somatic pathophysiological equivalence and implications for the integrative-unity rationale. Spinal Cord 1999;37:313-24.

[8] Shewmon DA. The brain and somatic integration: Insights into the standard biological rationale for equating "brain death" with death. J Med Philos 2001;26(5):457-78.

[9] Tononi G, Edelman GM. Consciousness and complexity. Science 1998; 282(5395):1846-51.

[10] Plum F. Coma and related global disturbances of the human conscious state. In: Peters A, ed. Cerebral cortex. New York: Plenum, 1991:359-425.

# Section one: Consciousness

In: Considering Consciousness Clinically
Editors: Gerry Leisman and Joav Merrick

ISBN: 978-1-63484-260-0


*Chapter 2*

# NETWORKS OF CONSCIOUS EXPERIENCE: COMPUTATIONAL NEUROSCIENCE IN UNDERSTANDING LIFE, DEATH AND CONSCIOUSNESS

***Gerry Leisman, MD, PhD[1,2]* and Paul Koch, PhD[3]***

[1]The National Institute for Brain and Rehabilitation Sciences, Nazareth, Israel
[2]Institute for Neurology and Neurosurgery,
Universidad de Ciencias Médicas de la Habana,
Facultad Manuel Fajardo, Havana, Cuba
[3]Retired, Sienalunga, Italy

## ABSTRACT

We demonstrate brain locations appearing to correlate with consciousness, but not being directly responsible for it. Technology reveals that brain activity is associated with consciousness but is not equivalent to it. We examine how consciousness occurs at critical levels of complexity. Conventional explanations portray consciousness as an emergent property of classical computer-like activities in the brain's neural networks. Prevailing views in this camp are that patterns of neural network activities correlate with mental states, that synchronous network oscillations in the thalamus and cerebral cortex temporally bind information, and that consciousness emerges as a novel property of computational complexity among neurons. A hard-wired theory is enigmatic for explaining consciousness because the nature of subjective experience, or 'qualia'- 'inner life' is a "hard problem" to understand; binding spatially distributed brain activity into unitary objects, and a coherent sense of self, or 'oneness' is difficult to explain as is the transition from pre- to conscious states. Consciousness is non-computable and involves factors that are neither random nor algorithmic - consciousness cannot be simulated; explanations are also needed for free will and for subjective time flow. Convention

* Correspondence: Professor Gerry Leisman, Director, The National Institute for Brain and Rehabilitation Sciences, Biomechanics Laboratory, Department of Mechanical Engineering, ORT-Braude College of Engineering, Snunit 51 Street, POBox 78, IL-21982 Karmiel, Israel. E-mail: gerry.leisman@staff.nazareth.ac.il

argues that neurons and their chemical synapses are the fundamental units of information in the brain, and that conscious experience emerges when a critical level of complexity is reached in the brain's neural networks. The basic idea is that the mind is a computer functioning in the brain. In fitting the brain to a computational view, such explanations omit incompatible neurophysiological details including: widespread apparent randomness at all levels of neural processes (is it really noise, or underlying levels of complexity; glial cells (which account for some 80% of brain); dendritic-dendritic processing; electrotonic gap junctions; cytoplasmic/cytoskeletal activities; and, living state (the brain is alive!); absence of testable hypotheses in emergence theory. There is no threshold or rationale specified; rather, consciousness "just happens." Consciousness then involves an awareness of what we are sensing or experiencing and some ability to control or coordinate voluntary actions. These issues of life, death, and consciousness are discussed in the context of Mike, the headless chicken, who survived for 18 months, and in the context of consciousness with high degrees of intellectual and cognitive function in a congenitally anencephalic brain, additionally in the reanimation work of the 1920-30's Soviets, and in auditory sentence processing in patients in comatose, vegetative, and minimally conscious states.

## INTRODUCTION

While consciousness has been variously defined in the literature as or even as, that annoying time between naps, its operational definition in the neurosciences is largely problematic for a variety of reasons. Convention portrays consciousness as an emergent property of classical computer-like activities in brain's neural networks. The prevailing views in this camp are that patterns of neural networks correlate with mental states, that synchronous network oscillations in the thalamus and cortex temporally bind information, and that consciousness emerges as novel property of computational complexity among neurons (1).

What we mean by "death" that includes the absence of consciousness in a physiological sense is puzzling. While we know a dead body when we see one and. death appears to us as a real event; being dead as an indisputable condition. Yet it turns out that even the dead body retains, for a while, some residual processes of life. Some individual cells still live; some "nests of cells" still communicate. But no one would argue that the human being is still alive just because every isolated process that might be called life has not yet ceased.

Much more complicated are those cases when a crucial part of the body-the brain-has died, yet the rest of the body, including the heart, is maintained by our technological interventions. In the past, whole-brain death led imminently and irreversibly to the death of the whole person; the entire body shut down. In the age of modern medicine, this process of shutting down is potentially suspended, making it difficult to know when or whether death has occurred.

## THE NEED FOR CONCEPTUALIZATION

The brain can lose function or be irreversibly damaged in a variety of ways. Certain insults will destroy the actual brain tissue anatomy, while others will lead to loss of function due to anoxic "starvation" of cells in the brain. While we can generate rules based on the interaction between environmental and anatomical circumstances, exceptions to those rules make the development of universals and therefore a definition of death difficult, as we shall see.

Anoxic conditions typically result from lack of oxygenated blood flow, which is often a direct result of cardiac arrest (asystole), severe brain swelling, drug intoxication and strokes. Under ischemic or anoxic conditions, the different parts of the brain succumb at different rates. After only a few minutes (~ 2-4), the cerebrum and cerebellum may suffer irreparable damage. The brainstem is much more resilient, however, and may be revived after many minutes (~ 15-20) of anoxia. It is this resilience that enables the condition known as the "persistent vegetative state," in which a person's brainstem continues to function after the upper brain has been destroyed or rendered non-functional. Such an individual entirely lacks cerebral functions of self-awareness or purposeful communication. "Awake but unaware," (see Figures 2 and 3) he exhibits brainstem functions of spontaneous breathing, reflexes to light and pain stimulus, and sleep-wake cycles. This is in contrast to wholly "brain dead" patients who have no functional brainstem and exhibit none of these traits. If anoxia persists, the brainstem too will eventually become damaged beyond the possibility of revival. At this point, the entire brain has died, and lacking medical intervention the body will undergo rigor mortis and putrefaction. However, if a mechanical ventilator is instituted quickly enough to a victim who has suffered death of the whole brain, the heart may be resuscitated and circulation and other bodily functions may be restored, including brain function, as we shall later see. This individual, sustained on a respirator and exhibiting total and irreversible lack of all functions of the entire brain, is considered by clinicians to be "brain dead."

Clinicians generally employ the term "brain death" to refer to a person whose whole brain has died and who is thus declared dead within standard medical practice. This usage has been criticized widely including by the Institute of Medicine (IOM), since it seems to present an ambiguity between a "dead organism," i.e., a person who is declared dead due to brain injury, and a "dead organ," i.e., the brain itself. When discussing donation from those who have normally been called "brain dead," the IOM recommends the modified term "donation after neurological determination of death," or DNDD (2). The question in dispute is precisely whether those who are brain dead should in fact be declared dead.

For organ donation that occurs after death is declared due to the permanent and irreversible cessation of heart and lung function, we will also use the most widely accepted term "donation after cardiac death," or DCD. Here, the IOM proposes the following new locution: "donation after cardiac determination of death," or DCDD. The usefulness of this innovation seems to be entirely tied up with the parallel between it and the proposed new term for the declaring death by neurological criteria, which for this inquiry we have chosen to avoid.

With the need for organs to transplant and an Ad Hoc Committee of the Harvard Medical School (3) provided a definition of irreversible coma providing a basis for the harvesting of organs based on a statistical judgment of coma irreversibility. This notion is certainly not a worldwide consensus definition of death. These guidelines form the basis of the "diagnosis" of death that is based on a clinical judgment and not on an effective operational definition of same. The guidelines indicates that the cause of death should be reasonably established and be reasonably irreversible with the concept of irreversibility being statistical in it methodology. The clinical criteria for this determination included: 1) nonreceptivity and nonresponsivity to externally applied stimuli and inner need; 2) the absence of spontaneous muscular movements or spontaneous respiration; and 3) no brainstem reflexes that can be elicited. The report stated that patients who passed these tests should be considered already dead, notwithstanding the continued function of their circulatory system. Since they were dead, treatment could be stopped (unilaterally) and organs could be procured even while the heart was still beating, including the heart itself.

The cause may result from a primary brain injury (i.e., trauma or hemorrhage) or from non- neurological illness (e.g., cardiac arrest with anoxia to brain). This diagnosis may be confounded of course by drug intoxication, metabolic/endocrine disturbance, severe facial trauma, pre-existing pupillary abnormalities, chronic $CO_2$ retention, and hypothermia. The basis for this definition unfortunately is not universal.

This wording was also promulgated by the President's Commission for the Study of Ethical Problems in Medicine and Biomedical and Behavioral Research, which issued an influential 1981 report entitled Defining Death: Medical, Legal and Ethical Issues in the Determination of Death (4). The first version of the Uniform Anatomical Gift Act (UAGA) in the United States was promulgated in 1968 (5) and then revised in 1987 (6). These acts allowed an individual to specify that he desired to be an organ donor after his death and that the determination of death was maintained as a separate statutory matter from the specification of who may become an organ donor in turn resulting in the treating of brain dead individuals as dead as the standard clinical paradigm, as it remains to this day. The clinical paradigms based on legal reports or on legislation do not alter the meaning of “life” and “death,” but only the consequences of transplant, burial, autopsy, transfer of property to the heirs, and so forth (7).

## DEVELOPMENT OF A CONTINUUM OF CONSCIOUSNESS IN THE CONTEXT OF DEATH?

As thinkers began to wrestle with the new problems of death that confront us in the age of ventilators, a salient distinction was made between death of the organism as a whole and death of the whole organism. The latter term would imply that all processes that could be called “life” have ceased in an individual for whom they once were operative. It is that absolute lifelessness that happens sometime after the human person has died. The death of the “organism as a whole,” by comparison, is a much more difficult concept to grasp. To say that there is an organism as a whole implies that there is something (someone) that (who) exists over and above the organism's individual material parts. This entity that exists “over and above its parts” is mortal in a way that the parts of which it is composed are not. Put differently, the death of the organism as a whole can leave behind living components that contributed, perhaps crucially, to the organism's “alive-ness” while it was still living, but those components taken separately are not “a” living organism.

Once this notion of a mortal organism as “a whole” is accepted, the task is set to determine what life-like activities of its component parts can persist without being absolute indicators of continuing organismal life. No one has trouble with positing the co-existence of life in isolated cells with death of the organism as a whole. Yet the advent of the ventilator introduces a much more difficult case: continued function in some of the living parts of an organism after the organism, itself, may already have died.

This leaves us with a series of rather difficult questions: Is the death of the person equivalent to the death of the integrated organism functioning as a whole? Is the wholly brain dead person still functioning as a whole organism? Are there other physiological failures besides that of the whole brain that might signal that death has occurred? What functions of the body are necessary for the human person to continue living? Can we really ever know? And if not, is death better defined "the old-fashioned way," as the permanent and irreversible cessation of breathing and heartbeat, when the individual is indisputably dead as seen through the prism of ordinary human experience? While these are not physiological questions alone, we cannot address them philosophically without a more detailed understanding of modern physiology-that is, of how the parts of the body relate to the human whole.

The "brainstem" formulation and the "higher brain" formulation of the definition of death both challenge the standard paradigm by suggesting that it has not adequately articulated the basic concept of death. The practical consequence of a successful challenge from either of these camps would be an expansion-either small or large-of the class of patients considered to be dead by neurological criteria, i.e., dead despite the continuation of ventilator-supported somatic functioning. A third challenge to the standard paradigm is of a much different sort. Shewmon (8-10) reports an understanding that has thrown the standard paradigm of the physiological and philosophical understanding of death into uncertainty. Shewmon (8) argues that that if we accept the definition of death as the loss of integrative function of the organism as a whole, then we cannot consider brain dead patients to be dead. And, conversely, if we maintain that brain dead patients are indeed dead, then we must abandon the loss of integrative functioning as the underlying definition.

Shewmon has shown that neither bodily disintegration nor asystole necessarily follow imminently after brain death (8). Over one hundred documented cases demonstrate chronic survival past a week's time, with one extreme case surviving over 14 years. Furthermore, he demonstrates that factors such as age, etiology, and underlying somatic integrity variably affect the survival probability of brain dead patients. Thus, not only is asystole not necessarily imminent upon brain death, but also it is the integrity of the rest of the body (the underlying somatic plasticity) and not the condition of the brain that most strongly influences survival.

Shewmon also argues against the consensus that the somatic disintegration that is observed in brain dead patients has as its cause the loss of neural regulatory centers; instead, he presents clinical evidence that dis-integration may be explained by the condition known as "spinal shock." Spinal shock is a transient condition that occurs following a sudden acute spinal cord injury, resulting in the temporary loss of function of the spinal region below the lesion. Such functions may be regained after 2 to 6 weeks, and include autonomic reflexes, sympathetic and parasympathetic tone, and thermoregulation. In several brain dead patients in whom life-support is sustained long enough, this loss and subsequent recovery of spinal cord regulation has been observed (8, 9). Shewmon (10) builds on these arguments in a 2001 paper that looks directly at the issue of integration and integrative unity. His philosophical exploration of these notions leads him to the following conclude that the body has no integrator but rather the holistic property of integration. In support of this idea, Shewmon discusses the various functions of the organism that qualify as integrative. Some of these seem to warrant the designation "brain-mediated," but many others do not. Among those that do not are, for example, wound-healing, immunological defense of "self" against "non-self," proportional growth, and even successful gestation of a fetus. These functions, and many others he names, have been exhibited by at least some brain dead bodies. Shewmon is careful to point out that calling these functions "non-brain-mediated" does not mean that the brain has nothing to do with them in an intact organism. We can better support Shewmon's understanding in the section on continuum theory.

## COMA

While the content of consciousness is a function of the higher brain, the capacity for consciousness resides in the brainstem. The brainstem and the higher brain play an important role in directing the integrative functions of an organism. Integrative functions are those complex processes and spontaneous innate activities that involve communication, coordination, and regulation of several subsystems within the body. Examples include respiration, heartbeat, blood pressure, temperature regulation, coordinated muscle movement, neuroendocrine control, and response to light and sound. Yet while some of these integrated functions directly correspond to a function in the brain (such as the ability to moderate the depth and pace of breathing), others (such as blood-pressure and body temperature regulation) are less clearly dependent on the brain's regulation. The extent to which brainstem regulation is necessary for somatically integrative functioning is a central matter of controversy. Clearly, however, the ability to behave in an integrative way is the some and substance of the argument to follow. That is while there may well be profound anatomical compromises to the nervous system, if the individual's nervous system can behave in an integrative fashion, then there is no functional compromise and there is a possibility of recovery through plasticity. This notion will be examined more fully in the discussion of persistent vegetative states below. We can easily measure and quantify stages of the continuum of consciousness, at least from coma to states of elation exemplified in Figure 1.

Laureys and colleagues (11) had conveniently produced a flow chart relating the nomenclature of (see Figure 2) and clinical compromises to (represented in Figure 3) conscious states. It is understood that critical damage to the reticular system produces coma, defined customarily as a pathological state of eyes-closed-unresponsiveness where the individual lacks both wakefulness and awareness, and exemplified in Figures 1 and 2 above. Critical damage to the thalamus, cerebral cortex, or its connections, while sparing the reticular system, produces a vegetative state, in which the patient is awake but unaware. The use of the concept of brain death is an ambiguous term that cannot be operationally defined and therefore has no place in a discussion of the science of death. Mollaret and Gouan in 1959 (13) coined the notion *le coma depasse* or "state beyond coma." They went on to define that state as based on an irreversible loss of the clinical function of the whole brain, including cortical (upper brain motor and cognitive), mid-brain (integrative), and brain stem (vegetative) function. The concept of brain death is relatively recent then.

The current clinical examination of death is exemplified in table 1 and is based on bedside and apnea testing. Table 2 provides sensitivity and specificity data on additional confirmatory clinical testing to support a determination of death. Steven Gould best states the problem with all of these approaches when he noted: We still carry the historical baggage of a Platonic heritage that seeks sharp essences and definite boundaries. Thus we hope to find an unambiguous "beginning of life" or "definition of death," although nature often comes to us as irreducible continua.

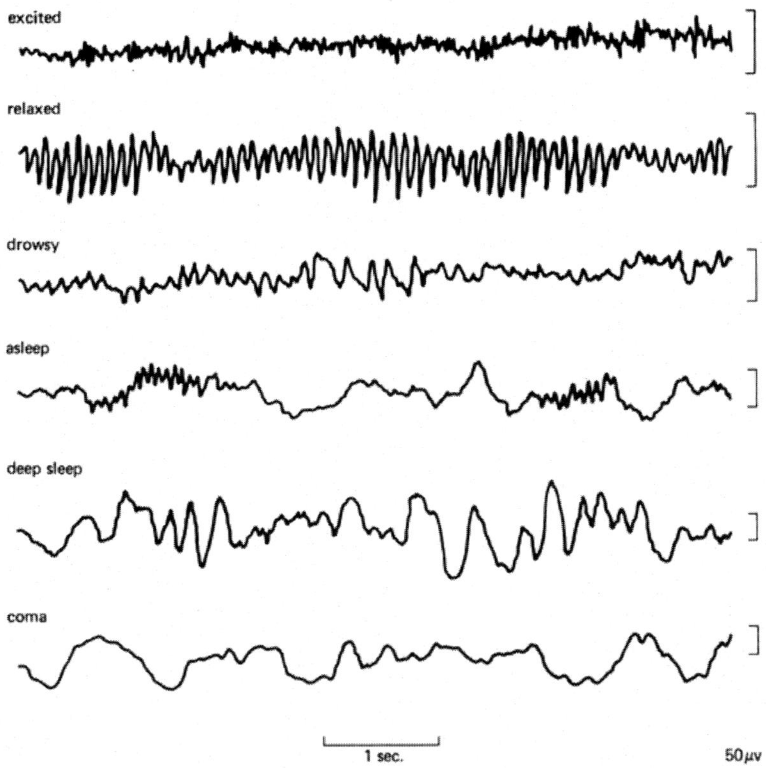


Figure 1. Quantifiable Altered States. Neural activity (EEG's) and the corresponding behavioral states accompanying arousal levels including those associated with an awake excited person, the alpha rhythm associated with relaxation with eyes closed, the slowing in frequency associated with a drowsy condition, the slow high amplitude waves of sleep, the larger slow waves associated with deep sleep, and the further slowing of EEG waves associated with coma.

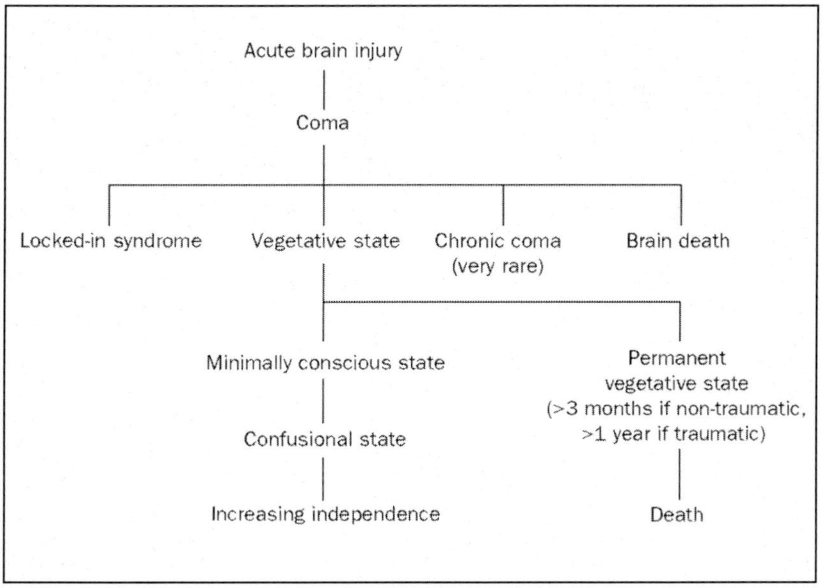


Figure 2. Clinical Levels of Arousal and Awareness (11).

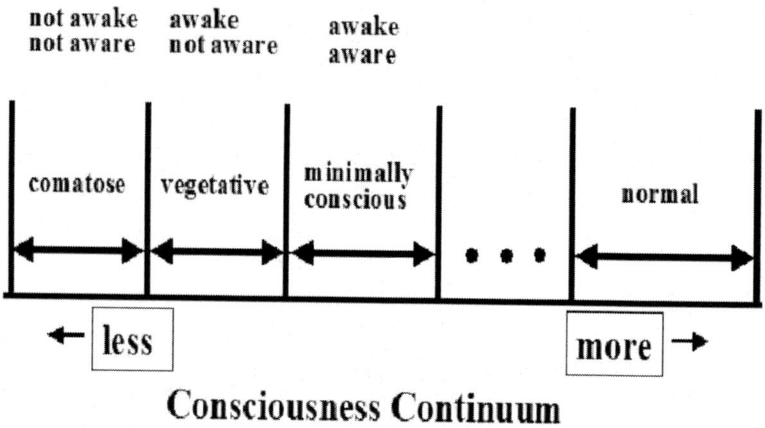


Figure 3. Clinically compromised altered states of consciousness (12).

**Table 1. Clinical Brain Death Testing Protocol Synopsis**

| Clinical bedside testing of the determination of death |
|---|
| Absent grimace or withdrawal response to pain |
| Pupils unresponsive to light |
| Absent corneal reflex |
| Absent gag reflex |
| Absent cough reflex to suctioning |
| Absent oculocephalic response - the eyes turn with the head - no eye movement -"doll's eye" |
| Absent vestibulo-ocular (caloric) response - the eyes fail to deviate away from the side you irrigate with ice water - no eye movement |

| Apnea confirmatory testing of death |
|---|
| Pre-test criteria: euvolemia, Temp $\geq$ 36.5° C, SBP $\geq$ 90, $pCO_2 \geq 40$ |
| Pre-oxygenate with 100% $O_2$, to achieve $pO_2 > 200$, disconnect the ventilator (or set rate at 0), deliver 100% $O_2$ at 6 L/min by cannula into the ET tube |
| ABG at 8 - 10 minutes |
| Test is positive if no respiratory movement and $pCO_2 \geq 60$ |
| Inconclusive if $pCO_2 < 60$, SBP < 90, $O_2$ sat < 80%, or cardiac arrhythmia |

**Table 2.**

| Test | Sensitivity (%) | Specificity (%) |
|---|---|---|
| EEG | +/-90 | +/- 90 |
| Somatic evoked potentials | 100 | +/- 95 |
| Brainstem auditory evoked potentials | 100 | 94 |
| Arteriogram | <96 | 100 |
| Transcranial doppler | 95 | 99 |
| Radionuclide perfusion scan | 95 | 100 |

Adding insult to injury in arguing for an operational definition of death palatable to philosophers, neuroscientists, physicians, and ethicists each with a profoundly different framework from which they conceive of death is the famous story of Mike the Chicken who survived headless for eighteen months maintaining all bodily functions including sex with a surviving brainstem.

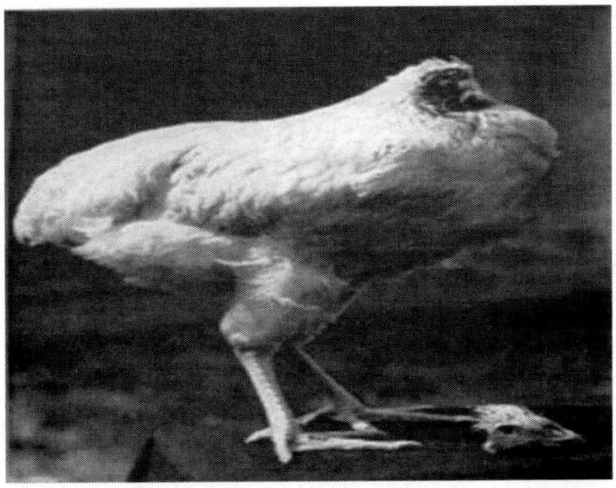

Figure 4. Although most of his head was in a jar, most of his brain stem and one ear was left. Since most chicken reflex actions are controlled by the brainstem, Mike was able to remain quite healthy. In the 18 months that Mike lived since beheading he grew from 2 1/2 lbs. to nearly 8 lbs.

## PERSISTENT VEGETATIVE STATE

Persistent Vegetative State (PVS) can be superficially described as eyes-open unconsciousness. In reviewing a recent history of the concept, it was first described by Jennet and Plum in 1972 (14). Eyes open unconsciousness is a dissociation between aware and awake states as diagrammed in Figure 1. The upper brain fails to receive or project information as well as evidence that exists of a lack of integration between the upper and mid-brain. The brainstem, however, is generally intact. This would adequately explain Mike's sexual prowess, but not his consciousness. In the human condition, this state would be more characteristic of the states of Karen Ann Quinlan, Nancy Cruzan, and Teri Schiavo.

Again as in coma, the concept of PVS is based on the judgment of a clinician in turn based on the 1994 Multi Society Task Force on PVS (15) with the criteria being the demonstration of sleep-wake cycles without the awareness of self or of others when awake. No apparent comprehension or expression of language is noticed, and no sustained and reproducible voluntary or purposeful response to external stimuli. The individual may demonstrate limb spasticity, but those movements are likely to be non-purposeful. Reports of some emotive events have been made including smiles and grimaces but not reproducible response to stimuli.

The cause of injury, co-morbid conditions and the length of time in the vegetative state determine the recovery from PVS. "Persistent" is defined as duration of greater than one month represented in Table 3. When the cause in non-traumatic (e.g., anoxic brain injury post CPR), a duration of greater than three months is termed "permanent." Duration of greater than 12 months post traumatic injury is considered "permanent" and is represented in table 4.

**Table 3. 1-Year Outcome in *Post-Traumatic* Vegetative State**

| | % Dead 1 year later | % Vegetative 1 year later | % Conscious 1 year later |
|---|---|---|---|
| Vegetative at 1 month | 28% | 18% | 54% |
| Vegetative at 3 month | 31% | 30% | 39% |
| Vegetative at 3 month | 28% | 53% | 19% |

**Table 4. 1-year Outcome in *Non-traumatic* Vegetative State**

| | % Dead 1 year later | %Vegetative 1 year later | % Conscious 1 year later |
|---|---|---|---|
| Vegetative at 1 month | 47% | 39% | 14% |
| Vegetative at 3 months | 36% | 58% | 6% |
| Vegetative at 6 months | 18% | 81% | 1% |

One might think that the anatomy itself might define a comatose, persistent, or permanent vegetative state when one sees an individual who is in that state and has the attendant anatomical or structural involvement. Immediately, additional explanations are necessary to counter the following situations.

Figure 5A left indicates a CT of a "normal" brain and the rightmost image of 5A indicates a CT of the well-known Terry Schiavo case indicating hydrocephalus and central loss of brain tissue.

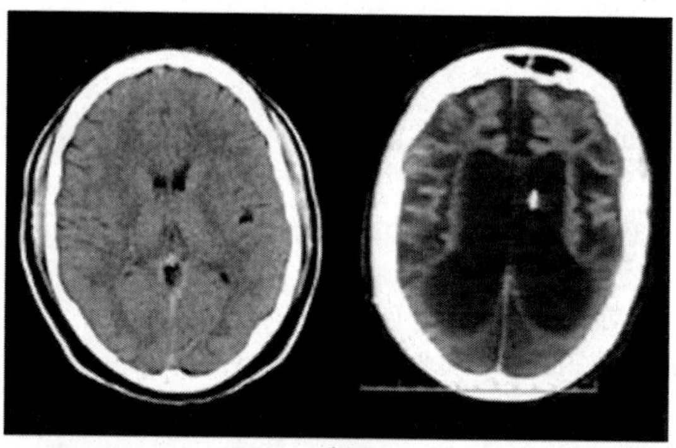

A

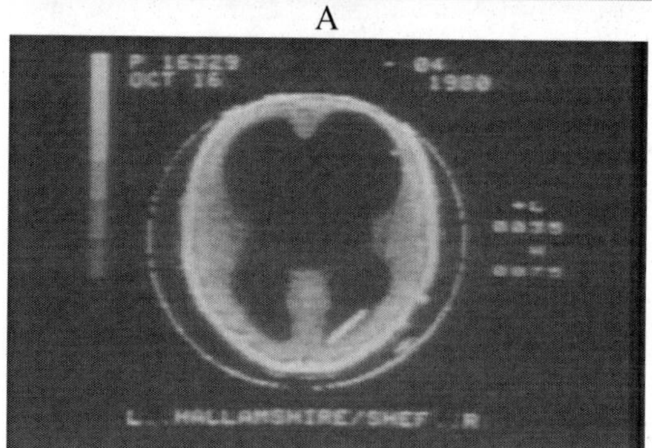


B

Figure 5. (Continued)

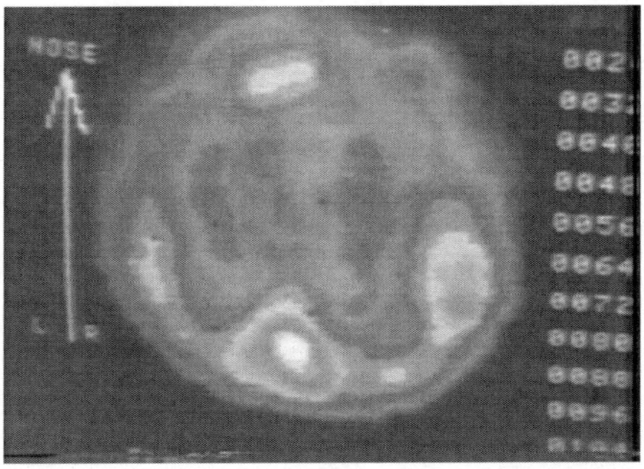


C

Figure 5. Does the Anatomy Define the PVS or is there a case for plasticity? (A) (left) CT of normal brain (right) Terry Schiavo's 2002 CT showing hydrocephalus & loss of brain tissue. (B) CT of congenitally hydrocephalic female aged 18 (C) Image of rCBF of congenitally hydrocephalic female aged 18.

However, Figure 5B represents a CT of a high normally functioning yet congenitally hydrocephalic female with an anatomical presentation not significantly distant from that represented in Figure 5A. Figure 5C represents the same young ladies rCBF indicating areas of function. The likely functional differences between these two cases are likely the result of one case being congenital and the other being the result of adult-onset trauma.

In examining the effect on fMRI of temporal lobe function on patients in PVS, Owen and colleagues (16) read sentences to an individual 13-months after a stroke. Functional magnetic resonance imaging revealed bilateral activation in his superior temporal lobes represented in Figure 6 (top) similar to the activation found in healthy controls (bottom). The patient later emerged into a minimally conscious state. (From A. M. Owen et al., (16)).

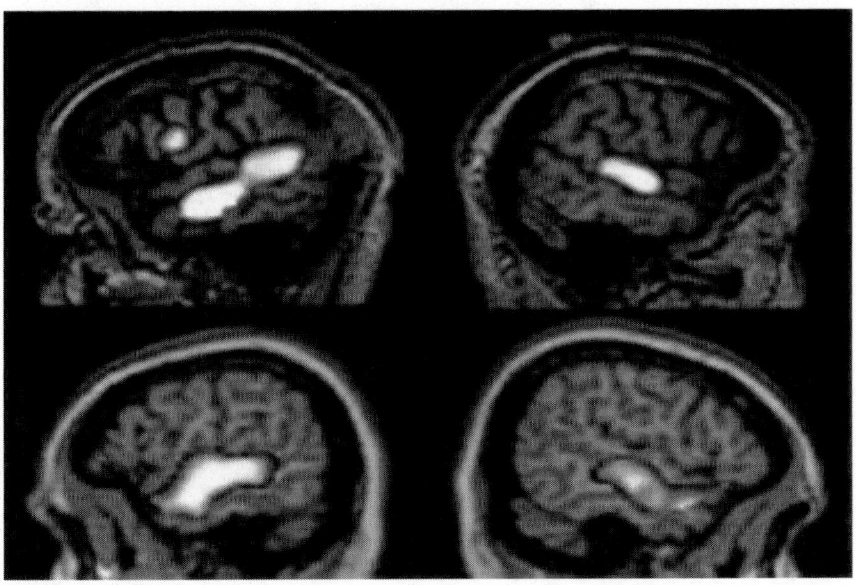

Figure 6. PVS and fMRI activation to sentences.

In attempting to additionally indicate the ability to measure different states of consciousness leading to attempts to objectify various clinical states including PVS and death, Laureys and colleagues (12) present in Figure 7 a representation of global cerebral metabolism in percent as a function of varying clinical states. We learn that PVS has an associated global metabolism of between 40-65 percent of normal being similar to deep anesthesia (17). Then again, individuals with congenital anencephaly who are of normal intellectual ability demonstrate similar significant reduction in global cerebral metabolism.

The implications of the nature of global cerebral metabolism in PVS includes the fact that such metabolic hypoactivity has precedent only in deep anesthesia and supports clinical evidence that cerebral cognitive function is lost in the vegetative state, leaving a body that can no longer think or experience pain according to Levy and colleagues (18). The pain-suppressing effect of general anesthesia is likely due primarily to its depressant effect on brain stem rather than on cerebral function in coma but not in PVS as the brainstem is functional in PVS. There is also no logical connection between such data and experience of pain.

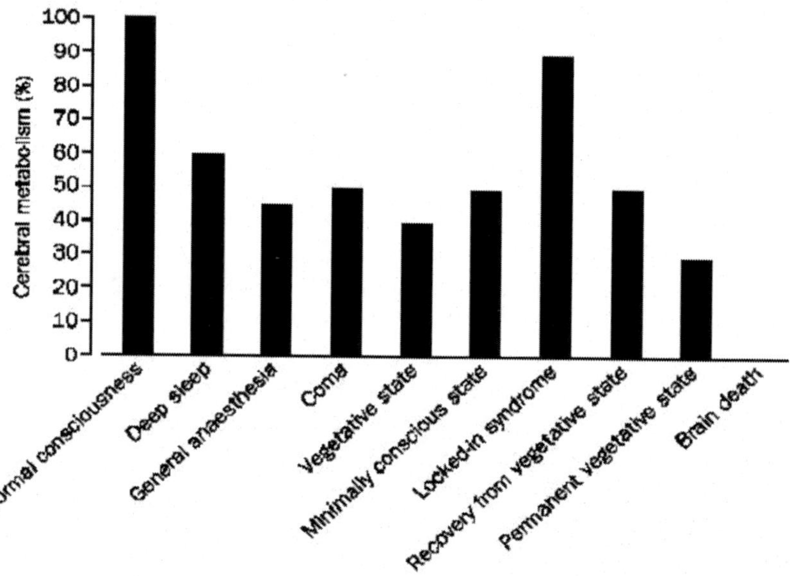


Figure 7. Global cerebral metabolism as a function of state of consciousness (after Laureys et al. (21)).

An additional view of why the Shiavo case was functionally different than the case of congenital hydrocephalus reported in Figures 11 is largely a result of connectivities represented in Figure 8.

The elevated CMRGlc observed during ages 3-10 yrs. corresponds to an era of exuberant connectivity that is needed for energy needs of neuronal processes. In childhood it is measurably greater by a factor of 2 compared to adults. PET scans show the relative glucose metabolic rate. We see the complexity of dendritic structures of cortical neurons consistent with the expansion of synaptic connectivities and increases in capillary density in the frontal cortex.

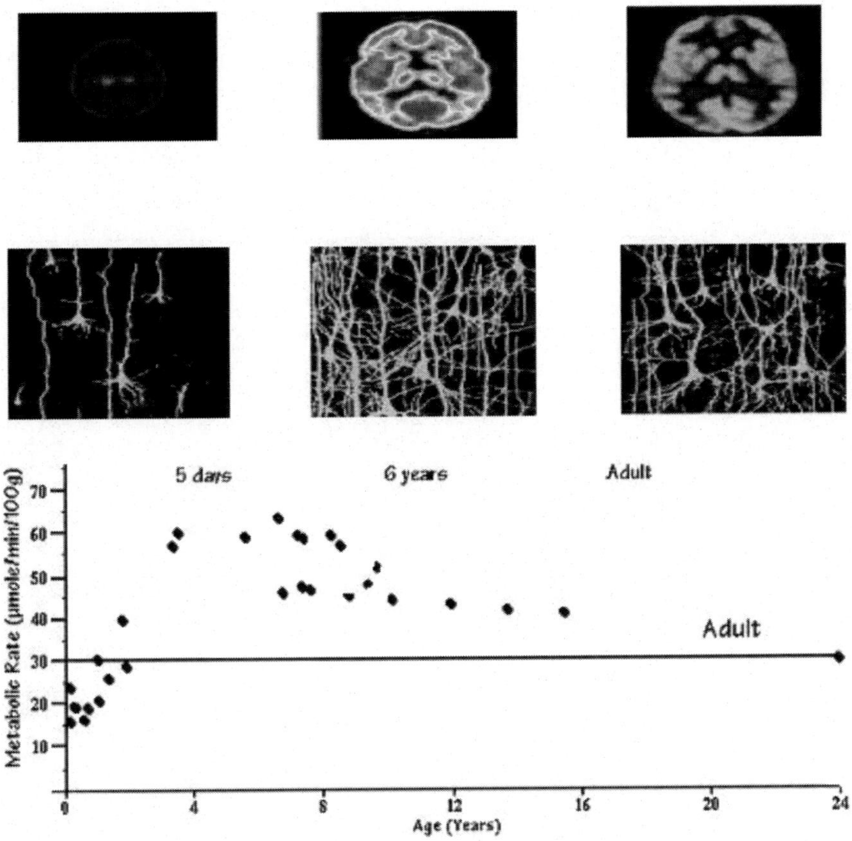


Figure 8. Cerebral metabolic rate as a function of age.

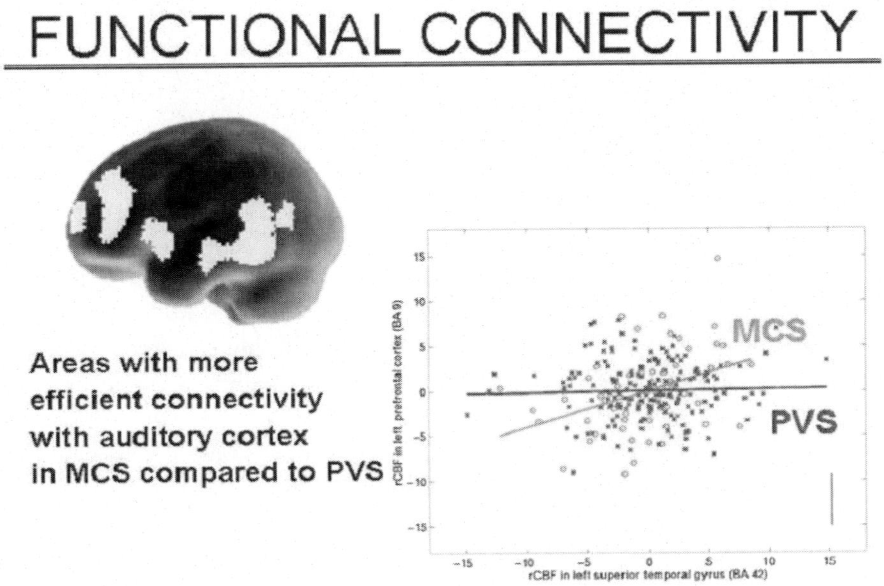


Figure 9. Functional disconnectivities in PVS.

Figure 9 represents the comparison on rCBF in the left superior temporal gyrus compared with activity in the left prefrontal cortex and demonstrates areas with more "efficient" connectivity with the auditory cortex in individuals with PVS as compared to those with Minimally Conscious States (MCS). The relationship is presented as representative of the concept of functional disconnectivity and follows from the notion earlier reviewed by Leisman and Melillo (19).

We therefore see PVS as a functional disconnection syndrome represented in a way similar to neonatal normal activation and similar to our functional disconnection syndromes (e.g., autism) (9, 20) There also exists in PVS a non-activation of higher-order association cortices, with impaired functional connections between distant cortical areas, including the thalamus and cortex, with the recovery of consciousness paralleled by the restoration of cortico-thalamo- cortical interaction.

We can actually see these functional disconnectivities in sleep (21). In sleep, brain areas loose ability to communicate with each other as compared to awake subjects who create responses in different destinations unlike sleep subjects who are more likely to create responses to single or fewer destinations. Reduced brain consciousness is associated with breakdown into non-coherent activity. Consciousness then could be considered to be the ability of the brain to integrate information with consciousness being the coherent communication between brain areas. PVS seems to be a compromise in that integration process. The result is in some cases that PVS can be seen as a locked-in syndrome with severe cognitive deficits but with primitive awareness of self and environment.

The unity of consciousness is based on a "centrencephalic system" that includes the reticular formation & thalamus. While it is not known which portions of the brain are responsible for cognition and consciousness; what little is known points to substantial interconnections among the brainstem, subcortical structures and the neocortex. Thus, the 'higher brain' may well exist only as a metaphorical concept, and not in reality. The role of cortex allows for the interface between world, the individual's body and the conscious self as well as well as in the integration of sensory input and motor output. Functional disconnectivities represent the behavioral traits observed and reconnection may be engineered.

To emphasize this point, we can provide a *gedanken* experiment on the so called Sprague Effect (22). The complete removal of posterior visual areas of a hemisphere in the cat (parietal areas too) renders the animal profoundly and permanently unresponsive to visual stimuli in the half of space contralateral to the cortical tissue removal. The cat is blind in the same way as would a human with radical damage to the geniculostriatal system. If one were then inflict additional damage on such a severely impaired animal at midbrain level, then the ability of the cat to orient and localize stimuli in the formerly blind field would be restored. This would be accomplished by removing the contralateral superior colliculus or by severing fibres in the central portion of the collicular commissure. Adding damage in the brainstem to the cortical damage "cures" a behavioral effect of massive cortical damage. The Sprague Effect is a consequence of secondary effects generated at the brainstem level by unilateral cortical removal. The damage deprives the ipsilateral superior colliculus of its normal cortical input. Damage unbalances collicular function via indirect projection pathways, those chiefly from the substantia nigra to the colliculus, which crosses the midline in a narrow central portion of the collicular commissure. The "restorative" interventions partially correct this imbalance, allowing the collicular mechanism to resume at least part of its normal functional contribution to behavior, with partial restoration of vision as a result. Minimally Conscious States (MCS).

To make the diagnosis of MCS, limited but clearly discernible evidence of self or environmental awareness must be demonstrated on a reproducible or sustained basis by any or all of the following including: following simple commands, gestural or verbal yes/no responses regardless of accuracy), intelligible verbalization, purposeful behavior, including movements or affective behaviors that occur in contingent relation to relevant environmental stimuli and are not due to reflexive activity. Some examples of qualifying purposeful behavior include: appropriate smiling or crying in response to the linguistic or visual content of emotional but not to neutral topics or stimuli, vocalizations or gestures that occur in direct response to the linguistic content of questions, reaching for objects that demonstrates a clear relationship between object location and direction of reach, touching or holding objects in a manner that accommodates the size and shape of the object, pursuit eye movement or sustained fixation that occurs in direct response to moving or salient stimuli. Although it is not uncommon for individuals in MCS to demonstrate more than one of the above criteria, in some patients the evidence is limited to only one behavior that is indicative of consciousness. Clinical judgments concerning a patient's level of consciousness depend on inferences drawn from observed behavior. Thus, sensory deficits, motor dysfunction, or diminished drive may result in underestimation of cognitive capacity.

Recovery from MCS to higher states of consciousness occurs along a continuum in which the upper boundary is necessarily arbitrary. Consequently, the diagnostic criteria for emergence from MCS are based on broad classes of functionally useful behaviors that are typically observed as such patients recover. Thus, emergence from MCS is characterized by reliable and consistent demonstration of one or both of the following: Functional interactive communication, functional use of two different objects, functional interactive communication may occur through verbalization, writing, yes/no signals, or use of augmentative, communication devices. Functional use of objects requires that the patient demonstrate behavioral evidence of object discrimination.

Giacino (23) has distinguished the MCS from the PVS by the presence of behaviors associated with conscious awareness. In MCS, cognitively mediated behavior occurs inconsistently, but is reproducible or sustained long enough to be differentiated from reflexive behavior. The reproducibility of such evidence is affected by the consistency and complexity of the behavioral response. Extended assessment may be required to determine whether a simple response that is observed infrequently is occurring in response to a specific environmental event or on a coincidental basis.

MCS has recently be shown to be alterable by physiological manipulation providing us with and additional *gedanken* experiment this time on elucidating the nature of MCS with deep brain stimulation. Electrodes receive pulses from pacemaker surgically placed (24) under the skin of patient's chest. Electrodes transmitted pulses from pacemaker to thalamus, for 12 hours after which the patient became significantly more alert and aware and had the capacity to express pain return. The patient reportedly kept his eyes open most of the time during the day and followed others with his eyes as they moved. The MCS patient, according to Schiff and colleagues communicated reliably with gestures and audible phrases of up to six words. He also took all meals orally and drank from a cup.

Schiff and colleagues have assumed and we support the notion that widespread loss of cerebral connectivity is assumed to underlie the failure of brain mechanisms that support communication and goal-directed behavior following severe traumatic brain injury. We had indicated earlier in Tables III and IV that disorders of consciousness that persist for longer than 12 months are considered to be immutable and no treatment is likely to accelerate recovery or improve functional outcome. Schiff and colleagues have shown otherwise Recent studies have demonstrated unexpected preservation of large-scale cerebral networks in patients in MCS indicating residual functional capacity in some patients that could be supported by therapeutic interventions. These individuals were thought by Schiff's group to be limited by chronic underactivation of potentially recruitable large-scale networks. Schiff and colleagues had demonstrated that in a 6-month double-blind alternating crossover study, bilateral deep brain electrical stimulation (DBS) of the central thalamus modulated behavioral responsiveness in a patient who remained in MCS for 6 years following traumatic brain injury before the intervention. The frequency of specific cognitively mediated behaviors (primary outcome measures) and functional limb control and oral feeding (secondary outcome measures) increased during periods in which DBS was on as compared with periods in which it was off. Logistic regression modeling demonstrated a statistical linkage between the observed functional improvements and stimulation history.

## Continuum Theory

In attempting to portray consciousness, thinking and memory and its skills as we have elsewhere, (1, 25-27) we could easily demonstrate how imaging technologies show brain locations appearing to correlate with consciousness, although not directly responsible for it. This is exemplified in Figure 10.

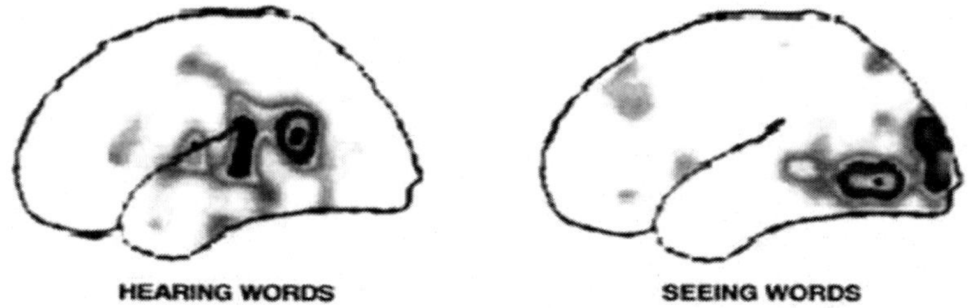


Figure 10. Imaging technologies show brain locations appearing to correlate with consciousness but perhaps not directly responsible for it. Technology reveals brain activity associated with consciousness but is that activity equivalent to it.

We have theorized earlier about how neural firings lead to thoughts and feelings (25-30). Conventional (i.e., functionalist, reductionist, materialist, physicalist, computationalist) approaches argue that neurons and their synapses are the fundamental units of information in the brain, and that conscious experience emerges when a critical level of complexity is reached in the brain's neural networks as exemplified in Figure 11.

In our previous thinking, we have examined activity waves in a layered neural continuum. With arborization facilitating synaptic connectivities, upon stimulation, neural cells become active and trigger excitatory and inhibitory signals through synaptic connectivities. If a given cell receives a sufficient preponderance of excitatory over inhibitory synaptic inputs it fires in turn and sends signals to other cells.

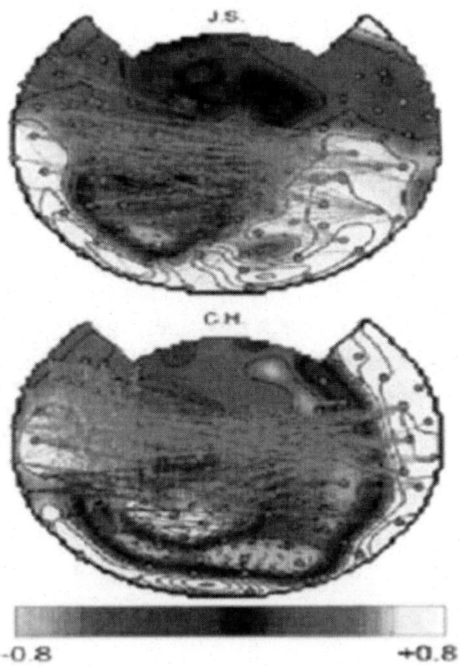


Figure 11. Electrophysiological consequences of consciousness as a function of increasing levels of system complexity. Is this how and when consciousness occurs? (21).

Recent years have seen a proliferation of work in neuroscience, computer science, physics, and biology concerning neurons and their connections. This stems from the dual motivations of understanding mental function in terms of its material constituents and emulating its aspects artificially. The latter effort has achieved some success, (31, 32) but progress in the larger endeavor has been slower, up against the size discrepancy between artificial neural networks (about 104 cells at most (33) and mammalian brains (109-1011 cells) (34, 35). It is clear that the type of analysis used to design, for example, conditionable pattern recognizers must be supplemented by an approach that can account for the organization of large numbers of neurons into what we call the "mind."

Our model of consciousness as a basis for a definition of death does not conceive, as do other theories, especially neural network models, that the mind is a computer-like entity. Other models dealing with interconnectivities omit details including: widespread apparent randomness at all levels of neural processes (is it really noise, or underlying levels of complexity?); glial cells account for approximately 80 percent of the brain; the effects of dendritic-dendritic processing; the effects of electrotonic gap junctions; the effects of cytoplasmic/cytoskeletal activities. Single cell paramecia swim & avoid obstacles with their cytoskeletons for example. Neuronal complexity is generally not accounted for. Many motile single-celled organisms lacking neurons swim, find food, learn, & multiply through internal cytoskeleton and the brain's living state (the brain is alive!). Invariably, no threshold or rationale is specified, rather, consciousness "just happens. "Our approach, which can be conveniently called continuum neural dynamics, was first proposed by Wilson and Cowan (35). They stated that a differential element of neural tissue (which in the continuum approximation still contains many cells) could be characterized completely by the connections it has with other such elements. As a consequence of the neglect of the details of near-neighbor connections interior to the elements, neurons themselves can be replaced by figurative "cells" which are of two species, "excitatory" (e-cells), and "inhibitory" (i-cells). Then neural activity on the macroscopic level is described by a field variable A(s,x,t) (s = e,i), which is the active fraction of species s at position x and time t. Connections are of four types, viz. e-e, e-i, i-e, i-i, where in each case the first-named is the afferent or pre-synaptic species and the second is the efferent or post-synaptic species; these connections are probabilistic, the probabilities decreasing with distance. (It is essential to this theory that the probabilities and their spatial ranges be different for the different connection types). The activity field A obeys an integro-differential equation (30), which expresses the fact that the change in activity in a region of the continuum is a nonlinear (i.e., sigmoid) function of synaptic input. This in turn is proportional to the algebraic sum of the activity in all other regions, weighted by the connection probabilities as is exemplified in Figure 12.

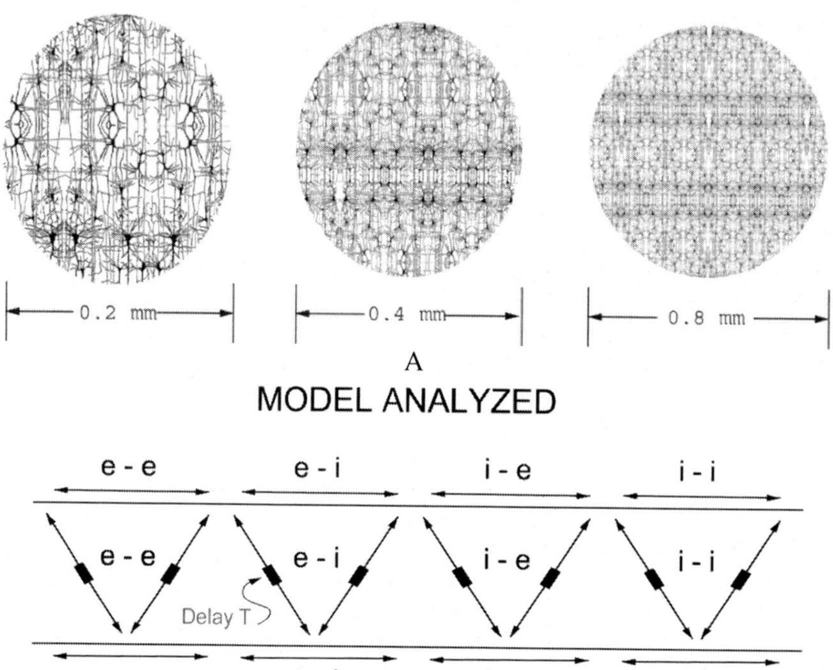


Figures 12. The Neural continuum (A) As we zoom out, our field of vision contains more and more, seemingly smaller and smaller cells. Eventually the distinctions among the individual cells blur. We have analyzed the properties of the material as a *neural continuum*. (B) Schematic of simplified cortical model: Two layers each consisting of excitatory and inhibitory cells. Synaptic connections within a layer are instantaneous; those between layers are subject to a (variable) delay, without dissipation in activation strength. There is a simplifying assumption of *axial uniformity* where the connection probabilities, ranges, time delays depend on axial or interlayer distance only. The neural continuum can be described as an assembly of cells, either purely excitatory (*e*-species) or purely inhibitory (*i*-species). The cells of each species within a continuum element send their respective collective signals to the other elements. Communications between the individual cells are provided by axons. Although many of these axons are quite long, their average length is less than 1 mm. In the continuum approximation this fact is represented by a mean connection range, over which the probability of connection between continuum elements decreases exponentially.

We consider here the application of this theory to a model, which we believe is a first approximation of cortical tissue. It consists of two identical layers, each containing both types of cell. Connections between cells in different layers are subject to a time delay without dissipation. The presence of e-e connections denotes a source of free energy in the medium, which can thus be described as "active." Active media amplify small signals, and this work concerns itself with determining the characteristics of disturbances that are preferentially amplified, the "fastest-growing normal modes" in other words.

Because the signals under consideration are initially small, a linear analysis suffices; the growing disturbances can then be described in terms of waves. For example, for relatively small delay the response of the two-layer system to an impulsive (delta-function) stimulus at one of the layers is a growing, propagating wave with narrowly determined wavelength and frequency. As delay increases the structure of the response becomes more complex, with two or more such waves being simultaneously excited. The delay acts as a control, determining both the spectral location of the resonances and the qualitative nature of the response (36). The preferentially amplified wavelengths are always large compared with the synaptic connection ranges.

Linear theory predicts that growth proceeds without limit. Therefore limitation to the growth must come from factors outside the theory. Nonlinear saturation, which has been studied to some extent, (28-30, 32, 35, 37, 38) is one possible limiting factor. It suits our purposes instead to postulate that growth at a particular wavelength stops when the delay time changes, so that growth at that wavelength is no longer favored. (The presence of a uniform decay ensures the disappearance of non-growing disturbances.) A change in delay, over times long compared with itself (and the periods of the resonant waves), can come about if the delay results from reentrant neuronal circuits (39).

Karl Pribram's holonomic theory reviews evidence that the dendritic processes function to take a "spectral" transformation of the "episodes of perception." This transformed "spectral" information is stored distributed over large numbers of neurons. When the episode is remembered, an inverse transformation occurs that is also a result of dendritic processes. It is the process of transformation that gives us conscious awareness.

We suggest below a mental phenomenology in which various aspects of "consciousness" consist of the simultaneous activation of elements of the continuum distant from each other by a multiple of some currently favored wavelength. At small delays this large-scale organization by wavelength is reproducible as a function of delay only. For larger delays, phase relations among the several activated modes cause the details of the resonant pattern to be functions as well of the spatiotemporal location of the initial signal. The elements under discussion contain enough cells to be complex neural networks, and a single "neural cascade" can involve, from inception to termination, some millions of neurons.

The Figures 13 and 14 depict how resonantly growing waves simultaneously activate distant modules into patterns of greater or lesser complexity. These patterns, the normal modes of our model of cortical tissue, may well be expressions of "mental" phenomena. For example, consider a case where the modules contain feature-recognition information. At low delays, when a single wavelength is resonantly excited, modules spaced at a distance equal to an integral multiple of the resonant wavelength will be simultaneously active or inactive. They can thus represent information that associates perhaps a face a voice and a name. A memory search then would involve changing the delay until the correct pattern is achieved.

As previously indicated, the longer the delay remains constant, the greater the exponential growth in the proportion of cells firing that is the number recruited into the search. Note that the figures depict the response to a single small local disturbance; there is no reason why it should occur in isolation unless there exists a fundamental dys-communication or functional disconnectivity between parts of the system.

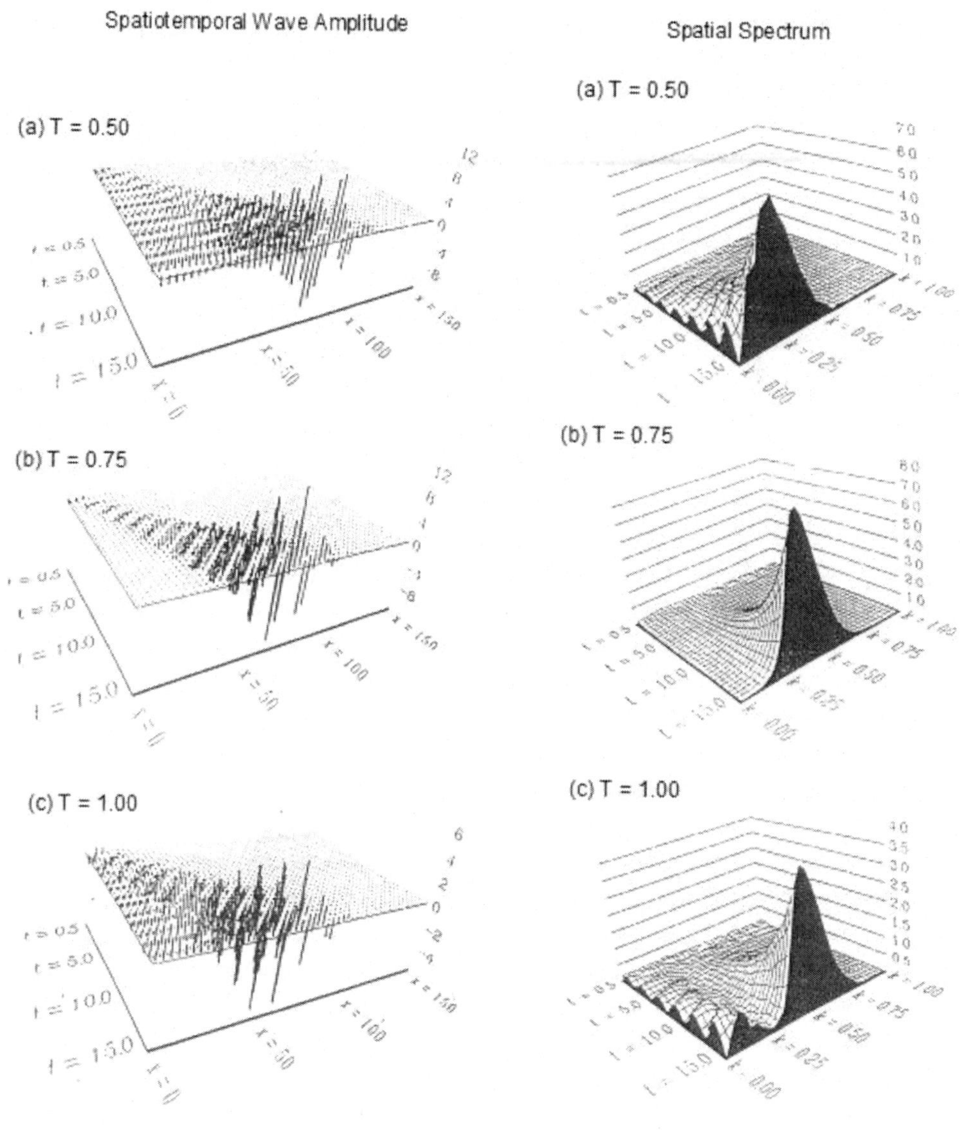


Figure 13. (Continued)

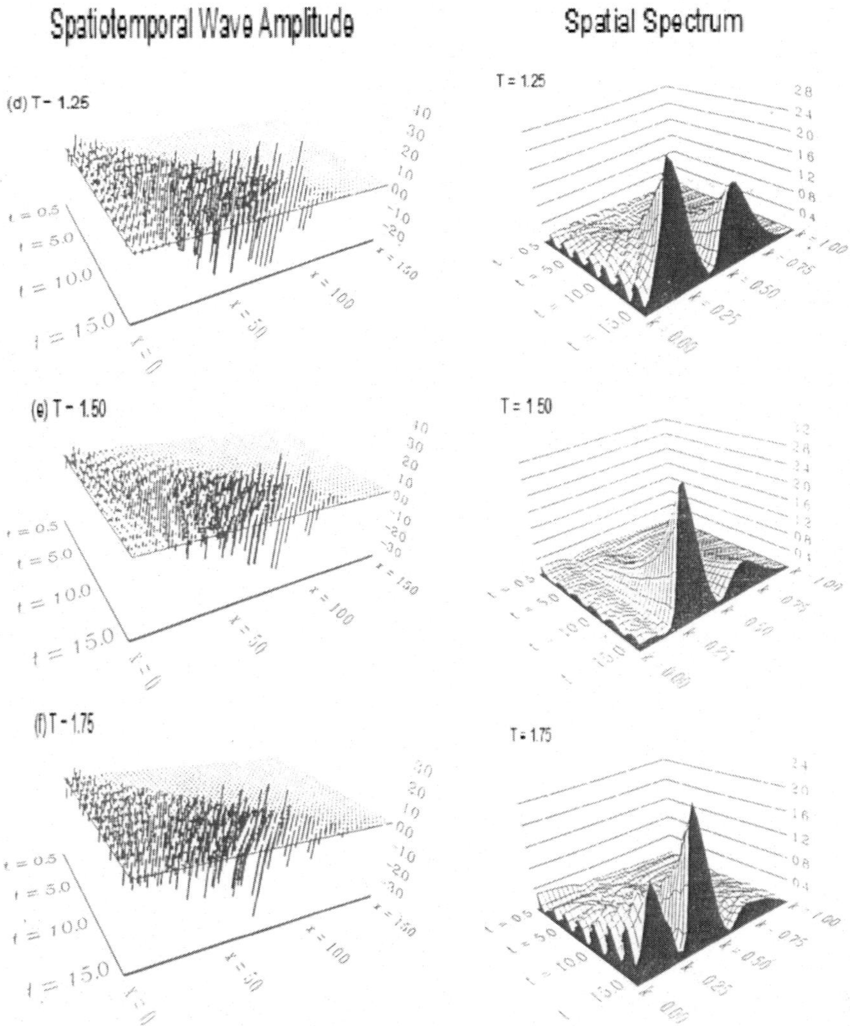


Figure 13. The neural medium contains stored electro-chemical energy and therefore can be described as *active*. Under a wide range of conditions, neural tissue amplifies initially small increments in collective neuronal activity; when this occurs, the amplified signal takes the spatio-temporal form of waves, and the amplification occurs at selected wavelengths. In our model the delay time T is the parameter most instrumental in determining the dominant wave or waves, whose wavelengths are about an order of magnitude greater than the average synaptic connection ranges. In our model the delay time T is the parameter most instrumental in determining the dominant wave or waves, whose wavelengths are about an order of magnitude greater than the average synaptic connection ranges. In this figure we see the spatiotemporal response of the model in Figure 3B to a unit impulsive stimulus to one layer at lateral position x = 0 and time t = 0. (Distances are normalized to the excitatory connection range and times to the uniform neural activity decay rate.) The response of the stimulated layer is shown for various values of interlayer time delay T: (a) T = 0.50, (b) T = 0.75, (c) T = 1.00, (d) T = 1.25, (e) T = 1.50, (f) T = 1.75. To avoid showing the infinite (delta function) stimulus, the earliest time shown is t = 0.5. For purposes of scaling, the graphs in this figure terminate at t = 15. The response at later times are shown in Figure 5. Parameters are given in Koch and Leisman (25).

Several disturbances separated from each other in space and time can give rise to a pattern more like a standing than a propagating wave. Growing standing waves may be useful in explaining "Tip-of-the-Tongue" and related phenomena in relatively normal situation and conditions such as persistent vegetative states or minimally conscious states in more egregious compromises to the status of brain functional integration.

When the delay is such that several wavelengths are simultaneously resonant, the location of the original disturbance is significant, since the phase relations among the excited waves in any particular region lead to interference patterns. For example at T = 1.25 (see Figure 5d), there are several adjacent modules simultaneously active near x = 150 and t = 25. Since the spatial origin of the figure represents the disturbance location, change in this location would change the position at which the large activity occurs. It is not far-fetched to draw a connection between this feature of the theory and the Proustian observation that memories of the same experience are never exactly the same. Furthermore, in the cortex, which can be represented by six layers (40), there are in general six waves that can be activated, so that the number of possible simultaneous resonances is larger than depicted here. This allows for enough complexity to explain some aspects of intelligence and certainly conscious awareness.

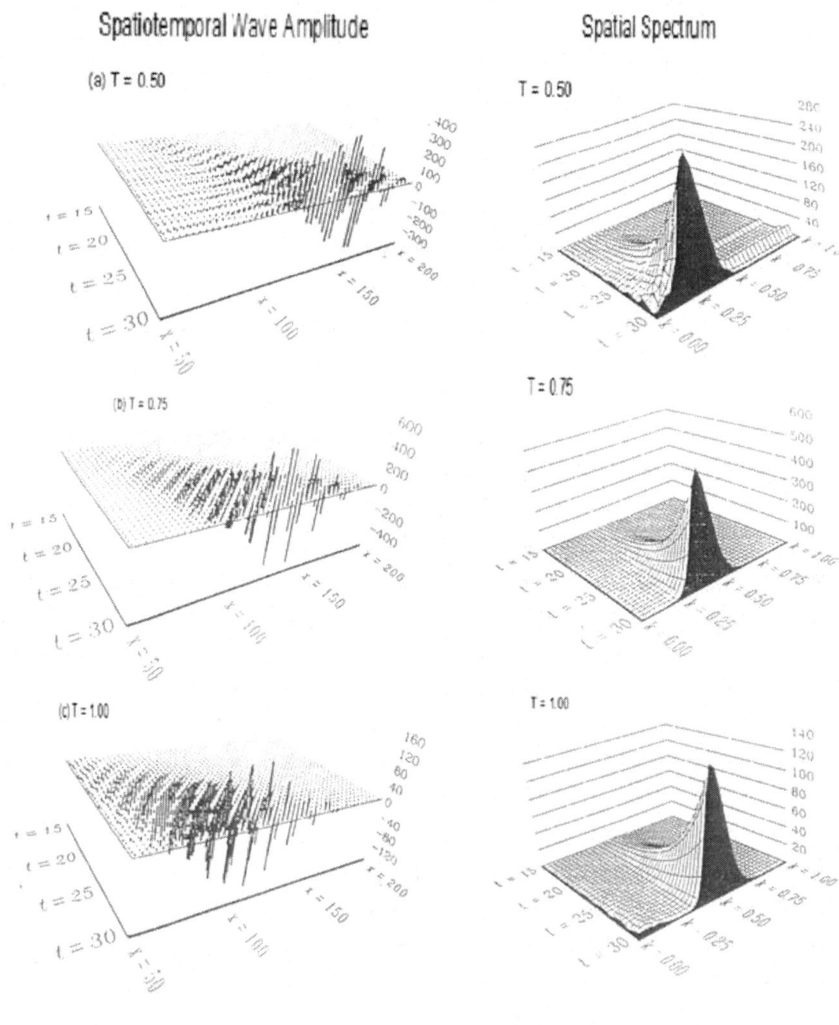


Figure 14. (Continued)

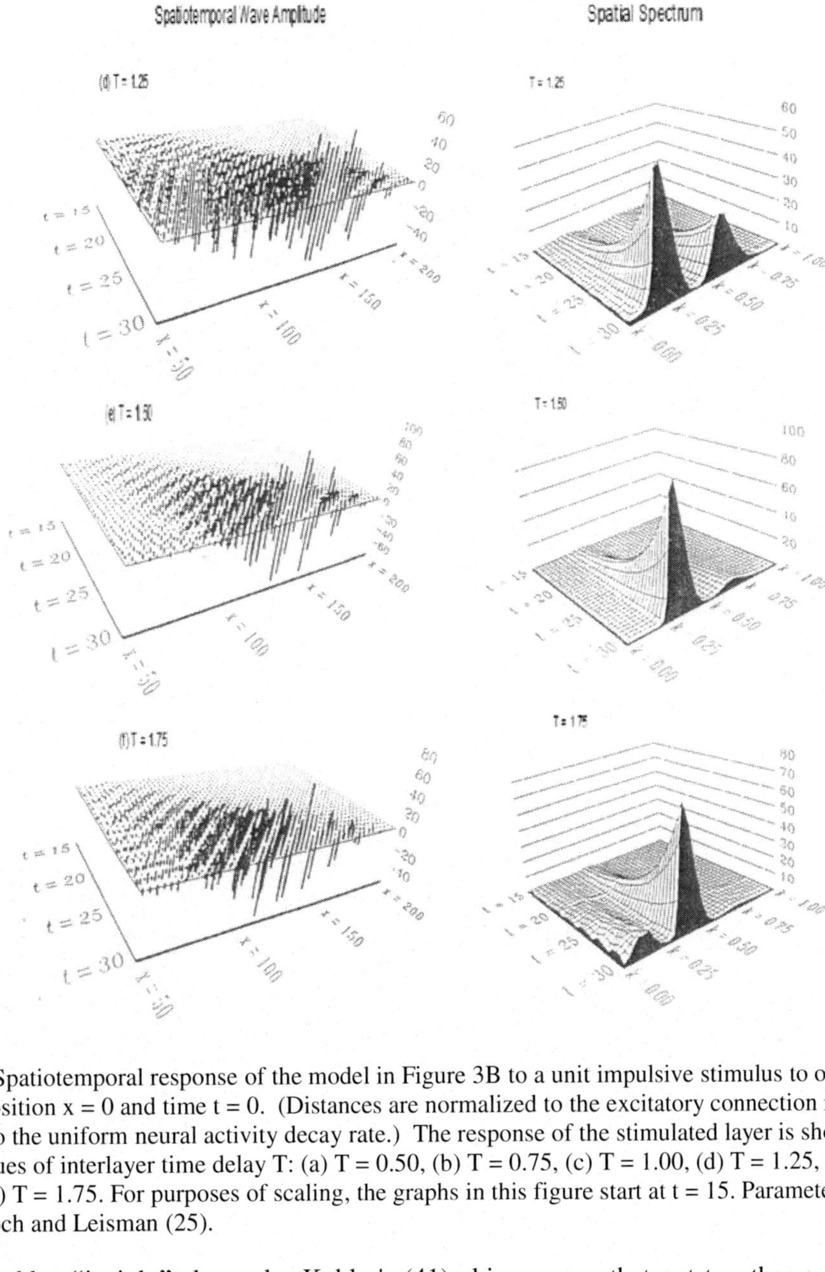


Figure 14. Spatiotemporal response of the model in Figure 3B to a unit impulsive stimulus to one layer at lateral position x = 0 and time t = 0. (Distances are normalized to the excitatory connection range and times to the uniform neural activity decay rate.) The response of the stimulated layer is shown for various values of interlayer time delay T: (a) T = 0.50, (b) T = 0.75, (c) T = 1.00, (d) T = 1.25, (e) T = 1.50, (f) T = 1.75. For purposes of scaling, the graphs in this figure start at t = 15. Parameters are given in Koch and Leisman (25).

The sudden "insight" shown by Kohler's (41) chimpanzee, that put together a platform and a stick to retrieve a banana inaccessible with either alone can be explained by the simultaneous activation of resonant patterns representing the two pieces of the puzzle. For this to be accomplished delay must be controlled, but an uncertainty is introduced through disturbance location and its effect on the positions of the interference patterns. In general large delay with its consequent complication of the resonant pattern is likely to be a favorable condition for such "creative thinking" to occur and its opposite for functional disconnectivities.

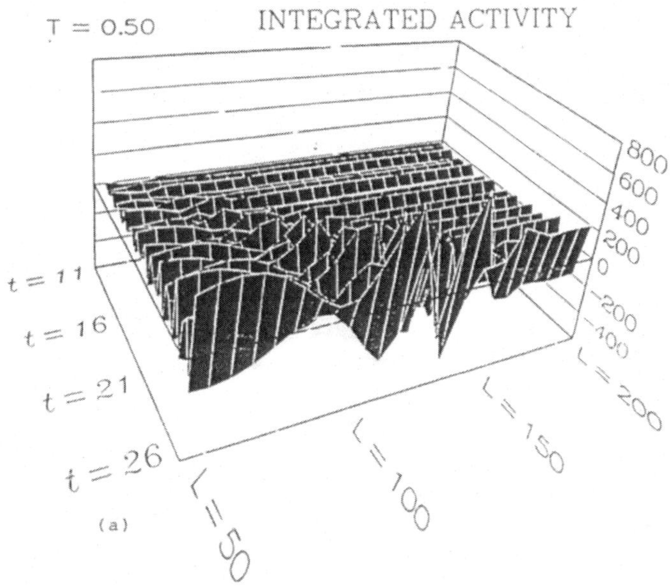


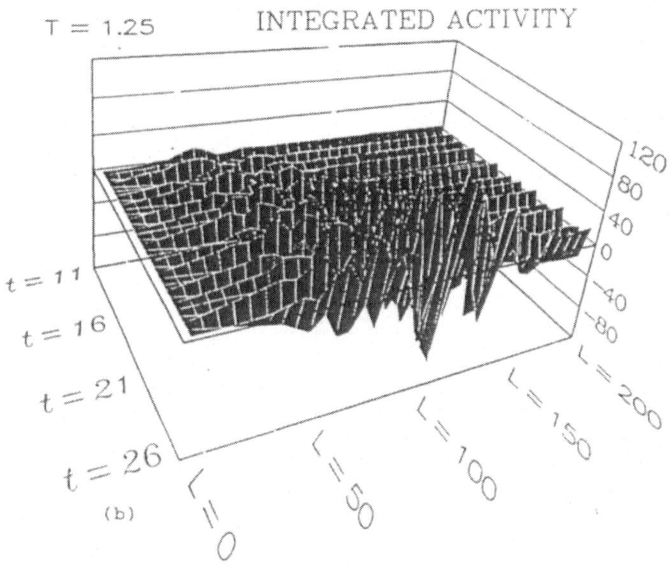


Figure 15. The total activity within a lateral region of the model in Figure 3B caused by a unit impulsive stimulus at time t = 0, as a function of distance L of the boundary of the region from the location of the impulse. (Distances are normalized to the excitatory connection range and times to the uniform neural activity decay rate.) The response of the stimulated layer between times t = 11 and t = 26 is shown for two values of interlayer time delay T: (a) T = 0.50, (b) T = 1.25. Parameters are given in Koch and Leisman (25).

The assumption that the delay changes before nonlinear effects set in is an expression of the familiar mental phenomenon of shifting attention. The wave forms in Figure (5) terminate at t = 30 decay periods, at which time the maximum amplitude shown is about 500 times the amplitude of the initial delta function disturbance. By then the wave has propagated about

200 excitatory connection lengths from the point of disturbance, so that about 107 cells (42), 0.1 to 1 percent of the (two-layer) cortex (18), have been involved. This is reasonable for a typical "mind moment."

In connection with attention shifts, we point out that in previous work (25-30) we have modeled the attentional center of the brain, and concluded that it communicates with the higher centers through a spatial-frequency signal. Attention integrates systems, and functional disconnectivities reflect impairment in that spatial frequency signal or signals. We speculate that shifts in attention occur as the delay in the cortex adjusts itself so that one of the cortical resonant wavelengths is equal to the wavelength of the attentional signal. The inability to adequately perform such operations to varying degrees creates functional disconnectivities.

Although we think that we can explain much of the problems of consciousness in the context of functional disconnectivities through a continuum neurophysics of wavelength propagation, a number of problems immediately arise in being able to use such a paradigm in creating a bounded continuum with death on one end of the spectrum and possibly hypervigilant states on the other.

## REFERENCES


[1] Leisman G, Koch P. Continuum model of mnemonic and amnesic phenomena. J Int Neuropsychol Soc 2000;6:589-603.

[2] Institute of Medicine. Organ donation: Opportunities for Action. Washington, DC: National Academies Press, 2006.

[3] Report of the ad hoc committee of the Harvard Medical School. A definition of irreversible coma. JAMA 1968;205(6):337-40.

[4] President's Commission for the Study of Ethical Problems in Medicine and Biomedical and Behavioral Research. Defining death: Medical, legal, and ethical issues in the determination of death. Washington, DC: US Government Printing Office, 1981.

[5] National Conference of Commissioners on Uniform State Laws. Uniform Determination of Death Act; 1980.

[6] URL: http://www.law.upenn.edu/bll/ulc/fnact99/1980s/udda80.htm.

[7] National Conference of Commissioners on Uniform State Laws. Uniform Determination of Death Act; 1987.

[8] URL: http://www.law.upenn.edu/bll/archives/ulc/fnact99/uaga87.pdf

[9] Capron AM, Kass LR. A statutory definition of the standards for determining human death: An appraisal and a proposal. Univ PA Law Rev 1972;121:87-118.

[10] Shewmon DA. Chronic "brain death": Meta-analysis and conceptual consequences. Neurology 1998;51(6):1538-45.

[11] Shewmon DA. Spinal shock and "brain death": Somatic pathophysiological equivalence and implications for the integrative-unity rationale. Spinal Cord 1999;37:313-24.

[12] Shewmon DA. The brain and somatic integration: Insights into the standard biological rationale for equating "brain death" with death. J Med Philos 2001;26(5):457-78.

[13] Laureys S, Owen AM, Schiff ND. Brain function in coma, vegetative state, and related disorders. Lancet Neurol 2004;3(9):537-46.

[14] Laureys S, Faymonville ME, De Tiege X, Peigneux P, Berre J, Moonen G, et al. Brain function in the vegetative state. In: Machado C, Shewmon DA, eds. Brain death and disorders of consciousness New York: Kluwer, 2004:229-38.

[15] Mollaret P, Goulan M. Le coma depasse. Rev Neurol (Paris) 1959;101:5-15.

[16] Jennett B, Plum F. Persistent vegetative state after brain damage. Lancet 1972;I:734-7.

[17] Multi-Society Task Force on PVS. Statement on medical aspects of the persistent vegetative state. New Engl J Med 1994;330:1499-1508,1572-9.
[18] Owen AM, Coleman MR, Menon DK, Johnsrude IS, Rodd JM, Davis MH, et al. Residual auditory function in persistent vegetative state: a combined PET and fMRI study. Neuropsychol Rehab 2005;15:290–306.
[19] Beuthien-Baumann B, Holthoff VA, Rudolf J. Functional imaging of vegetative state applying single photon emission tomography and positron emission tomography. Neuropsychol Rehabil 2005;15(3-4): 276-82.
[20] Levy DE, Sidtis JJ, Rottenberg DA, Jarden JO, Strother SC, Dhawan V, et al. Differences in cerebral blood flow and glucose utilization in vegetative versus locked-in patients. Ann Neurol 1987;22(6):673-82.
[21] Leisman G, Melillo RM. Functional brain organization in developmental dyslexia. In: Tobias, HD ed. Focus on Dyslexia Research. Hauppauge, NY: Nova Science, 2004:105-49.
[22] Leisman G, Melillo RM. Cortical asymmetry and learning efficiency: A direction for the rehabilitation process. In: Randall SV, ed. Learning disabilities: New research. Hauppauge, NY: Nova Science, 2006:1-24.
[23] Tononi G, Edelman GM. Consciousness and complexity. Science 1998; 282(5395):1846-51.
[24] Sprague JM. Interaction of cortex and superior colliculus in mediation of visually guided behavior in cat. Science 1966;153(3743):1544–7.
[25] Giacino JT, Ashwal S, Childs N, Cranford R, Jennett B, Katz DI, et al. The minimally conscious state. Neurology 2002;58:349-53.
[26] Schiff ND, Giacino JT, Kalmar K, Victor JD, Baker K, Gerber M, et al. Behavioral improvements with thalamic stimulation after severe traumatic brain injury. Nature 2007;448(7153):600-3.
[27] Koch P, Leisman G. Wave theory of large-scale organization of cortical activity. Int J Neurosci 1996;86:179-96.
[28] Koch P, Leisman G. A layered neural continuum architecture in attentional and seizure disorders. Int J Neurosci 2000;107(3-4):199-232.
[29] Koch P, Leisman, G. Effect of local synaptic strengthening o global activity-wave growth in the hippocampus. Int J Neurosci 2001;108(1-2): 127-46.
[30] Koch P, Leisman G. Wavelength coding of mental processes as an emergent property of the neural continuum. In: IEEE Proceedings of the International Conference of Neural Networks, vol I., Dordrecht, The Netherlands: Kluwer, 1990:471-4.
[31] Koch P, Leisman G. A continuum model of activity waves in layered neuronal networks: computer models of brain-stem seizures. In: Proceedings of the third annual IEEE symposium on computer-based medical systems, Los Alamitos, CA: IEEE Computer Society Press, 1990:525-31.
[32] Koch P, Leisman G. A continuum model of activity waves in layered neuronal networks: a neuropsychology of brain-stem seizures. Int J Neurosci 1990;54(1/2):41-62.
[33] Grossberg S, ed. Neural networks and natural intelligence, Cambridge, MA: MIT Press, 1980.
[34] Kohonen T. The self-organizing map. Proceedings of the IEEE, 1990;78: 1464-80.
[35] Traub RD, Miles R, Wong RKS. Large scale simulations of the hippocampus. IEEE Eng Med Biol Mag 1988;7:31-8.
[36] Jensen D. The principles of physiology, New York: Appleton, 1976:324.
[37] Wilson HR, Cowan JD. A mathematical theory of the functional dynamics of cortical and thalamic nervous tissue, Kybebernetic 1973; 13:55-80.
[38] MacDonald N. Biological delay systems: Linear stability theory. New York: Cambridge University Press, 1989.
[39] Brisyuk R. Quantitative investigation of the neural net model of two homogeneous populations. Moscow: Academy of Soviet Science, Scientific Center for Biological Research, 1982.
[40] Ermentrout GB, Cowan JD. Large scale spatially organized activity in neural nets. SIAM J Appl Math 1980;38:1-21.
[41] Desmond JE, Moore JW. Adaptive timing in neural networks: The conditioned response. Biol Cybern 1988;58:405-15.

[42] Krone W, Mallot H, Palm G, Schuz A. Spatiotemporal receptive fields: a dynamical model derived from cortical architectonics, Proc R Soc Lond B Biol Sci 1986; B226:421-4.

[43] Köhler W. The mentality of apes. New York: Harcourt, 1925:125.

[44] Traub RD, Miles R, Wong RKS. Models of synchronized hippocampal burst in the presence of inhibition. I. Single population events. J Neurophysiol 1988;58:739-51.

In: Considering Consciousness Clinically
Editors: Gerry Leisman and Joav Merrick

ISBN: 978-1-63484-260-0


*Chapter 3*

# AROUSAL AND CONSCIOUSNESS: EFFECTS OF TOTAL CORTICAL EXTIRPATION IN THE MAMMAL

***Hugh Staunton, PhD, FRCPI, FRCP (deceased)****

Department of Clinical Neurological Sciences,
Royal College of Surgeons in Ireland, Dublin, Ireland

## ABSTRACT

The experiments described in this chapter establish that a mammal without a cerebral cortex or striatum and with a damaged diencephalon is capable of a general mindless arousal, simulating wakefulness, with opening of the eyes, standing and walking, clambering over objects placed in its path, associated with a lowered threshold to sensory stimulation. It seems that during evolution of the mammal, a primitive arousal mechanism remains where it was, namely, at a reptilian anatomical level, and that true waking and awareness are grafted onto and integrated with it as the thalamus and cortex develop.

## INTRODUCTION

A description of waking without awareness in the human who has sustained brain damage was first offered by Kretschmer in 1940 (1). He used the term apallic, by which he meant a non-functioning cortex. The state could be temporary, resulting in death, or could emerge in the reacquisition of some degree of awareness. In some cases it may become permanent (referred to by some as persistent). A sleep-waking cycle has come to be an accepted and diagnostic feature of the vegetative state, differentiating it from coma (2).

* Correspondence: Professor Gerry Leisman, Director, The National Institute for Brain and Rehabilitation Sciences, Biomechanics Laboratory, Department of Mechanical Engineering, ORT-Braude College of Engineering, Snunit 51 Street, POBox 78, IL-21982 Karmiel, Israel. E-mail: gerry.leisman@staff.nazareth.ac.il

In 2002, a closely allied state, the 'minimally conscious state,' was coined (3) to describe those patients with who show 'inconsistent but reproducible signs of awareness, including the ability to follow commands,' but remaining unable to communicate interactively.

Concerning the vegetative state, it has become realised that some such patients can volitionally and reliably modulate their functional MRI responses, reflecting preserved awareness. In a recent study (4), 4 of 23 patients in a clinical vegetative state showed responses on either a motor imagery task, spatial imagery task, or both. This nevertheless left 19 patients who did not respond. The EEG in such patient is rarely flat, though not so consistently piloting the wake/sleep behavioral state with a clearly desynchronized/ synchronized EEG of the normal subject (5). The question is therefore begged 'what is happening in the non-responsive patients when they are in the waking (or indeed sleeping) state?' The terms are used clinically in this context and without precision. No necessary and sufficient criterion is offered for what constitutes 'waking' and 'sleeping.'

Jennett and Plum (6) for instance write as follows: 'they (the patients) have periods when, without any provocation they lie for periods with their eyes open; at other times they seem to sleep ----- it may be difficult to determine whether their sleep/wake rhythms have a normal diurnal pattern ----- the eyes are open and may blink to menace, but they are not attentive ----- it seems there is wakefulness without awareness.'

## Activation of 'Waking,' 'Attention,' Arousal

A canon of knowledge has accumulated since the 1930's on the anatomico-physiological basis for waking, or what Moruzzi and Magoun (7) have referred to (amongst other descriptions) as 'arousal.' From Berger (8) on, a number of investigators, including among them Adrian (9), Adrian and Mathews (10), Bremer (11, 12), Walter and Walter (13) have produced a constellation of evidence showing that the activation of 'waking' or 'attention' by afferent stimulation of the unspecific thalamocortical system is accompanied by a desynchronized EEG and is dependent for its expression on the cerebral cortex. This is predicated on believing that the cortex is necessary for these states to exist. To this sensory system must now be added projections from the ventral *tegmentum*, *raphé* nucleus, *locus ceruleus*, posterior hypothalamus and the basal forebrain (for review of the different neurochemically mediated 'arousal' systems see Jones (14)). Given the constraining effect of the experimental situation in the foregoing body of work, the behavioral effects could perforce not be closely observed, much reliance being placed on eye opening.

The clinical neurological world still believes that some degree of functional integrity of the cerebral cortex and its relationship with deeper nuclei is necessary for waking and sleeping (see e.g., (15)). What therefore constitutes the behavioral state in mammals in whom the cerebral cortex has been removed?

## What Constitutes the 'Waking' (or 'Sleeping') State of the Human in a Vegetative State?

The above question prompted a review of the animal literature on the behavioral effects of cortical extirpation, and this, with its implications in general is the subject of the present communication. There is a body of literature available ranging from 1892 to the late nineteen thirties (just overlapping with the Magoun era), which describes the long-term behavior of animals in whom the entire cortex, with or without the striatum, has been removed, with variable accompanying thalamic damage (Bard and Rioch (16), Dresel (17), Dusser de Barenne (18), Golz (19), Karplus and Kreidln (20), Rademaker and Winkler (21), Rothmann (22), Schaltenbrand and Cobb (23) Kleitman and Camille (24)). The species examined include cat, dog and macaque monkey. In these studies, which were afterwards anatomically documented, there is usually complete or almost complete removal of the six-layered isocortex (neocortex), with commonly a remnant of the piriform area left behind. This area, in which terminates the lateral olfactory stria, includes part of the amygdala, the uncus and anterior end of the parahippocampal gyrus, all three-layered non-isocortex. In most cases striatum was removed, except where electively preserved, as in one case of Schaltenbrand and Cobb's two experimental animals (23). When not completely removed, the striatum was commonly severely damaged The thalamus was usually significantly damaged, due to a combination of direct operative damage and later significant retrograde and anterograde degeneration. The description of the behavior of all these animals is consistent. They are described as awakening at irregular intervals (not specifically diurnal), commonly when 'hungry,' though also spontaneously. This 'awakening' appears to be part of a general arousal. The animal will open its eyes, stand up and walk about purposelessly (they are for the most part blind and deaf and lack sensory localizing ability). Figure 1 illustrates this phenomenon in a 'thalamic' cat of Schaltenbrand and Cobb. Figure 2 illustrates the post-mortem brain of this animal juxtaposed with a normal cat brain (reproduced from Brauer and Schober (25).

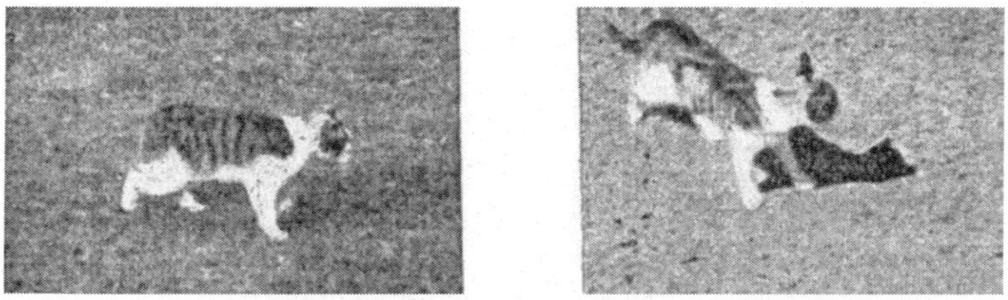

Figure 1. Cat following total bilateral cortical extirpation (from Schaltenbrand and Cobb (23)).

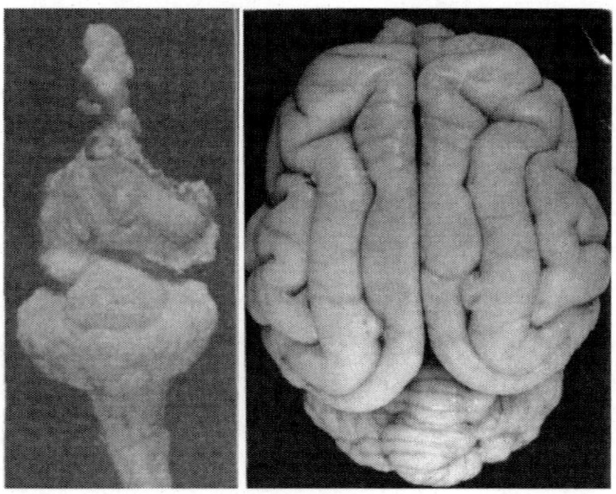

Figure 2. Post mortem brain of cat in Figure 1 juxtaposed with normal cat brain (adapted from Brauer and Schober (25).

Figure 3 illustrates a dog in whom a similar procedure has been performed (reproduced from Rothmann (22). The animal will eat when food is put into contact with its mouth. Some will take up the food spontaneously. Others will require it to be put in the mouth. Some will actually reject certain foods. The following are some descriptions by the authors (where German, translated by this author): 'quietly curled-up, sleeping --- regular quiet breathing, closed eyes, and no movement of limbs or head --- the same means will awaken it as those which will waken a normal dog --- walks around in circles' (Goltz); 'clear change between a more somnolent and more waking condition'(Karplus and Kreidl); 'walks up and down stairs --- dog walks in a lively fashion about the garden and walks successfully over obstacles --- dog lies and sleeps with the prevailing heat --- quite awakened, he walks frequently in little right-sided circles, also directly ahead and to the left side' (Rothmann). The animal reacts to pain in a general, non-specifically localizing fashion. It may exhibit rage (16, 23). If given a painful stimulus, the animal may snap at the air somewhere in the region of the stimulus, without accurate localization.

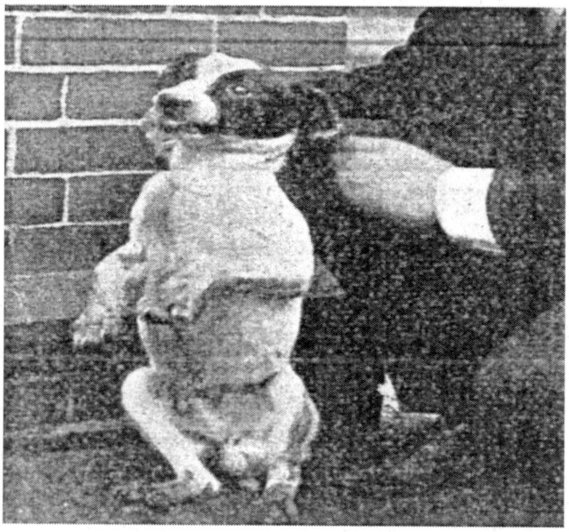

Figure 3. Dog following total bilateral cortical extirpation (from Rothmann (22)).

## DISCUSSION

Very little reference has been made to these experiments in the subsequent literature. Given the current restraints imposed by ethics committees, it is unlikely that such procedures will be repeated. Thus they warrant perhaps closer attention than has been given them in the past. The authors without exception refer to states of waking and sleeping, despite the absence of a cerebral cortex. If one is to adhere to the view that the cortex is indispensable for waking and sleeping, the animals cannot be truly awake (conscious) or in any form of sleep. What appears to occur is a state of generalized physiological arousal, simulating consciousness but without conscious content. The state may ready the intact mammal for purposive conscious activity. Remembering that most cases of vegetative state do not reveal evidence of cognitive activity, (4) the eye opening and general 'arousal' of the decorticated animal have similarities to the motor behavior which occurs in the vegetative state. Given the greater degree of motor specialization, the sophisticated (though unconscious) motor behavior of the decorticated animal would not be expected in the 'vegetative' human. These data would suggest that, in the absence of a functioning cerebral cortex, it is questionable whether the terms waking and sleeping, implying active organized cortical activity, should be applied as a routine in a description of behavior in the vegetative state.

The experiments cited here establish that a mammal without a cerebral cortex or striatum and with a damaged diencephalon is capable of a general mindless arousal, simulating wakefulness, with opening of the eyes, standing and walking, clambering over objects placed in its path, associated with a lowered threshold to sensory stimulation. It seems that during evolution of the mammal, a primitive arousal mechanism remains where it was, namely, at a reptilian anatomical level, and that true waking and awareness are grafted onto and integrated with it as the thalamus and cortex develop.

## ACKNOWLEDGMENTS

Hugh Staunton passed away in 2012. He was a former eminent clinical neurologist. He began his career by studying in Dublin. He went on to work at the University of Edinburgh, where he published many papers and obtained his PhD. He then spent a number of years at The National Hospital, Queen's Square in London, followed by the Max Planck Institute in Frankfurt. He returned to Dublin in 1970 to work as a clinical neurologist at the Beaumont Hospital and the Mater Hospital and took an academic interest in a variety of neurological topics, including amyloidosis, epilepsy surgery and definition of anatomy by brain imaging, headache and language. During his time in Dublin, he was the dean of the Richmond Institute for Neurology and Neurosurgery, a clinical lecturer in the Royal College of Surgeons and editor of the Irish Medical Journal from 1983 to 1986. Upon his death, Dr Staunton donated his collection of books to the Dublin Neurological Society. This collection is a diverse and extensive one encompassing not only medical texts, but also literature on physics, linguistics, psychology and neuropsychology and dream studies. The library comprises 245 books in total.

## REFERENCES

[1] Kretschmer E. Das apallische Syndrom. Z Gesamte Neurol Psychiatr 1940;169:576-9. (German)

[2] Multi-Society Task Force on PVS. Medical aspects of the persistent vegetative state. Part 1. N Engl J Med 1994;330(21):1499-508.

[3] Giacino JT, Ashwal S, Childs N, Cranford R, Jennett B, Katz DI, et al. The minimally conscious state: definition and diagnostic criteria. Neurology 2002;58:349-53.

[4] Monti MM, Vanhaudenhuyse A, Coleman M, Boly M, Pickard J, Tshibanda L, et al. Willful modulation of brain activity in disorders of consciousness. N Engl J Med 2010;362(7):579-89.

[5] Brenner RP. The interpretation of the EEG in stupor and coma. Neurologist 2005;11(5):1-14.

[6] Jennett B, Plum F. Persistent vegetative state after brain damage. Lancet 1972;1: 734-7.

[7] Moruzzi G, Magoun H. Brain stem reticular formation and activation of the EEG. Electroencephalogr Clin Neurophysiol 1949;1:455-73.

[8] Berger H. Über das elektrenkephalo gramm des Menschen II. J Psychologie Neurologie 1930;40:160-79. (German)
[9] Adrian ED. Afferent discharges to the cerebral cortex from peripheral sense organs. J Physiol 1941; 100:159-91.
[10] Adrian ED, Matthews BHC. Berger rhythm: potential changes from the occipital lobes in man. Brain 1934;57:355-85.
[11] Bremer F. Cerveau isolé et physiologie du sommeil. Comptes rendus des séances de la Societé de biologie et de ses filiales 1935;118:1235-42. (French)
[12] Bremer F. L'activité électrique de l'écorce cérébrale. Paris: Hermann, 1938. (French)
[13] Walter WG, Walter VJ. The electrical activity of the brain. Annu Rev Physiol 1949;11:199-230.
[14] Jones BE. Arousal systems. Front Biosci 2003;8:s438-51.
[15] Staunton H. Mammalian sleep. Naturwissenschaften 2005;92:203-20.
[16] Bard P, Rioch D. A study of four cats deprived of neocortex and additional portions of the forebrain. Bull Johns Hopkins Hosp 1937;60(2):73-125.
[17] Dresel K. Die Funktionen eines grosshirn- und striatumlosen Hundes. Klin Wochenschr 1924;49: 2231-3.(German)
[18] Dusser de Barenne JG. Recherches expérimentale sur les functions du système nerveux central, faites en particulier sur deux chats dont le néopallium avait été enlevé. Archiv Neerl Physiol Homme Anim 1920;4:31-123. (French)
[19] Golz F. Der Hund ohne Grosshirn. Siebente Abhandlung über die Verrichtungen des Grosshirns. Pflugers Arch gesamte Physiol. Menschen. Tiere 1892;51:570-614. (German)
[20] Karplus J, Kreidl A. Über Total exstirpationen einer und beider Grosshirnhemisphären an Affen (Macacus rhesus). Arch Physiologie 1914;30:155-212. (German)
[21] Rademaker G, Winkler C. Annotations on the physiology and the anatomy of a dog, living 38 days, without both hemispheres of the cerebrum and without cerebellum. Proc R Acad Sci Amsterdam 1928; 31:332-8.
[22] Rothmann H. Zusammenfassender Bericht über den Rothmannschen grosshirnlosen Hund nach klinischer und anatomischer Untersuchung. Z Gesamte Neurolog Psychiatr 1923;87:247-313. (German)
[23] Schaltenbrand G, Cobb S. Clinical and anatomical studies on two cats without neocortex. Brain 1931; 53:449-88.
[24] Kleitman N, Camille N. Studies on the physiology of sleep. VI. The behavior of decorticated dogs. Am J Physiol 1932;100:474-80.
[25] Brauer K, Schober W. Katalog der Säugetiergehirne. Jena: Gustav Fischer Verlag, 1970. (German)

In: Considering Consciousness Clinically
Editors: Gerry Leisman and Joav Merrick

ISBN: 978-1-63484-260-0


*Chapter 4*

# THE DIAGNOSIS OF BRAIN DEATH: APNEIC-OXYGENATION AS A SELF-FULFILLING DIAGNOSTIC TEST

***James Tibballs* and Ari R Joffe***

The University of Melbourne and Royal Children's Hospital Melbourne, Victoria, Australia, University of Alberta, Stollery Children's Hospital, Alberta and John Dossetor Health Ethics Center Edmonton, Alberta, Canada

## ABSTRACT

Current medical practice does not satisfy the legal, ethical and moral requirements for certifying death of the whole brain as required before organ procurement. The uncomfortable truth is that organ donors may not have been dead. Use of currently available technology to determine brain blood flow has not been adopted routinely. One of us argues that although these techniques cannot guarantee 100% accuracy, they represent the best current medical practice available. Lack of recommendations to use these techniques in organ procurement guidelines appears to continue a long history of favoring organ procurement from persons not dead but dying from devastating brain injury. Labeling a body as dead under bedside clinical tests alone is a pretentious fiction. On the other hand, one of us argues that, with more empirically validated testing for brain death as a state of devastating brain injury, abandoning the dead donor rule and donating organs with informed consent may be justifiable, and would more accurately reflect the facts of the situation. Either way, continuing with doing the apnea test is not defensible.

* Correspondence: James Tibballs, The University of Melbourne and Royal Children's Hospital Melbourne, Victoria, Australia. E-mail: james.tibballs@rch.org.au

# INTRODUCTION

The medical, legal and ethical circumstances under which organs may be procured for the purpose of transplantation continue to be debated. The determination of "brain death" has only been necessary for the purpose of organ procurement. In this paper, we argue that current clinical testing for "brain death" is not only unreliable but also harmful and that the medical criterion of "brain death" itself cannot represent death. The responsibility of diagnosing "brain death" rests with doctors who may, as some do for organ procurement after cardiac death (1), consider diagnosis of death to be neither an ontological nor moral issue, but merely a question of acceptable medical practice and thereby, by this means only, satisfying the "dead donor rule." Indeed, the authors of the American Academy of Neurology brain death guidelines (2) have said exactly this, when they claim that "the gold standard (of death) is not the UDDA (Uniform Determination of Death Act) but a neurological examination and irreversible loss of all brainstem function…The medical community acknowledges that a permanently ventilated, apneic (patient)…is dead."

## Problems in current practice of determining brain death using the apnea test

### *The apnea test*

According to established practice (3-9), the determination of brain death is merely a clinical exercise consisting of tests. In essence, these tests consist of findings of coma and lack of brain stem reflexes in the absence of confounding factors. However, at best, such examinations can only determine that the prospective donor is dying, not dead. The *sine qua non* of these tests is the apneic-oxygenation test.

### *Rationale of the apneic-oxygenation test*

Essentially, if the prospective organ donor cannot breathe spontaneously in the presence of coma and absence of other brain stem reflexes, "brain death" is declared.

The test may be performed in a variety of ways but essentially it allows the accumulation of carbon dioxide in blood, hypercarbia, which is a powerful stimulant to the respiratory center. If any sign of respiratory effort is observed, the respiratory center is deemed not dead and organ procurement disallowed.

### *Performance of apneic-oxygenation test*

Invariably, the test is conducted when the prospective organ donor is receiving mechanical ventilation. After ensuring that no confounding factors, such as hypothermia, hypotension, sedation, muscle relaxation, electrolyte or metabolic abnormalities are present, the mechanical ventilation is disconnected. Passive oxygen therapy is supplied with or without CPAP to ensure that hypoxemia does not occur. A stringent watch is made for any spontaneous respiratory effort and arterial blood gas analysis performed at intervals.

The test is terminated if any spontaneous respiratory effort is observed or, in the circumstance of continued apnea, the $PaCO_2$ attains a pre-determined level. In United States, Canada, Australia and New Zealand that level is 8.0 kPa (60 torr) and in United Kingdom 6.7 kPa (50 torr), or an increase of 2.7 kPa (20 torr) above the pre-test level. Although at first consideration the test appears soundly based, it has numerous flaws which should preclude its use.

## Flaws of the apneic-oxygenation test

### *Fatal harm from hypercarbia*

The most obvious problem is that the test may theoretically cause brain death (10, 11). Obviously, it is not harmful if the patient is already dead; however, the purpose of performing the test is to determine if the prospective organ donor is alive or dead. According to well-known neuro physiological principles (12), any increase in $PaCO_2$ will result in cerebral vasodilation permitting an increase in cerebral blood volume and a resultant increase in intracranial pressure which in turn may compromise blood flow to the brain. Areas of ischemia will become irreversible, and areas of penumbra will convert to irreversible ischemia if exposed to intracranial hypertension associated with hypercarbia during the test (13). In other words, performance of the test in a person not dead may well cause the very condition the test is purported to diagnose, brain death. The test is thus a self-fulfilling one. Further support for this claim comes from cases of recovery of some brainstem function in adults diagnosed with brain death (14). The claim was that these patients did not have an apnea test, and therefore were not proven dead. A more likely explanation is that the process of brain ischemia had not progressed to irreversible completion because these patients had not been subjected to the harmful apneic-oxygenation test.

### *Hypercarbia may itself be a confounder*

In addition to being harmful, the test is unreliable. The necessary level of $PaCO_2$ to be attained to exclude respiratory center function is itself brain depressive. In the fully conscious state, carbon dioxide causes sedation ($CO_2$ narcosis) at approximately 10.0 kPa (75 torr) (15) and unconsciousness at 12.0 kPa (90 torr) (16). Sensitivity to hypercarbia would be expected to increase in coma, that is, depressive effects of hypercarbia may be observed at lower levels of hypercarbia than in the fully-conscious state. In other words, hypercarbia may depress the respiratory center rather than stimulate it. These data suggest the apnea test may lack sensitivity in diagnosing brain death, and there are other reasons to support this claim (see below regarding medullary function).

### *The apnea test has been empirically refuted*

Levels of $PaCO_2$ attained during routine performance of the test often exceed the threshold levels required for declaration or exclusion of brain death. Empirical data show that the apnea test lacks specificity (excluding brain death). Case reports exist of observations of the onset of spontaneous respiration at $PaCO_2$ far in excess of the level at which brain death may be declared (14, 17-21). In these circumstances, had the test been terminated at the lower $PaCO_2$ level required in organ procurement guidelines, these persons would have been declared dead when in truth they were alive and may have been subjected to organ procurement. In addition, there are several reported cases of clinically diagnosed brain death followed later by spontaneous respirations (14, 22). These cases should not be a surprise given what is known about respiratory physiology. Chemosensation of pH (and hence $PaCO_2$) is widespread in brainstem, including multiple sites in medulla and pons that *together* maintain the normal thresholds of sensitivity to $PaCO_2$ (23). When *only* lower medullary function remains, the level of $PaCO_2$ needed to stimulate breathing can be expected to exceed 60mmHg. Moreover, lesions made in the pre-Botzinger complex of the rostral medulla in animals result in fatal apneas on exposure to hyperoxia (as in the apnea test), despite breathing when not exposed to hyperoxia (24). Acute lesions to the pre-Botzinger complex can cause apnea, but eupnea often resumes over days as the brainstem respiratory network reconfigures (25). This event would rarely be possible to detect given the usually rapid withdrawal of life support or organ donation after the diagnosis of brain death. Given that it is widely accepted that diagnosis of death should have 100% specificity, even rare cases of misdiagnosis are of great concern.

***Potential harm from complications of the apnea test***

The apneic-oxygenation test poses other dangers to the prospective organ donor, even when performed well. Systemic hypotension (26-30), dysrrhythmias (26) and pulmonary hypertension are common (31-34) and are presumably related to hypercarbia. If performed improperly, hypoxemia and barotrauma may occur (28, 35-37). Variability in performance of the test, including its complete lack, are widespread even in countries with well-developed health-care systems (38-45). Even in an expert center where the test is performed well (46), 10 of 207 (5%) tests were aborted because of hypoxemia or hypotension or both (47). Despite dogged defence of the test (48), its nocuous nature and lack of reliability suggest that it is time to remove it from practice and organ procurement guidelines. Since the only proven interventions in the intensive care of the acute brain injury patient are those to prevent hypotension and hypoxemia (49), acceptance of such results during apneic-oxygenation is not justifiable and is self-fulfilling.

***The apnea test does not test medullary respiratory center function***

The apnea test is done to test lower medullary function, the innate drive to breathe, and the completion of the cascade of brainstem injury, on the hypothesis that all brainstem function must be lost in death. The physiological study of respiration shows that after ponto-medullary transection, eupnea is transformed into a markedly altered two phase respiratory pattern, and after transection in the rostral medulla, between the Botzinger and pre-Botzinger complexes, only a gasping, slow, one phase respiratory pattern occurs (25, 50, 51). Indeed, gasping is the one respiratory pattern that can be reproducibly obtained in medullary preparations (25). Gasping is not sensitive to hypercarbia (25, 50, 51). Gasping is recruited in severe hypoxia, and is a respiratory effort aimed at sustaining life, necessary for autoresuscitation from hypoxic coma and apnea in animals and humans (52). The fact is that eupnea, stimulated by hypercarbia, is dependent on pontomedullary circuits, and altered two phase breathing stimulated by hypercarbia is dependent on the entire medulla with chemosensory input from pons. Gasping is dependent on only the medulla caudal to the Botzinger complex and is a sign of the organism attempting autoresuscitation. Hypercarbic hyperoxia will not stimulate gasping in even an intact organism. To really test for medullary function, and apnea, would require severe hypoxia, which is unacceptable due to its harmful global effects.

***Confounders to performing an apnea test are usually present***

Several confounders of the clinical examination for brain death are vaguely described, unvalidated, and left to highly variable clinical judgment (11). Two confounders are often present that are, remarkably, rarely considered. First, cervical spinal cord injury with acute quadriplegia and apnea is often reported with brain herniation, and sometimes reversible; indeed, high cervical cord injury is found in 50-100% of patients with brain death (52). Cervical spinal cord injury would invalidate the exam for consciousness (motor response), and for apnea. Second, endocrine dysfunction occurs theoretically in all brain death cases due to hypothalamic and pituitary injury. This means that central adrenal and thyroid deficiency should be routinely present in those suspected of brain death. The problem is that adrenal and thyroid deficiency states can cause coma and apnea (11, 53). Curiously, endocrine dysfunction is mentioned as a confounder in most guidelines on testing for brain death (7, 54), but the fact that it should be present in suspected brain death is ignored.

## IMPLICATIONS AND POTENTIAL SOLUTIONS

In the light of the above criticisms, the question is posed - why have we been seemingly content to procure organs under the guise of so-called "brain death." Quite obviously, procured organs are needed for those with fatal illnesses and whose continued existences are dependent upon their availability. For this reason, the definition of death has been adjusted serially over the years to overcome perceived difficulties. In essence, we have been procuring organs from those individuals who have no possibility of meaningful recovery or who may in crude terms be, "as good as dead." This is grounded in the clinical observation of failure to breathe but unfortunately eschewal of other signs of persistent brain function such as continued hypothalamic/pituitary function, electro encephalogram activity, and evoked potential activity (55).

### Alternatives to the apneic-oxygenation test

***Brain blood flow testing***

The basis for performing a test of brain perfusion is simple – if the brain has no blood flow, no part of the brain can be alive. Nonetheless, difficulties exist with selecting the appropriate tests and determining their reliability (48). Despite such caution, such tests are curiously recommended as optional, or required when some clinical tests cannot be performed. Unlike the apneic-oxygenation test, some tests of brain blood flow carry only small risks for the prospective organ donor.

The "gold standard" test for brain blood flow is a 4-vessel angiographic study but its use is probably declining because it is invasive and more difficult to perform than non-invasive tests which are readily available. Of these, radionuclide scintigraphy using brain-lipid-soluble technetium 99m-hexamethyl propyleneeamineoxime (HMPAO) or technetium 99m-ethylcysteinate dimer (ECD) are considered the most reliable (56). However, only two studies with 16 patients in one (57) and 20 patients in the other (58) have compared radionuclide scintigraphy with 4-vessel angiography. Combining results of these studies yields specificity (excluding brain death) of 1.00, but with wide 95% confidence intervals (0.37-1.00) and a sensitivity of 1.00 also with wide 95% confidence intervals (0.92-1.00). A recent review of diffusible radionuclide brain blood flow testing found that specificity for clinical brain death is based on only 41 patients, and for single photon emission computed tomography blood flow testing this specificity is based on only 12 patients, both with wide 95% confidence intervals (59). It has been shown that electroencephalographic activity can remain in cases with clinical brain death and absent brain blood flow on four-vessel angiography, suggesting the angiogram did not rule out residual blood flow sustaining viability of parts of the brain (60, 61). One study found that 13/43 (30%) of clinically brain-dead patients with absent four vessel angiographic brain blood flow had persistent cerebral perfusion by computed tomography (62). Clearly, more research is needed to determine reliability of scintigaphic studies, and they should be compared to a four-vessel angiographic study, in addition to clinical tests of brain death (which are erroneously assumed to be reliable).

Despite the exhortation that determination of "brain death" can be based on a determination of absence of brain blood flow rather than clinical tests, pituitary function may continue even when cerebral angiography excludes blood flow. In 6 patients meeting clinical criteria for brain death, 3 had neither cerebral nor hypophyseal flow, whereas 3 had no cerebral flow but evidence of hypophyseal flow (63). In another study (64), of 22 children with clinical brain death but without diabetes insipidus (presumed preserved hypophyseal function), 12 underwent 4-vessel cerebral angiography which demonstrated no flow and 4 had radionuclide perfusion scans which also demonstrated no flow.

Thus, it is apparent that hypophyseal function can persist even though angiography and radionuclide scanning fails to identify blood flow. One could argue that persistent pituitary function does not exclude a diagnosis of brain death since the pituitary's blood supply is extradural and may escape the effects of intracranial hypertension. However, it is undeniable that pituitary function is a brain function - which should be extinguished to satisfy a legal requirement of cessation of *all* brain function before organ procurement. Furthermore, it is unclear how extradural blood flow to intracranial contents (such as pituitary) can continue if the pathophysiology of brain death is lack of brain blood flow due to intracranial pressure exceeding arterial pressure. Continued pituitary function relies on hypothalamic function as well, which should be extinguished if brain blood flow was truly stopped.

Thus, although a test of cerebral blood flow using radionuclide scanning may provide the best possible information about the viability of the whole brain in comparison to clinical tests including the apneic-oxygenation test, such a test is also probably not totally accurate. But practically, what more can we do other than rely upon the most accurate testing available? The question then arises – can we ever determine total brain death? If the answer is no, which we claim, the question becomes - in what state of brain inactivity of the prospective organ donor should we undertake organ procurement?

### *Abandon the dead donor rule, or abandon organ donation*

We have argued that the apnea test is neither safe nor reliable in diagnosing total brain failure. Furthermore, the literature is not able to support the claim that absent detectable brain blood flow on an ancillary test proves lack of brain blood flow and inevitable brain necrosis. Moreover, brain blood flow is detected in at least 5-40% of patients currently declared dead based on accepted clinical testing (55). That this is so is supported by the finding that lack of pathological brain destruction, or even severe brain injury, is found in over 40% of autopsies of brain dead patients that had ongoing circulation for over 24-48 hours (46, 65). These data suggest that a test of brain blood flow is neither sensitive enough (many potential organ donors would be lost because they have blood flow), nor specific enough (some with absent detectable flow still have brain blood flow and brain function) to prove the state of brain death.

One of us has argued that brain death is a neurologically devastating state with a very poor prognosis, but not death itself (65). In this state of brain death, arguably, the patient no longer has a future like ours, a future of value, or what makes life worth living (65). Accordingly, with informed consent of patient or surrogate, organ donation prior to withdrawal of life support may be justifiable. This admittedly may be considered active euthanasia. Nevertheless, it has been argued that this is not morally different from withdrawal of life support at the end of life in other patients (66, 67). When a ventilator is withdrawn with consent, the physician's action (removal of the ventilator) causes the effect (patient's death). Both removal of the ventilator and organ harvest are acts that cause the death, and the informed consent is what makes them justified acts. It is a moral fiction that withdrawal of life support is simply allowing a natural death. By this line of argument, abandoning the dead donor rule, and allowing vital organ donation prior to death when in the clinical state of brain death, with informed consent, may be justifiable.

This potential solution requires open debate. The law accepts that withdrawal of life support with consent is not killing, attributing the death to the underlying condition (a legal fiction); whether the law will accept that organ harvest prior to death is similarly acceptable is unclear. Continuing to do the apnea test is not the solution, as it ignores our arguments that it is an unreliable and self-fulfilling diagnostic test. Ignoring the fact that brain blood flow testing has not been shown to be accurate is also not the solution. It is time to face up to the uncomfortable conclusion that we can only diagnose a devastating state of neurological injury. With empirically validated longer periods of observation, empirical clarification of confounding conditions, and empirical clarification of brain blood flow test specificity, abandoning the dead donor rule may be the best solution. Abandoning organ donation and its benefits to society is much less desirable.

## Conclusion

Current medical practice does not satisfy the legal, ethical and moral requirements for certifying death of the whole brain as required before organ procurement. The uncomfortable truth is that organ donors may not have been dead. Use of currently available technology to determine brain blood flow has not been adopted routinely. One of us argues (10) that although these techniques cannot guarantee 100% accuracy, they represent the best current medical practice available. Lack of recommendations to use these techniques in organ procurement guidelines appears to continue a long history of favoring organ procurement from persons not dead but dying from devastating brain injury. Labeling a body as dead under bedside clinical tests alone is a pretentious fiction. On the other hand, one of us argues (55) that, with more empirically validated testing for brain death as a state of devastating brain injury, abandoning the dead donor rule and donating organs with informed consent may be justifiable, and would more accurately reflect the facts of the situation. Either way, continuing with doing the apnea test is not defensible.

## REFERENCES


[1] Bernat JL, Capron AM. Defining death in donation after circulatory determination of death protocols: A bluish shade of purple (author's reply). Crit Care Med 2010;38:1761-2.

[2] Wijdicks EFM, Varelas PN, Gronseth GS, Greer DM. Evidence-based guideline update for determining brain death in adults. Reply from the authors. Neurology 2010; e-letter 31 August, available online at: http://www.neurology.org/cgi/eletters/74/23/1911 , accessed Oct 6, 2010.

[3] Wijdicks EFM. Current concepts: the diagnosis of brain death. N Eng J Med 2001;344:1215-21.

[4] American Academy of Neurology. Practice parameters for determining brain death in adults. Neurology 1995;45:1012-4.

[5] American Academy of Pediatrics. Guidelines for the determination of brain death in children. Pediatrics 1987;80:298-300.

[6] Wijdicks EFM, Pfeifer EA. Neuropathology of brain death in the modern transplant era. Neurology 2008;70:1234-7.

[7] Shemie SD, Doig C, Dickens B, Byrne P, Wheelock B, Rocker G, et al. Brain arrest: the neurological determination of death and organ donor management in Canada. CMAJ 2006;174(6):S1-S30.

[8] Australian and New Zealand Intensive Care Society. The ANZICS statement on death and organ donation, 3rd ed. Melbourne: ANZICS, 2008.

[9] Pallis C, Harley DH. ABC of brain stem death, 2nd ed. London: BMJ, 1996.

[10] Tibballs J. A critique of the apneic oxygenation test for the diagnosis of "brain death." Pediatr Crit Care Med 2010;11:475-8.

[11] Joffe AR, Anton NR, Duff JP. The apnea test: rationale, confounders, and criticism. J Child Neurol 2010. DOI: 10.1177/0883073810369380.

[12] Guyton AC, Hall JE. Textbook of medical physiology. Philadelphia, PA: Elsevier, 2006.

[13] Coimbra CG. Implications of ischemic penumbra for the diagnosis of brain death. Braz J Med Biol Res 1999;32:1479-87.

[14] Joffe AR, Kolski H, Duff J, de Caen AR. A 10-month-old infant with reversible findings of brain death. Pediatr Neurol 2009;41:378-82.

[15] Refsum HE. Relationship between state of consciousness and arterial hypoxemia and hypercapnia in patients with pulmonary insufficiency, breathing air. Clin Sci 1963;25:361-7.

[16] Lumb AB. Nunn's applied respiratory physiology, 5th ed. Oxford: Butterworth, 2000.

[17] Levin SD, Whyte RK. Brain death sans frontières. N Eng J Med 1988;318: 852.

[18] Haun SE, Tobias JD, Deshpande JK. Apnea testing in the determination of brain death: is it reliable? Clin Intensive Care 1991;2:182-4.

[19] Brilli RJ, Bigos D. Altered apnea threshold in a child with suspected brain death. J Child Neurol 1995;10:245-6.

[20] Okamoto K, Sugimoto T. Return of spontaneous respiration in an infant who fulfilled current criteria to determine brain death. Pediatrics 1995;96: 518-20.

[21] Vardis R, Pollack MM. Increased apnea threshold in a pediatric patient with suspected brain death. Crit Care Med 1998;26:1917-9.

[22] Roberts DJ, MacCulloch KAM, Versnick EJ, Hall RI. Should ancillary brain blood flow analyses play a larger role in the neurological determination of death? Can J Anesth 2010. DOI 10.1007/s12630-010-9359-4.

[23] Feldman JL, Mitchell GS, Nattie EE. Breathing: rhythmicity, plasticity, chemosensitivity. Annu Rev Neurosci 2003;26:239-66.

[24] Gray PA, Janczewski WA, Mellen N, McCrimmon DR, Feldman JL. Normal breathing requires pre-Botzinger complex neurokinin-1 receptor-expressing neurons. Nat Neurosci 2001;4(9):927-30.

[25] St-John WM. Noeud vital for breathing in the brainstem: gasping – yes, eupnea- doubtful. Phil Trans R Soc B 2009;364:2625-33.
[26] Goudreau JL, Wijdicks EFM, Emery SF. Complications during apnea testing in the determination of brain death: predisposing factors. Neurology 2000;55:1045-8.
[27] Vivien B, Amour J, Nicolas-Robin A, et al. An evaluation of capnography monitoring during the apnea test in brain-dead patients. Eur J Anaesthesiol 2007;24:868-75.
[28] Saposnik G, Rizzi G, Vega A, Sabbatiello R, Deluca JL. Problems associated with the apnea test in the diagnosis of brain death. Neurol India 2004;52:342-5.
[29] Jeret JS, Benjamin JL. Risk of hypotension during apnea testing. Arch Neurol 1994; 51: 595-9.
[30] Wu XL, Fang Q, Li L, Qiu YQ, Luo BY. Complications associated with the apnea test in the determination of the brain death. Chin Med J 2008;121: 1169-72.
[31] Lahana A, Costantopoulos S, Nakos G. The local component of the acute cardiovascular response to simulated apneas in brain-dead humans. Chest 2005;128:634-9.
[32] Combes JC, Nicolas F, Lenfant F, Cros N, Athis PD, Freysz M. Haemodynamic changes during the apnea test in patients with brain death. Ann Fr Anesth Reanim 1996;15:1173-7.
[33] Ebata T, Watanabe Y, Amaha K, Hosaka Y, Takagi S. Haemodynamic changes during the apnea test for diagnosis of brain death. Can J Anaesthiol 1991;38:436-40.
[34] Ohno M. Cardiovascular effects of apnea test in the diagnosis of brain death. Jpn J Anesthesiol 1990;39:822-6.
[35] Burns JD, Russell JA. Tension pneumothorax complicating apnea testing during brain death evaluation. J Clin Neurosci 2008;15:580-2.
[36] Monterrubio-Villar J, Cordoba-Lopez A. Barotrauma during apnea testing for brain death determination in a five-year-old boy. Anaesth Intensive Care 2008;36:462-3.
[37] Vivien B, Haralambo MS, Riou B. Barotraumatisme lors du test d'apnée chez des patients en état de mort encéphalique. Ann Fr Anesth Reanim 2001;20:370-3.
[38] Earnest MP, Beresford HR, McIntyre HB. Testing for apnea in suspected brain death: method used by 129 clinicians. Neurology 1986;36:542-4.
[39] Mejia RE, Pollack MM. Variability in brain death determination practices in children. JAMA 1995;274:550-3.
[40] Mathur M, Petersen L, Stadtler M, Rose C, Ejike JC, Petersen F, et al. Variability in pediatric brain death determination and documentation in Southern California. Pediatrics 2008;121:988-93.
[41] Wijdicks EFM. The clinical criteria of brain death throughout the world: why has it come to this? Can J Anaesth 2006;53:540-43.
[42] Powner DJ, Hernandez M, Rives TE. Variability among hospital policies for determining brain death in adults. Crit Care Med 2004;32:1284-8.
[43] Greer DM, Varelas PN, Haque S, Wijdicks EFM. Variability of brain death determination guidelines in leading US neurologic institutions. Neurology 2008;70:284-9.
[44] Choi EK, Fredland V, Zachodni C, Lammers JE, Bledsoe P, Helft PR. Brain death revisited: the case for a national standard. J Law Med Ethics 2008;36: 824-36.
[45] Chin KJ, Kwek TK, Lew TWK. A survey of brain death certification – an impetus for standardisation and improvement. Ann Acad Med Singapore 2007;36:987-94.
[46] Wijdicks EFM, Rabinstein AA, Manno EM, Atkinson JD. Pronouncing death. Contemporary practice and safety of the apnea test. Neurology 2008; 71:1240-4.
[47] Yee AH, Mandrekar J, Rabinstein AA, Wijdicks EF. Predictors of apnea test failure during brain death determination. Neurocrit Care 2010;12:352-5.
[48] Wijdicks, EFM. The case against confirmatory tests for determining brain death in adults. Neurology 2010;75:77-83.
[49] Bratton SL, Chestnut RM, Ghajar J, Hammond FFM, Harris OA, Hartl R, et al. Blood pressure and oxygenation. J. Neurotrauma 2007;24(Suppl 1):S7-S13.
[50] Abdala APL, Rybak IA, Smith JC, Zoccal DB, Machado BH, St-John WM, et al. Multiple pontomedullary mechanisms of respiratory rhythmogenesis. Respir Physiol Neurobiol 2009;168(1-2):19-25.

[51] Smith JC, Abdala APL, Rybak IA, Paton JFR. Structural and functional architecture of respiratory networks in the mammalian brainstem. Phil Trans R Soc B 2009;364:2577-87.
[52] Joffe AR, Anton N, Blackwood J. Brain death and the cervical spinal cord: a confounding factor for the clinical examination. Spinal Cord 2010;48:2-9.
[53] Coimbra CG. Are "brain dead" (or "brain-stem dead") patients neurologically recoverable? In: deMattei R, Byrne P, eds. Finis vitae: Brain death is not true death. Oregon, OH: Life Guardian Foundation, 2009:313-78.
[54] Wijdicks EFM, Varelas PN, Gronseth GS, Greer DM. Evidence-based guideline update: Determining brain death in adults. Neurology 2010;74: 1911-8.
[55] Joffe AR. Are recent defenses of the brain death concept adequate. Bioethics 2010;24:47-53.
[56] MacDonald A, Burrell S. Infrequently performed studies in nuclear medicine. J Nucl Med Technol 2009;37:1-13.
[57] Wieler H, Marohl K, Kaiser KP, Klawki P, Frössler H. Tc-99m HMPAO cerebral scintigraphy. A reliable noninvasive method for determination of brain death. Clin Nucl Med 1993;18:104-9.
[58] Munari M, Zucchetta P, Carollo C, Gallo F, De Nardin M, Marzola MC, et al. Confirmatory tests in the diagnosis of brain death: Comparison between SPECT and contrast angiography. Crit Care Med 2005;33:2068-73.
[59] Joffe AR, Lequier L, Cave D. Specificity of radionuclide brain blood flow testing in brain death: case report and review. J Intensive Care Med 2010;25:53-64.
[60] Ashwal S, Schneider S. Failure of electroencephalography to diagnose brain death in comatose children. Ann Neurol 1979;6:512–7.
[61] Paolin A, Manuali A, DiPaola F, Boccaletto F, Caputo P, Zanata R, et al. Reliability in diagnosis of brain death. Intensive Care Med 1995;21:657–62.
[62] Combes JC, Chomel A, Ricolfi F, d'Athis P, Freysz M. Reliability of computed tomographic angiography in the diagnosis of brain death. Transplant Proc 2007;39:16–20.
[63] Schrader H, Krogness K, Aakvaag A, Sortland O, Purvis K. Changes of pituitary hormones in brain death. Acta Neurochirg 1980;52:239-40.
[64] Fackler JC, Troncoso JC, Gioia FR. Age-specific characteristics of brain death in children. AJDC 1988;142:999-1003.
[65] Joffe AR. The neurological determination of death: what does it really mean? Issues Law Med 2007;23:119-40.
[66] Miller FG, Truog RD. Rethinking the ethics of vital organ donations. Hastings Cent Rep 2008;38:38-46.
[67] Miller FG, Truog RD, Brock DW. Moral fictions and medical ethics. Bioethics 2010;24(9):453-60. doi: 10.1111/j.1467-8519.2009.01738.x.

In: Considering Consciousness Clinically
Editors: Gerry Leisman and Joav Merrick

ISBN: 978-1-63484-260-0


*Chapter 5*

# DISRUPTED AXONAL FIBER CONNECTIVITY AS A MARKER OF IMPAIRED CONSCIOUSNESS STATES

***Rafael Rodriguez-Rojas[1,2], Karla Batista[1], Yasser Iturria[3], Calixto Machado[4], Gerry Leisman[5,6], Mauricio Chinchilla[7], Philip DeFina[8], Maylen Carballo[1] and Juan M. Morales[1]***

[1]Brain Imaging Group, International Center for Neurological Restoration, Havana, Cuba
[2]The Abdus Salam International Centre for Theoretical Physics, Trieste, Italy
[3]Neuroimaging Department, Cuban Neuroscience Center, La Habana, Cuba
[4]Institute of Neurology and Neurosurgery, Department of Clinical Neurophysiology, Havana, Cuba
[5]The National Institute for Brain and Rehabilitation Sciences, Nazareth, Israel
[6]Universidad de Ciencias Médicas de la Habana, Facultad Manuel Fajardo
[7]Neurology Department, Hermanos Ameijeiras Hospital, Havana, Cuba
[8]International Brain Research Foundation, New York, United States of America

## ABSTRACT

Persistent vegetative states (PVS) and locked-in syndrome (LIS) are well-differentiated disorders of consciousness that can be reached after a localized brain injury in the brainstem. The relations of the lesion topography with the impairment in the whole-brain architecture and functional disconnections are poorly understood. Methods: Two patients (PVS and LIS) and 20 age-matched healthy volunteers were evaluated using diffusion tensor imaging (DTI). Anatomical network was modeled as a graph whose nodes are represented by 71 brain regions. Inter-region connections were quantified through Anatomical Connection Strength (ACS) and Density (ACD). Complex networks properties such as local and global efficiency and vulnerability were studied. Mass univariate testing was performed at every connection using network based statistic approach. Results: LIS patients' network showed significant differences from controls in the brainstem-thalamus-frontal cortex circuitry, while PVS patients showed a widespread disruption of anatomical connectivity in both hemispheres. Both patients showed a reorganization of network attributes, with decreased global and local efficiency, significantly more pronounced in PVS. Conclusions: Our results suggest that DTI-based network connectivity combined with graph theory is useful to study the long-range effect of confined injuries and the relationship to the degree of consciousness impairment, underlying PVS and LIS.

## INTRODUCTION

The brainstem plays a key role in cerebral cortex activation as the origin of the ascending reticular activating system. Severe conditions can arise as a consequence of a traumatic or a non-traumatic injury in this area. Characteristic clinical symptomatology includes well-differentiated disorders of consciousness (DOC) such as "vegetative states" (VS) and "locked-in syndrome" (LIS). The VS encompasses a spectrum of patients who have emerged from coma to exhibit basic orienting response but show no indication of awareness (1, 2). By contrast, LIS is marked by tetraplegia and anarthria but consciousness and somatosensory perception are preserved (3, 4). Because patients with LIS show paralysis of all voluntary motor function except eye movements, they may be mistakenly thought to be in VS. Behavioral deficits in these patients can be as severe as those produced by diffuse damage to the cortical areas underlying high-level processing, indicative of awareness. The specific contribution of individual regions to the clinical performance is determined by their topological integration into brain networks (2, 5). This highlights the need to delineate the connectivity pattern in specific patients in order to elucidate how each connection and sub-network is anatomically related to the injured area and makes specific contribution to the level of consciousness.

Advancements in neuroimaging techniques, such as diffusion tensor imaging (DTI), offer the potential to probe anatomical connectivity between remote neuronal populations. Recent studies have suggested that structural networks of the human brain can be characterized by using graph theoretical approaches (for review, see Bullmore and Sporns (6) and He and Evans (7). Even though DTI has provided unique insights on the underlying brain circuitry accounting for the presence of consciousness and its alterations (5), the relationship of the network topology and efficiency metrics with specific clinical states such as VS and LIS remains unclear.

On the other hand, recent studies in patients with DOC using functional MRI (fMRI) have shown impaired connectivity in the thalamo-cortical and fronto-parietal networks, possibly reflecting interruptions of higher-order processes (8, 9). However, these studies do not provide information about neuroanatomic connectivity between different network nodes. Furthermore, the complexities of the association between brain structure and function are not well understood.

To our knowledge, this work introduces for the first time, the use of graph theoretical approaches and DTI to differentiate the topological organization of white matter network in patients in VS and with LIS. In order to identify the characteristics properties of injured networks in comparison with healthy architectures we used network-based statistics. In this study, we therefore sought to suggest essential differences in reduced global network efficiency and altered nodal efficiency between these DOC.

# OUR STUDY

*Patient in VS:* We studied a 24-year-old female patient who suffered a meningoencephalitis when she was 3 years old, and developed a hydrocephalus requiring several ventricular derivations to peritoneum, pleura and gallbladder. Four years ago, she suffered an acute hydrocephalus due an obstruction of the ventricular derivation, causing a central and uncal herniation with a compression of the brainstem. After being in coma during 4 weeks she was diagnosed as been in a persistent vegetative state (PVS). Magnetic resonance imaging showed destruction of the rostral part of the pons, the mesencephalon, and both thalami.

## Patient with LIS

We studied a 47-year-old male patient who developed an acute stroke of the basilar artery territory with sudden loss of consciousness. The patient remained in coma for 3 weeks, but afterwards opened his eyes and showed sleep-wakefulness cycles. He was diagnosed as having been in a PVS state. Nonetheless, when our group clinically examined him we noted that we were able to establish communication with him using through coded messages by blinking or vertical eye movements, indicating answers of YES or NO. We diagnosed him as being in a Locked-in syndrome (LIS). The patient demonstrated quadriplegia and the inability to speak, but he was undoubtedly conscious and aware, with no loss of cognitive function. He only preserved vertical eye movements and the blink responses. MRI showed ischemic lesions of the pons, corresponding to the basilar artery territory.

### *Controls*

Twenty healthy subjects (13 male, 11 female, age: 35.0 ± 12.1) were selected from the Cuban Human Brain Mapping Project database (10). Volunteers reported no history of psychiatric or neurological disorders. Those studies were selected so as to coincide with the average age of the patients and the age of these were within the standard deviation of the controls database.

### *Image Acquisition and Preprocessing*

All images were acquired using a MRI scanner Siemens Symphony 1.5 T (Erlangen, Germany). Using a standard diffusion gradient direction scheme (twelve diffusion-weighted images and a b=0 image), DW-MRI data were acquired using a single shot EPI sequence. To each subject, two interleaved sets of 25 slices of 6 mm thickness with a distance factor of 100% were acquired with the following parameters: b = 1200 s/mm$^2$; FOV = 256×256 mm$^2$; acquisition matrix=128 × 128; corresponding to an 'in plane' spatial resolution of 2×2 mm$^2$; TE/TR = 160 ms/7000 ms. Two interleaved sets were necessary because it was impossible to cover the whole head with a good spatial resolution using a single set due to a pulse sequence limitation (max: 35 slices). Both sets were joined to form a volume of 50 contiguous slices of 3 mm thickness covering the whole brain for each subject. The aforementioned acquisition was repeated 5 times to improve signal to noise ratio (SNR). In order to improve EPI quality, magnitude and phase difference images of a T2 gradient echo field mapping sequence were acquired with TE = 7.71 ms and 12.47 ms.

Also, a 3D high-resolution T1-weighted MPRAGE pulse sequence covering the whole brain was acquired with the following parameters: 160 contiguous slices of 1-mm thickness in sagittal orientation; in plane FOV=256×256 $mm^2$, and matrix size 256×256 yielding an spatial resolution of 1×1×1 $mm^3$. The echo time, repetition time, and inversion time were set to TE/TR/TI = 3.93 ms/3000 ms/1100 ms with a flip angle FA = 15°. Lesion areas were manually segmented on the MPRAGE images using MRIcron software (http://www.sph.sc.edu/comd/rorden/mricron/) to create binary masks in native space.

### *Network Definition*

The graph framework used here has been widely described in Iturria-Medina et al. (11). In brief, the cerebral volume is represented as a non-directed weighted graph $G$ in which nodes $N$ correspond to anatomically defined regions and arcs $a_{ij}$ to the connections joining them. In DTI-based graphs, between-regions connectivity can be reasonably restricted to white matter tracts connecting voxels of the surfaces of the corresponding anatomical areas. This approach significantly reduces the computational cost of the procedure.

While definition of the network nodes is consubstantial with graph theory, standard image-matching algorithms to map atlas to brains are challenged in patients with brain injury. To overcome this inconvenience, MPRAGE volumes were spatially normalized to the T1-MNI template using the 'unified segmentation' approach, available in SPM8 (http://fil.ion.ulc.ac.uk/spm) (12).

This procedure combines segmentation, bias correction and spatial normalization in the non-linear deformation model. Lesioned area was excluded from the calculation using a cost function masking to improve normalization results. Lesion masks for each patient were created using rough drawings of lesion boundaries. Atlas was registered with the gray matter volume maps in native space and segmented into 71 regions, using the anatomically labeled template corresponding to the Jacob Atlas developed by the Montreal Neurological Institute (http://www.mni.mcgill.ca/) and the IBASPM toolbox (available at http://www.fil.ion.ucl.ac.uk/spm/ext/#IBASPM) (13). Thus, the topological properties of the brain anatomical networks were defined on the basis of the 71x71 binary graph $G$.

### *Fiber tracking and node-node connectivity*

Figure 1 shows an overview of the methodology used in this study to identify impaired connections and compromised sub-networks in patients. An iterative streamline fiber tractography algorithm is employed for finding the most probable trajectory between each pair of gray matter regions (11). Streamlines exceeding 20 mm and below 500 mm in length and a curvature threshold of ± 90° were used to generate the connectivity matrix for each subject.

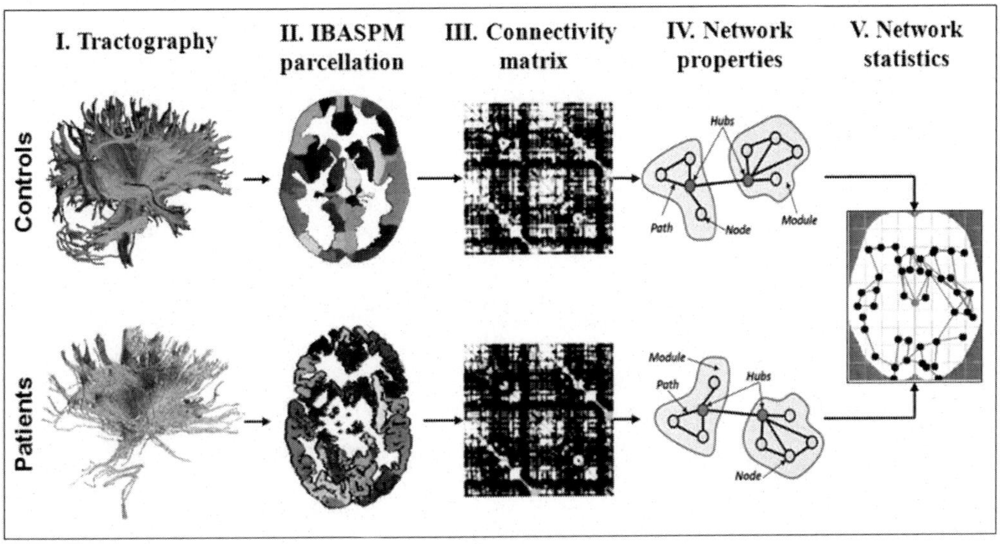


Figure 1. I. Streamline fiber tractography; II. Nodes definition using non-linear transformations and IBASPM toolbox; III. Anatomical network construction; IV. Calculation of network efficiency using graph theory; and V. Identification of impaired connections using network based statistic.

The connectivity between a pair of nodes was quantified by two different anatomical connectivity measures: Anatomical Connection Strength (ACS) and Anatomical Connection Density (ACD) (11). ACS is related to the amount of nervous fibers shared by regions $A_i$ and $A_j$ by counting the nodes on the surfaces involved in the connection:

$$C_{Zone}^{ACS}(A_i, A_j) = \sum w(a_{ij}) \quad (1)$$

where $w(a_{ij})$ quantifies the conditional weight of the arc $a_{ij}$. On the other hand, ACD is a measure of the fraction of the surface involved in the connection with respect to the total surface of both areas. Thus, it can be estimated as the ratio between ACS and the number of nodes $N_i$ and $N_j$ belonging to the surfaces of $A_i$ and $A_j$, respectively:

$$C_{Zone}^{ACD}(A_i, A_j) = \frac{C_{Zone}^{ACS}(A_i, A_j)}{|N_i| + |N_j|} \quad (2)$$

*Z* transformation was used to provide probability statements about the deviation of the connectivity measures from the normal values. *Z* scores of ACD and ACS were calculated by means of $Z = (x - \mu)/\sigma$, where $x$ represents the value of ACD or ACS in each patient, while $\mu$ and $\sigma$ are respectively the mean value and the standard deviation of $x$ in the population of normal subjects.

## *Graph analysis*

To characterize the effect of the lesions over the efficiency in information exchange in brain connectional architecture, we estimated the global and local efficiency of network as organizational attributes of integration and segregation, respectively. For a graph *G* with *N* nodes, the global efficiency can be computed as

$$E_{glob} = \frac{1}{N(N-1)} \sum_{(i \neq j) \in G} \frac{1}{d_{ij}} \tag{4}$$

where $d_{ij}$ is the shortest geodesic lengths between pair of nodes $i$ and $j$. On the other hand, the local efficiency $E_{loc}$ is measured as:

$$E_{loc} = \frac{1}{N} \sum_{i \in G} E_{glob}(G_i) \tag{5}$$

where $E_{glob}(G_i)$ is the global efficiency of the local subgraphs, neighbors of node $i$.

In order to identify disconnected subnetworks in the patients, mass univariate testing was performed at every connection using network based statistic (NBS) approach (14). Primary t statistic threshold for each link was set to 3.1 and 5000 permutations test were used to determine the statistical significance of differences in network parameters.

## FINDINGS

Fiber tractography localized connectivity disruption at different levels in the brainstem in patients in VS and with LIS, showing high consistency with lesion's topology (Figure 2). In VS patients, lesion in mesencephalon and rostral pons caused a disruption of cortico-spinal tract and cerebral peduncle, causing a widespread alteration of thalamus-subcortical and cortico-cortical connectivity. On the other hand, brain injury in LIS is confined to the ventral pons disrupting the cortico-spinal and spino-thalamic tracts, while cortical connectivity is preserved.

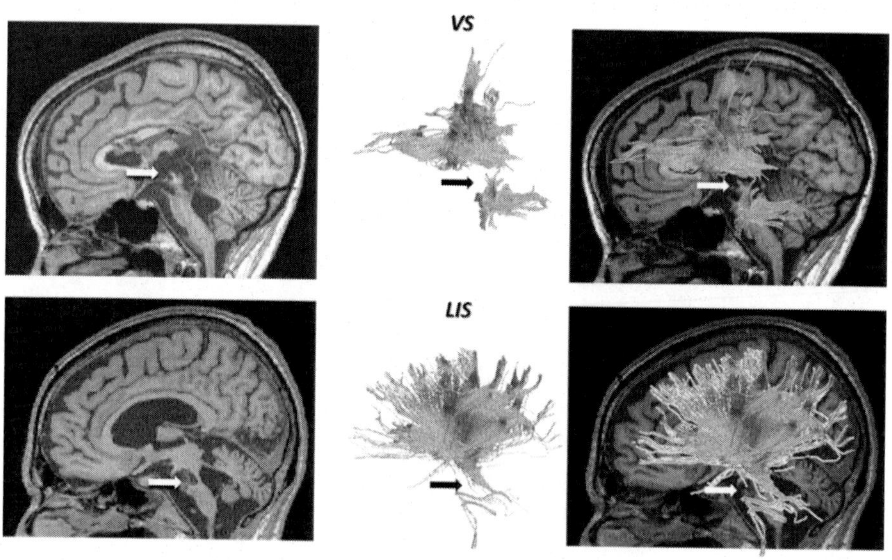


Figure 2. From left to right: anatomical damage, streamline fiber tractography and spatial correlation of impairments in patients. Upper: Patient in VS showing a widespread disruption in cortical and subcortical connectivity. Lower: Patient with LIS showing an injury in pontine crossing tracts and preserved cortical networking.

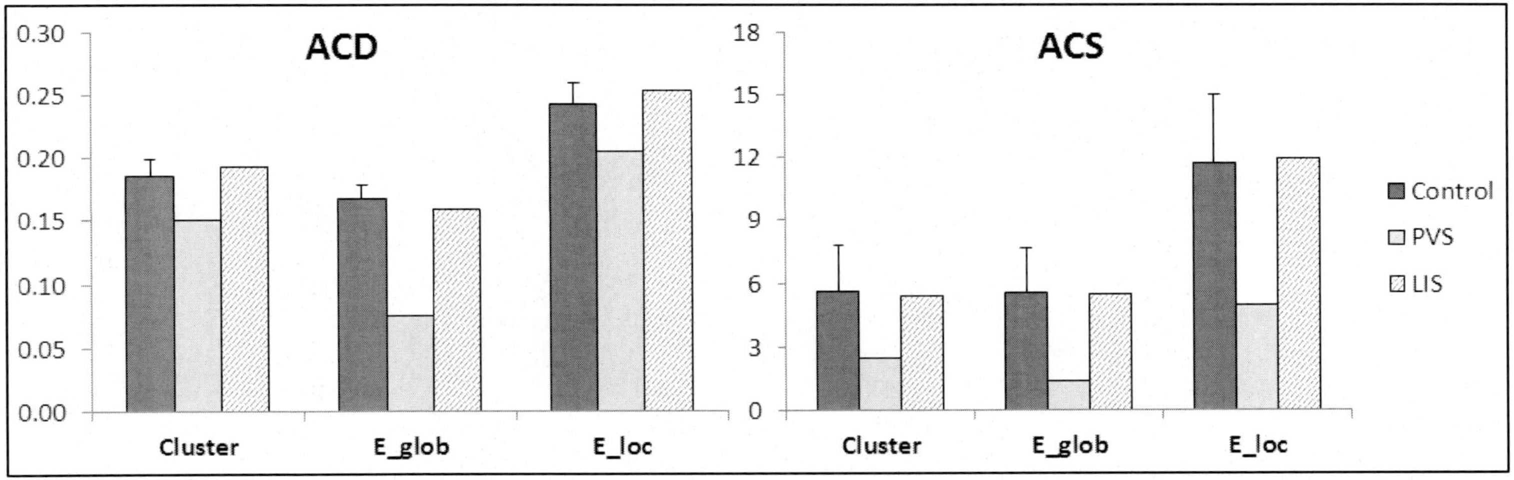


Figure 3. Differences in area under the global network properties curves: clustering index, global efficiency and local efficiency. The clustering and efficiency index differences between normal controls and patients for Anatomical Connection Density (ACD) and Anatomical Connection Strength (ACS) descriptors are depicted. Bars represent the mean of each network property and black lines represent standard deviations in control database.

**Table 1. Z scores of anatomical connectivity measures for both patients. Note that the patient with LIS shows a (non-significant) tendency to higher local properties than healthy controls**

| | ACD | | | | | | ACS | | | | | |
|---|---|---|---|---|---|---|---|---|---|---|---|---|
| | *Cluster* | | *E_glob* | | *E_loc* | | *Cluster* | | *E_glob* | | *E_loc* | |
| | % | *Z* | % | *Z* | % | *Z* | % | *Z* | % | *Z* | % | *Z* |
| ***PVS*** | -19.2 | 2.79* | -55.2 | 8.84* | -15.1 | 2.13* | -55.5 | 1.44 | -75.4 | 2.06* | -53.8 | 1.20 |
| ***LIS*** | 3.5 | -0.51 | -5.3 | 0.85 | 4.4 | -0.62 | -3.7 | 0.09 | -2.5 | 0.07 | 11.4 | -0.26 |

*Statistically significant (Z > 2).

As shown in figure 3, for Cluster, E_glob and E_loc the values of ACD and ACS in VS subject were lower than the corresponding mean values of control subjects, as expected. On the contrary, a trend toward increased clustering and local efficiency accompanied by reduced global efficiency was found for ACD in patients with LIS, but these differences were not significant.

The *Z* score test showed significantly lower ($Z > 2$) global and local efficiency, as well as clustering index in ACD network in patient in VS, while ACS network showed significant reduction only for global efficiency.

On the other hand, anatomical connectivity measures showed no differences in patients with LIS compared to controls (Table 1). Seeing together, these results suggest that balance between local specialization, provided by Cluster and E_loc, and global integration indicated by E-glob, has been spoiled in VS while remains essentially intact in LIS.

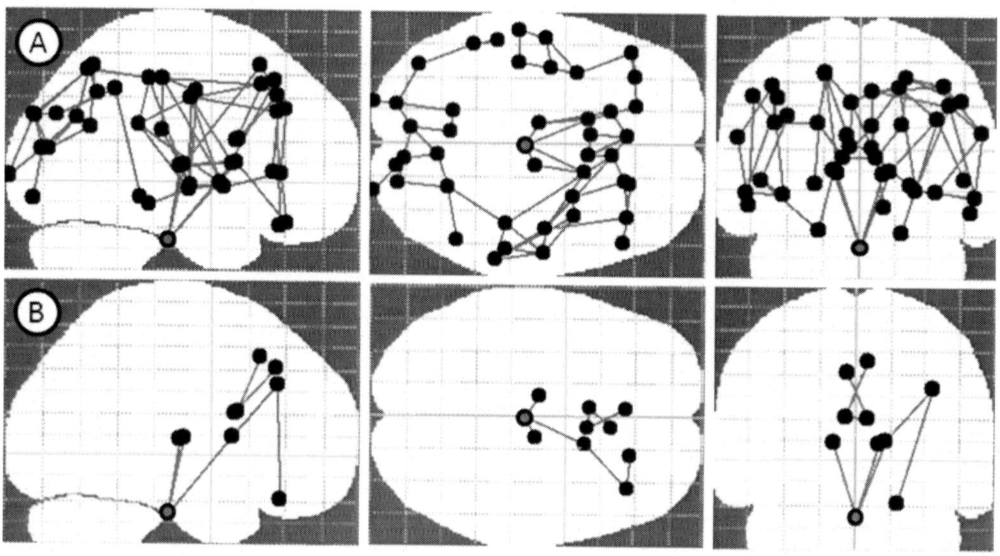


Figure 4. Nodes and streamline representation of impaired connections in VS (A), and LIS (B). Each node is depicted as a black circle positioned at its node's center of gravity. Gray circle is positioned in brainstem where structural injury is located. Significance of differences was calculated using network-based statistics.

A network based statistical analysis was used to identify particular node pairs that were abnormally connected in patients. NBS reveals that the architectural network presents anomalous organization in both patients compared with the corresponding healthy values, but is suggestively different between them. Streamlines interconnecting each of these node pairs are visualized in Figure 4. A widespread network was found to be significantly impaired in VS patient ($p < 0.05$, corrected) interconnecting several nodes comprising all cerebral lobes. Only two sub-networks were found to be significantly impaired in the patient with LIS ($p < 0.05$, corrected), corresponding to the basal ganglia-thalamus-frontal cortex circuitry.

## DISCUSSION

An accurate and reliable assessment of the level and content of consciousness in DOC is critical for the subsequent management and rehabilitation, as well as legal and ethical decision-making. To date, the gold standard for diagnosis of the level of consciousness is behavioral. However, the scope and reliability of available scales, examiner experience and overlapping of impairments in consciousness limit clinical diagnosis. These concerns may lead to misdiagnosis in patients with LIS, where cortical functions are preserved but the inability of production of voluntary motor behavior may resemble patients in VS.

This study provides supports that DTI is a potent tool for dissecting the complex neuroanatomic substrate of different DOC. Although the result of brain fiber tracking was not necessarily parallel to the clinical symptoms, essential differences between patients in VS and LIS are evidenced in Figure 4. Viewed as a network disorder, vegetative state has been found widespread impairment in cortico-cortical connectivity in addition to the brainstem connections. This result suggests that the loss of awareness in patients with lesions in the brainstem might be associated with aberrant neuronal connectivity among widely distributed brain regions, and provide structural evidence for the notion of VS as a disconnection syndrome. Significant reduction of all structural network attributes in this pathological condition might be interpreted as a considerable decline in the amount of possible nervous information that can be exchanged over the brain, and how deficiently it can be managed at local and global levels.

On the contrary, patient with LIS showed a cortical connectivity pattern that was comparable with that observed in healthy controls. This is in agreement with previous studies showing a near-to-normal functional connectivity in LIS (15, 16). Disruption of connections between brainstem, basal ganglia and frontal motor regions is consistent with quadriplegia, aphonia and quadriplegia and paralysis of the cranial nerves, while cortical networks supporting consciousness remain intact. Those results are highly consistent with remarkable functional and cognitive differences between these pathological states, extensively reported in previous studies (1, 3, 16-20).

Curiously, ACD shows a higher sensitivity to differentiate network properties of pathological states, especially VS, from healthy connectivity patterns. This is an unexpected result, considering that differences in ACS exceed 50% for all the network parameters. More likely, this apparent contradiction could be a result of the comparison of single subject against a normalized database. The relatively large range of age in a small population of healthy subjects induces an overstated standard deviation, which decreases the predictive ability of the *Z* score. A seminal study made by Iturria et al. (11) found significant correlations among these connectivity matrixes. However this high correlation was obtained between gray matter structures of healthy subjects, which may support our conclusion. By definition, ACD is searched as a measure of the fraction of the surface involved in the connection with respect to the total surface of both areas, while ACS give an estimate of the amount of nervous fibers shared by these areas (11). Thus, ACD normalize for the differences in surface area and volume of brain regions (network nodes) related with normal inter-subject variability and/or aging (21).

Our MRI configuration allows for acquisition in 12 isotropically distributed diffusion-encoding directions. This limitation determines the capacity of a tensor to model properly multiple fiber tracts in one voxel. For that reason we applied the fiber assignment by continuous tracking (FACT) streamline tracking algorithm (22). This algorithm is computationally inexpensive and has been demonstrated to be able to robustly reproduce brain circuitry. Figure 2 illustrate the performance of the tractography method and the high topological association between damaged tissue and fiber disruption in both patients. Application of advanced tractographic algorithms with high angular resolution can avoid limitations inherent to streamline tracking. However, they might not be computationally feasible as diagnostic tools in a clinical environment.

The main limitation to our study is that our findings are limited to two patients. However, large scale trials from patients with severe brain damage present challenging complexities related with acquisition, analysis and interpretation of neuroimaging data and inhomogeneities in lesion topology, which are unique for each patient. Our results suggest that DTI-based network connectivity combined with graph theory is useful to study the long range effect of confined injuries and the relationship with the degree of consciousness impairment, underlying PVS and LIS. The feasibility and reliability in the application of these techniques to characterize single cases have encouraging implications for use them as diagnostic and prognostic techniques in DOC.

Our results suggest that DTI-based network connectivity combined with graph theory is useful to study the long range effect of confined injuries and the relationship with the degree of consciousness impairment, underlying PVS and LIS. This is the first approach to characterize the dissimilarities in branching configuration underlying the clinical and behavioral differences between vegetative states and locked-in syndrome. More detailed comparisons between normal and pathological ACS and ACD maps combined with graphic theoretical tools could become a potential procedure to diagnose and distinguish different disorders of consciousness related to white matter injury in the pathways from brainstem to cerebral cortex.

## ACKNOWLEDGMENTS

RRR was partially supported by the "Abdus Salam" International Center for Theoretical Physics, Trieste, Italy. Authors would like to thank Andy Stanert for the revision of the manuscript.

## REFERENCES

[1] Monti MM, Laureys S, Owen AM. The vegetative state. BMJ 2010;341:c3765.

[2] Querol-Pascual MR. Clinical approach to brainstem lesions. Semin Ultrasound CT MRI 2010;31:220-9.

[3] Cardwell MS. Locked-in syndrome. Tex Med 2013;109(2):e1.

[4] Patterson J, Grabois M. Locked-in syndrome: a review of 139 cases. Stroke 1986;17(4):758-64.

[5] Edlow BL, Takahashi E, Wu O, Benner T, Dai G, Bu L, et al. Neuroanatomic connectivity of the human ascending arousal system critical to consciousness and its disorders. J. Neuropathol Exp Neurol 2012;71(6):531-46.

[6] Bullmore E, Sporns O. Complex brain networks: graph theoretical analysis of structural and functional systems. Nat Rev Neurosci 2009;10(3):186-98.

[7] He Y, Evans A. Graph theoretical modeling of brain connectivity. Curr Opin Neurol 2010;23(4):341-50.

[8] Crone JS, Ladurner G, Holler Y, Golaszewski S, Trinka E, Kronbichler M. Deactivation of the default mode network as a marker of impaired consciousness: an fMRI study. PLoS One 2011;6(10):e26373.

[9] Noirhomme Q, Soddu A, Lehembre R, Vanhaudenhuyse A, Boveroux P, Boly M, et al. Brain connectivity in pathological and pharmacological coma. Front Syst Neurosci 2010;4:160.

[10] Hernandez-Gonzalez G, Bringas-Vega ML, Galan-Garcia L, Bosch-Bayard J, Lorenzo-Ceballos Y, Melie-Garcia L, et al. Multimodal quantitative neuroimaging databases and methods: the Cuban Human Brain Mapping Project. Clin. EEG Neurosci 2011;42(3):149-59.

[11] Iturria-Medina Y, Canales-Rodriguez EJ, Melie-Garcia L, Valdes HP, Martinez E, Aleman-Gomez Y, et al. Characterizing brain anatomical connections using diffusion weighted MRI and graph theory. Neuroimage 2007;36:645-60.

[12] Ashburner J, Friston KJ. Unified segmentation. Neuroimage 2005;26(3):839-51.

[13] Alemán-Gómez Y, Melie-García L, Valdes-Hernández P. IBASPM: toolbox for automatic parcellation of brain structures. Proceeding of 12th Annual Meeting of the Organization for Human Brain Mapping. Available on CD-Rom in NeuroImage, 2006;27(1).

[14] Zalesky A, Fornito A, Bullmore E. Network-based statistic: Identifying differences in brain networks. Neuroimage 2010;53:1197-1207.

[15] Soddu A, Vanhaudenhuyse A, Bahri M, Bruno M, Boly M, Demertzi A, et al. Identifying the default-mode component in spatial IC analyses of patients with disorders of consciousness. Hum Brain Mapp 2012;33:778-96.

[16] Vanhaudenhuyse A, Noirhomme Q, Tshibanda LJ, Bruno MA, Boveroux P, Schnakers C, et al. Default network connectivity reflects the level of consciousness in non-communicative brain-damaged patients. Brain 2010;133(Pt 1):161-71.

[17] Guldenmund P, Vanhaudenhuyse A, Boly M, Laureys S, Soddu A. A default mode of brain function in altered states of consciousness. Arch Ital Biol 2012;150(2-3):107-121.

[18] de Jong BM. "Complete motor locked-in" and consequences for the concept of minimally conscious state. J. Head Trauma Rehabil 2013;28(2):141-3.

[19] Bardin JC, Schiff ND, Voss HU. Pattern classification of volitional functional magnetic resonance imaging responses in patients with severe brain injury. Arch Neurol 2012;69(2):176-81.

[20] Bruno MA, Vanhaudenhuyse A, Thibaut A, Moonen G, Laureys S. From unresponsive wakefulness to minimally conscious PLUS and functional locked-in syndromes: recent advances in our understanding of disorders of consciousness. J Neurol 2011;258(7):1373-84.

[21] Hedman AM, van Haren N, Schnack H, Kahn R, Hulshoff Pol HE. Human brain changes across the life span: a review of 56 longitudinal magnetic resonance imaging studies. Hum Brain Mapp 2012;33(8):1987-2002.

[22] Mori S, Crain BJ, Chacko V, Van Zijl PC. Three-dimensional tracking of axonal projections in the brain by magnetic resonance imaging. Ann Neurol 1999;45:265-9.

In: Considering Consciousness Clinically
Editors: Gerry Leisman and Joav Merrick

ISBN: 978-1-63484-260-0


*Chapter 6*

# CHILDREN AND SEVERE TRAUMATIC BRAIN INJURY: PROGNOSTIC FACTORS OF THE GLASGOW OUTCOME SCALE AFTER 6 MONTHS

***Dovilė Grinkevičiūtė**, *Rimantas Kėvalas and Vaidotas Gurskis***
Department of Pediatrics, Lithuanian University of Health Sciences, Kaunas, Lithuania

## ABSTRACT

In this chapter, we aimed at determining the prognostic factors that have an impact on outcomes of children who sustained severe traumatic brain injury. A total of 109 children with severe traumatic brain injury, admitted to the Pediatric Intensive Care Unit, Hospital of the Lithuanian University of Health Sciences, during a 4-year period were included in the study. The median age of the patients was 10.4 years (range 0.2–18 years). As initial assessment tools, the Glasgow Coma Scale (GCS), Pediatric Trauma Score (PTS), and Pediatric Index of Mortality 2 (PIM2) were employed during the first hour after admission. Gender, age, injury mechanism, injury pattern, time to admission, multiple injuries, findings on initial CT, hematological and circulatory disorders, intracranial pressure, and cerebral perfusion pressure were evaluated and their impact on outcome was analyzed by means of univariate and multivariate logistic regression analysis. Outcome after 6 months was assessed by using the Glasgow Outcome Scale (GOS): GOS scores of 1, 2, and 3 were defined as poor outcome, and scores of 4 and 5, as good outcome. All children were treated according to the protocol of severe head trauma management. The survival rate was 86%. Poor and good outcomes were documented in 30 (27.6%) and 79 (72.4%) patients, respectively. Two independent predictive factors for poor outcome after 6 months were identified: PIM2 of $\geq$ 7.9% (OR = 11.1; 95% CI, 2.2–56.5) and serum lactate level of $\geq$ 3.03 mmol/L (OR = 5.4; 95%, CI 1.0–28.1). To sum up, the PIM2 and the serum lactate level were found to be independent predictive factors associated with poor outcome in children after severe traumatic brain injury.

---

* Correspondence: Dovilė Grinkevičiūtė, Department of Pediatrics, Lithuanian University of Health Sciences, Eivenių 2, Kaunas 50009, Lithuania. E-mail: dovilgrin@hotmail.com

## Introduction

Trauma remains one of the most important sources of disorders in childhood, accounting for serious, potentially lifelong morbidity and representing the most likely cause of death after the first year of life in developed countries (1, 2). Head trauma is one of the most common injuries in childhood. More than 80% of these injuries are mild, but traumatic brain injury is the leading cause of death due to trauma in children (3).

Head trauma is responsible for primary and secondary brain injury. Cerebral hypoxia and ischemia are the leading causes of secondary brain damage. These alterations can be seen by simple laboratory tests, though the role of metabolic changes has not been fully elucidated yet (4).

For patient evaluation after severe head trauma, several scales such as the Pediatric Trauma Score (PTS), Glasgow Coma Scale (GCS), or Pediatric Index of Mortality 2 (PIM2) can be used. Trauma scoring systems have played an essential role in the evolution of trauma care over the past 20 years; however, they remain poorly valued by many emergency physicians (5).

Understanding and appropriate use of trauma scoring systems and laboratory findings together with specific guidelines of treatment can make a significant contribution to improving the prognosis of children after severe head injury. Early recognition of factors predicting outcome is important for quality assessment and could contribute to more selective management of the most severe injuries (6).

In this study we tried to identify simple predictive factors of outcome in children after severe traumatic brain injury within the first hour of admission. The knowledge of these factors might be helpful in predicting and improving outcome by means of correct management of children after severe traumatic brain injury.

The aim of the study was to evaluate outcome and determine prognostic factors associated with poor outcome after 6 months in children who sustained severe head injury.

## Materials and Methods

All children with severe head injury admitted to the Pediatric Intensive Care Unit (PICU), Hospital of the Lithuanian University of Health Sciences (former Kaunas University of Medicine), Lithuania, from January 2003 to June 2008 were recruited to the study. The study population comprised 109 children: 68 (62.4%) boys and 41(37.6%) girls. The median age was 10.4 years (range from 0.2 to 18).

Most injuries occurred due to road traffic accidents: 41 (37.67%) sustained trauma as pedestrians; 29 (26.6%), passengers; and 16 (14.7%), bicyclists. Four (3.7%) were beaten by other people, 15 (13.8%) experienced falls, 1 (0.9%) was hit by a horse, and in 3 (2.7%) cases trauma circumstances were unclear. Only 29 (26.6%) patients were transported directly to our PICU from the accident scene. The majority (n = 80, 73.4%) of the patients were transferred from other hospitals by the pediatric transport team of our PICU. The mean admission time (time from the accident to arrival to the PICU) was 6.5 ± 7.4 hours, and it was longer in patients initially managed in a regional hospital than in patients directly transferred to our PICU (7.7 ± 7.0 vs 3.7 ± 5.6 hours, respectively; $P < 0.01$). Good outcome was identified in

60 (75.0%) patients from regional hospitals and 19 (65.5%) patients transported directly to the PICU ($P > 0.05$).

The severity of head injury was categorized according to the Glasgow Coma Scale (GCS): a score of ≤ 8 indicated severe head injury (7).

As initial assessment tools, the PTS, post-resuscitation GCS, and PIM2 were used. The GCS score and the PTS were calculated on arrival to the first hospital. The PIM2 for each patient was calculated from the information collected at the time a child was admitted to the PICU or recorded at the time of the first face-to-face contact between the patient and the doctor from a special pediatric transport team of the PICU in case of transporting the patient from the regional hospital. The PIM2 was evaluated based on the regression equation as published in the literature (8). Serum lactate, glucose, and sodium levels were measured during the first hour of admission.

For children under 1 year of age, the Pediatric Glasgow Coma Scale (PGCS) was applied instead of the GCS. The PGCS differs from the GCS only by the verbal response subscale.

All patients were treated according to the protocol of severe head injury management, which is based on intracranial pressure (ICP)-targeted therapy (9) and a set of guidelines for the acute management of severe traumatic brain injury in infants, children, and adolescents (10). ICP was measured in 63 (57.8%) cases.

Outcome was assessed at 6 months after trauma using the Glasgow Outcome Scale (GOS) (11, 12). An interview by phone was used as the method of follow-up. A GOS score of 1 was assigned to children who died; a GOS score of 2, to children who demonstrated persistent vegetative state with no obvious cortical function; a GOS score of 3, for severe disability (conscious but disabled); a GOS score of 4, for a moderate disability or mild neurological defect (disabled but independent); and a GOS score of 5, for good recovery (completely healthy child). The GOS scores of 1, 2, and 3 were defined as poor outcome, and the GOS scores of 4 and 5, as good outcome.

The study was performed with the permission of the Ethical Committee of Kaunas University of Medicine (No. BE-2-46; September 21, 2005).

Statistical data analysis was performed by using the SPSS 12 software package. Data were expressed as mean with standard deviation (SD) or median with interquartile range as appropriate. A significance level of 0.05 was chosen for testing statistical hypotheses. We used receiver operating characteristics (ROC) curves analysis to determine the threshold value of predictive factors, indicating a change in the outcome (poor or good). Having the threshold values of the scales, we evaluated their sensitivity and specificity.

Univariate and multivariate logistic regression was used to determine which factors had the greatest influence on outcome after 6 months.

## RESULTS

The mean glucose, serum lactate, and serum sodium levels on the first hour of admission were 9.6 (4.5) mmol/L, 3.1 (2.1) mmol/L, and 139 (4.3) mmol/L, respectively. The median PTS was 4 (–2; 10); GCS score, 6 (3; 8); and PIM2, 15.6% (0.8%; 92.2%).

The distribution of patients by the GOS score after 6 months is shown in Figure 1. Poor outcome was identified in 30 (27.5%) cases; good outcome, in 79 (72.5%) cases.

The threshold values of serum lactate and serum glucose levels for poor outcome after 6 months were 3.03 mmol/L (sensitivity of 80% and specificity of 65%) and 9.25 mmol/L (sensitivity of 70% and specificity of 78%), respectively.

Patients with a serum glucose level of ≥ 9.25 mmol/L and a serum lactate level of ≥ 3.03 mmol/L were 9.8 times ($P < 0.01$) and 7.3 times ($P < 0.05$), respectively, more likely to have poor outcome after 6 months than those with serum glucose or serum lactate levels of < 9.25 mmol/L and < 3.03 mmol/L, respectively. The serum sodium level had no impact on outcome after 6 months (Table 1).

The threshold value of the GCS score for poor outcome after 6 months was 5 (sensitivity of 65% and specificity of 64%). The corresponding values of the PTS and PIM2 scores for poor outcome after 6 months were 4 (sensitivity of 70% and specificity of 58%) and 7.9% (sensitivity of 75% and specificity of 81%), respectively.

**Table 1. Probability of poor outcome after 6 months according to laboratory findings and trauma scores (univariate analysis)**

| Prognostic factor (No/yes) | OR | 95% CI |
|---|---|---|
| Serum glucose ≥ 9.25 mmol/L | 9.8** | 2.9–33.3 |
| Serum lactates ≥ 3.03 mmol/L | 7.3** | 2.3–22.7 |
| Serum sodium (mmol/L) | 1.0 | 0.9–1.2 |
| PTS ≤ 4 | 3.2* | 1.1–9.5 |
| PIM2 ≥ 7.9% | 12.5** | 3.8–41.2 |
| GCS score ≤ 5 | 3.4* | 1.2–9.7 |

*$P < 0.05$; **$P < 0.01$.

The patients with a GCS score of ≤ 5, PTS of ≤ 4, and PIM2 of ≥ 7.9% were 3.4 ($P < 0.05$), 3.2 ($P < 0.05$), and 12.5 ($P < 0.01$) times, respectively, more likely of having poor outcome after 6 months than those with a GCS score of >5, PTS of > 4, and PIM2 of < 7.9% (Table 1).

**Table 2. Factors predicting poor outcome after 6 months in children with traumatic brain injury (multivariate analysis)**

| Prognostic factor (No/yes) | OR | 95% CI |
|---|---|---|
| PIM2 ≥ 7.9% | 11.1** | 2.2–56.5 |
| GCS score ≤ 5 | 1.9 | 0.3–10.8 |
| PTS ≤ 4 | 0.8 | 0.1–4.9 |
| Serum lactates ≥ 3.03 mmol/L | 5.4* | 1.0–28.1 |
| Serum glucose ≥ 9.25 mmol/L | 3.1 | 0.5–16.1 |

*$P < 0.05$; **$P < 0.01$.

In order to determine the predictive factors for poor outcome after 6 months in children who sustained severe traumatic brain injury, all factors significantly predicting poor outcome after 6 months were entered in the multivariate logistic regression model. Two independent predictive factors for poor outcome after 6 months were found: PIM2 of ≥ 7.9% and serum lactate level of ≥ 3.03 mmol/L. The PIM2 of ≥ 7.9% and the serum lactate level of

≥ 3.03 mmol/L were associated with a 11.1- and 5.4-fold greater risk of poor outcome, respectively, after 6 months ($P < 0.05$) (Table 2).

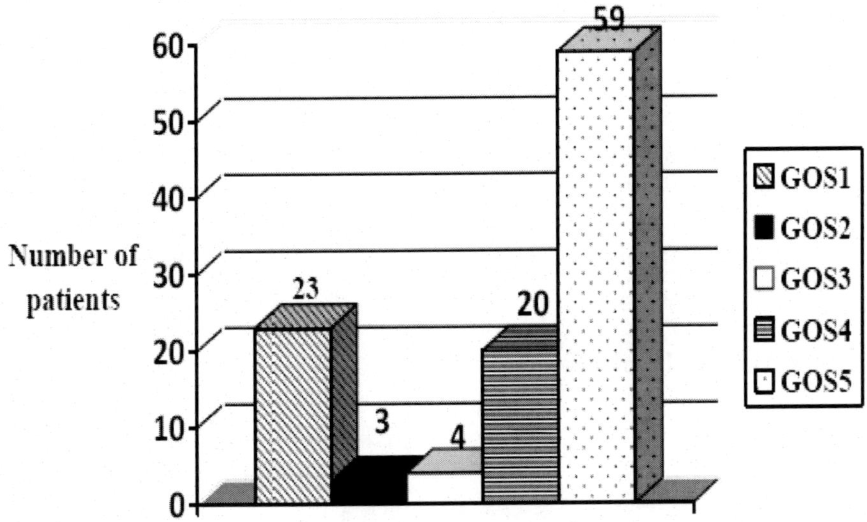


Figure 1. Distribution of children with severe traumatic brain by the Glasgow Outcome Scale score after 6 months in injury.

## DISCUSSION

In this study, we aimed at identifying the markers of unfavorable outcome within the first few hours of admission and to evaluate their relative importance in predicting outcome.

We used 3 scoring systems that are really easy to apply and a simple laboratory test that can be easily performed in any hospital. Trauma scoring systems can be classified into physiological, anatomical, and combined systems (5).

The GCS was first introduced in the 1970s to provide a simple reliable method of recording the level of patients' consciousness and monitor a change. This scale was developed to standardize the reporting of neurological findings and to provide an objective measure of the level of function of comatose patients. The GCS is one of the most common tools used by trauma care providers as it enables the gradation of head injury severity using simple observations rather than invasive or specialist techniques. In particular, the GCS is commonly used to predict the patient's outcome after trauma (7). The GCS has been modified for its use in children who are too young to have reliable language skills, producing the PGCS (5).

The GCS was developed to standardize the assessment of a patient's consciousness level. Only three behavior elements are evaluated: a) motor; b) verbal; and c) eye opening. This makes GCS easy to use, even in a prehospital setting. The GCS can assess the depth and predict the duration of coma. The aim of developing the GCS was to use simple terms that could be readily understood by a wide range of observers, including doctors, nurses, and others (13). The GCS is used as means of communication between different staff caring for patients from the scene of accident through to the ICU. Beyond the care of the patients, the

GCS has been used to classify head injured patients in epidemiological studies worldwide. Three grades of severity are recognized: severe (GCS 8 or less), moderate (GCS 9–12), and mild (GCS 13–15) (13).

The most appropriate time to assess the GCS for prognosis is therefore after resuscitation and stabilization. After resuscitation, however, many patients are often intubated and sedated, making the assessment on the full scale impossible. Clinicians vary in how they deal with this, but the evaluation of motor response alone is very useful under such circumstances (13). In some studies, the relationship between the GCS and the GOS in pediatric head trauma patients was found, but the threshold value of this scale was not determined (14). Some authors (4, 15) used the GCS as means of dividing pediatric head trauma patients into subgroups and found a statistically significant difference in outcome between the subgroups. Ducrocg et al. reported that a threshold value of GCS for death was 5 (16). In our study, we did not take into account brain ischemia- or hypoxia-associated lesions, the absence of which can lead to good functional outcome even when the GCS score is 3–5 (15).

The PTS is a combined trauma score. It was developed to predict the survival of injured children. Specifically designed for children, the PTS incorporates elements similar to those evaluated for adult trauma victims. The PTS evaluates only three anatomical and three physiological components, making it simple and quick to use.

Tepas et al. in their study documented a direct linear relationship between the PTS and injury severity and confirmed the PTS as an effective predictor of both injury severity and mortality already in 1988. The threshold value of the PTS in their study was 6 (17). Another study performed in 1998 by Orliaguet et al. determined that the threshold value of the PTS for mortality after severe injury was $\leq 4$. Cantais et al. reported that death was significantly associated with the PTS of $< 5$ in severely traumatized children. The occurrence of head trauma significantly influenced the mortality rate (15). Some authors attempted to define a predictive value of the Injury Severity Score (ISS) (16) and found it to be an independent predictor of death after severe trauma. However, the ISS is a strictly anatomical trauma score and is more suitable for patients with multiple injuries, while the PTS is a combined trauma score and is adjusted for the evaluation of pediatric trauma patients. Moreover, the PTS is simple enough to be used for the triage of pediatric trauma patients by any care providers with different levels of their professional competence. The calculation of this simple index, which is easy to perform, could be very useful in an emergency setting because it not only predicts injury severity , but also identifies the children at immediate risk of dying without appropriate and timely intervention (15). Although univariate analysis showed the GCS and the PTS to be good predictive factors for poor outcome, multivariate analysis did not find these two scales to be independent predictors of poor outcome in children with severe traumatic brain injury.

The PIM2 as a general score indicating the severity of illness in pediatric patients is not specifically dedicated for the evaluation of trauma patients. The validity of the PIM rests on how well it does what it is developed to do: to predict death for patients who die and survival for those who survive. The PIM2 is a score that represents well the patient's condition early after admission to the PICU. Taking this into account, the PIM appears to be superior to the PRISM (Pediatric Risk of Mortality) and the PRISM III. The PIM evaluates the condition of the patient directly on arrival to the PICU (e.g., when the patient's condition is least affected by therapeutic interventions) (19). One area where the PIM clearly outperforms the PRISM III is its ease of use. The PIM requires the collection of only 8 variables on admission, while the PRISM III requires the collection of the most abnormal (highest and lowest) values of 17 physiological variables during the first 24 h after admission plus 6 additional risk factors. The labor required to collect the data is obviously greater with the PRISM III unless automated data collection systems are present. The authors of the PIM emphasize that the coefficients for the PIM are freely available, whereas the use of the PRISM III requires the payment of a fee (20). Though the PIM2 is used for the prediction of mortality, our study has shown that it is an independent predictor of poor outcome after 6 months in severe pediatric traumatic brain injury.

The original publication of the GOS in 1975 (13) reviewed the term already used to describe survivors after severe head injuries. The GOS was introduced with the aim to have a limited number of exclusive categories that summarized the social capacity of the patient rather than listing specific disabilities (13). Studies have shown that changes on the 5-score outcome scale in the majority of patients occurred within the first 6 months. For this reason, many international studies evaluate the outcome after 6 months, which also proves to be an interval at which the majority of patients in a study can be successfully followed up (21).

The advantages of the GOS include its easy use on admission and appropriateness for any age group (22). In the study where the GOS was used to evaluate the short-term outcome of pediatric polytrauma patients at 6 weeks, 3 months, 6 months, and 1 year after injury, children demonstrated an improvement in function during the 12-month period according to the GOS, with statistically significant differences found between 6 weeks and 3 months, and 3 and 6 months after injury. These improvements appeared to slow during the next 6 months, with no statistically significant differences seen between 6 and 12 months (22). Based on the literature, we evaluated the GOS after 6 months, taking into account that later the changes in outcome are not significant.

No doubt, threshold values for poor outcome after severe pediatric head injury can vary depending on the differences of trauma care system of the country, region, or institution, but in general our study has shown that all the 3 trauma scoring scales are good predictive tools in pediatric trauma scoring.

However, as PTS is easy to apply, it is recommended to use for triage purposes: according to our study, the PTS of $\leq 4$ requires immediate intervention as the patient is at a high risk of poor outcome. Emergency physicians should be familiar with extant trauma scoring systems. The differences among systems should be taught during emergency medicine residency programs (5).

Though the pathophysiology of hyperglycemia in neurologic injury after head trauma remains unclear, some studies have reported that hyperglycemia is associated with death in children with head injury (23), and higher glucose levels are associated with worse outcome (4). An increased tissue lactate level in the regions of contusion and infarction of the injured brain was documented by means of proton magnetic resonance spectroscopy (24), but we failed in finding the studies reporting the serum lactate level as a predictor of late outcome in children with head trauma.

It is very important to remember that intensive care mortality models should only be used for patients' groups; they should never be used to guide the management of an individual patient. The PRISM and PIM scales are sensitive tools for the comparison of the actual number of deaths in the unit with the number predicted by one of the models, but not to decide that an individual patient is too sick to be worth treating (9).

New methods such as cerebral microdialysis (25), cerebral blood flow measurement (26, 27), and near-infrared spectroscopy (28) are helpful in monitoring the injured brain and prediction of secondary brain damage and outcome. However, most of them are invasive, can be easily misinterpreted, and have a limited clinical use (27).

We have shown that simple tools used within the first hour of admission in case of severe pediatric traumatic brain injury can be very helpful for evaluation of outcome and correct management in order to reduce morbidity and mortality. The PIM2 of $\geq 7.9\%$ and the serum lactate level of $\geq 3.03$ mmol/L were found to be independent predictive factors for poor outcome in children after severe traumatic brain injury.

## REFERENCES

[1] Soto-Ares G, Vinchon M, Delmaire C, Abecidan E, Dhellemes P, Pruvo JP. Cerebellar atrophy after severe traumatic head injury in children. Child Nerv Syst 2001;17(4-5):263-9.

[2] Holland AJA. Paediatric trauma. J Paediatr Child Health 2005;41:623-4.

[3] Gessler P. Evaluation of pediatric head trauma in the emergency department. Eur J Pediatr 2006;165(3):141.

[4] Chiaretti A, Piastra M, Pulitano S, Pietrini D, De Rosa G, Barbaro R, et al. Prognostic factors and outcome of children with severe head injury: an 8– year experience. Child's Nerv Syst 2002;18: 129-36.

[5] Fani-Salek MH, Totten VY, Terezakis SA. Trauma scoring systems explained. Emerg Med 1999;15:155-66.

[6] Ducrocq S, Meyer PG, Orliaquet GA, Blanot S, Laurent-Vannier A, RenierD, et al. Epidemiology and early predictive factors of mortality and outcome in children with traumatic severe brain injury: experience of a French pediatric trauma center. Pediatr. Crit Care Med 2006;7(5):461-7.

[7] Gabbe BJ, Cameron PA, Finch CF. The status of the Glasgow Coma scale. Emerg Med 2003;15: 353-60.

[8] Shann F. Paediatric index of mortality (PIM): a mortality prediction model for childen in intensive care. Neonat Pediatr Intensive Care 1997;23:201-7.

[9] Grinkevičiūtė D, Kėvalas R, Tamašauskas A, Matukevičius A, Gurskis V, Liesienė R. Sunki vaikų galvos smegenų trauma.Ar yra optimalus gydymo būdas? (Severe pediatric head injury: is there any optimal solution?). Medicina 2006;42(4):278-87.

[10] Adelson PD, Bratton SL, Carney NA, Chesnut RM, du Coudrey HM, Goldstein B, et al. Guidelines for the acute medical management of severe traumatic brain injury in infants, children and adolescents. Pediatr Crit Care Med 2003;4(Suppl):S1-S71.

[11] Jennett B. Development of Glasgow Coma and Outcome Scales. Nepal J Neurosci 2005;2:24-8.

[12] Willis CD, Gabbe BJ, Butt W, Cameron PA. Assessing outcomes in pediatric trauma populations. Injury 2006;37(12):1185-96.

[13] Jennett B, Bond M. Assessment of outcome after severe brain damage. Lancet 1975;1(7905):480.

[14] Odebode TO, Abubakar AM. Childhood head injury: causes, outcome and outcome predictors. Pediatr Surg Int 2004;20:348-52.

[15] Cantais E, Paut O, Giorgi R, Viard L, Camboulives J. Evaluating the prognosis of multiple, severely traumatized children in the intensive care unit. Intensive Care Med. 2001;27:1511-7.

[16] Ducrocq S, Meyer P, Orliaquet G, Blamot S, Laurent - Vannier A, Carli P. Epidemiology and early predictive factors of outcome in children with severe head injury. Crit Care 2001;5(suppl 1):243.

[17] Tepas JJ3rd, Ramenofsky ML, Mollitt DL, Gans BM, Ditchfield M. The pediatric trauma score as a predictor of injury severity: an objective assessment. J. Trauma 1988;28(4):425-9.

[18] Orliaquet GA, Meyer PG, Blanot S, Jarreau MM, Charon B, Buisson C, et al. Predictive factors of outcome in severely traumatized children. Anesth Analgesia 1998;87(537):542.

[19] Leteurtre S, Leclerc F, Wirth J, Noizet O, Magnenant E, Sadik A, et al. Can generic paediatric mortality scores calculated 4 hours after admission be used as inclusion criteria for clinical trials? Crit Care 2004;8:185-93.

[20] Randolph AG. Paediatric index of mortality (PIM): do we need another paediatric mortality prediction score? Intensive Care Med 1997;23:141-2.

[21] Jensen RL, Hahn YS, Ciro E. Risk factors of intracranial pressure monitoring in children with fiberoptic devices: a critical review. Surg Neurol 1997;47:16-22.

[22] van der Sluis CK, Kingma J, Eisma WH, ten Duis HJ. Pediatric polytrauma: short-term and long-term outcomes. J Trauma. 1997;43(3):501-6.

[23] Cohran A, Scaife ER, Hansen KW, Downey EC. Hyperglycaemia and outcomes from pediatric traumatic brain injury. J Trauma 2003;55(6):1035-8.

[24] Sutton LN, Wang Z, Duhaime AC, Costarino D, Sauter R, Zimmerman R. Tissue lactate in pediatric head trauma: a clinical study using 1H NMR spectroscopy. Pediatr Neurosurg 1995;22(2):81-7.

[25] Engstrom M, Polito A, Reinstrup P, Romner B, Ryding E, Ungerstedt U. Intracerebral microdialysis in severe brain trauma: the importance of catheter location. J Neurosurg 2010;102:460-9.

[26] Vajkoczy P, Roth H, Horn P, Lucke T, Thome C, Hubner U, et al. Continuous monitoring of regional cerebral blood flow: experimental and clinical validation of a novel thermal diffusion microprobe. J Neurosurg 2000;93:265-74.

[27] Steiner LA, Andrews PJ. Monitoring the injured brain: ICP and CBF. Br J Anaesth. 2006;97(1):26-38.

[28] Gupta AK. Monitoring the injured brain in the intensive care unit. J Postgrad Med 2002;48(3):218-25.

In: Considering Consciousness Clinically
Editors: Gerry Leisman and Joav Merrick

ISBN: 978-1-63484-260-0


*Chapter 7*

# TIMING OF ENTRY TO A MINIMALLY CONSCIOUS STATE RELATED TO PROGNOSIS FOR PEOPLE WITH SEVERE TRAUMATIC BRAIN INJURY

***Xuehai Wu and Jianghong Zhu, PhD****
Fudan University Huashan Hospital,
Department of Neurosurgery,
National Key Laboratory for Medical Neurobiology,
Institutes of Brain Science,
Shanghai Medical Collgee-Fudan University,
Shanghai, China

## ABSTRACT

In this chapter we explore the relationship between the timing of reaching a minimally conscious state and clinical prognosis in patients with severe traumatic brain injury (TBI). Sixty-five severe TBI patients who moved into a minimally conscious state (MCS) during rehabilitation were divided into two groups, the early MCS group and late MCS group, according to whether their MCS was detected within one month after head injury. The Glass outcome scale (GOS) was applied as a major parameter to compare the prognosis between the two groups at the end of six-month follow-up. The mean GOS in the early MCS group was 4.31 ± 0.92 at 6 months after injury, comparing to 2.50 ± 0.91 in late MCS group ($p < 0.001$), and indicating significant difference between two groups. For several TBI patients who entered MCS during rehabilitation, patients who moved into MCS within one month after injury displayed better prognosis than those who took a longer time to reach MCS. Results support the necessity to differentiate early MCS and late MCS for severe TBI patients.

* Correspondence: Jianhong Zhu, MD, PhD, Fudan University Huashan Hospital, Department of Neurosurgery, 12 Wulumuqi Zhong Rd. Shanghai, 200040, China. E-mail: jzhu@fudan.edu.cn

## INTRODUCTION

The development of neurosurgical intensive care has greatly decreased the mortality of patients with severe traumatic brain injury (TBI), though the number of patients with severe consciousness disorders arises as an accompanying issue. Coma, vegetative state (VS), and the minimally conscious state (MCS) patients were major and common forms of conscious disorder in severe TBI patients. While patients in coma have complete failure of the arousal system and VS characterized by the complete absence of behavioral evidence for self or environmental awareness, MCS is a state of consciousness inconsistent but clearly discernible.

It has been indicated that patients who are in MCS have preserved brain networks that retain the potential for activation. For example, functional MRI studies have suggested that patients in MCS can retain nearly integral auditory and visual network (1, 2). However, a fact is that the prognosis of patients in MCS varies greatly, and there have been few studies on this phenomenon. Based on our experience and previous work, we have noticed that there is great variability in when a severe TBI patient may enter an MCS. Some patients may recover from coma within several days after brain injury, while others could take much longer. Therefore, the question arises here is whether the time at which such patients enter MCS is related to the prognosis of patients with severe TBI. To address this issue, we conducted a prospective and observational study between January 2005 and August 2010 involving 65 patients who entered MCS after severe brain injury.

## OUR STUDY

The diagnosis of MCS was identified by behavioral criteria (3). MCS patients show inconsistent but discernible evidence of consciousness. Under behaviorally diagnostic criteria, patients may in minimally conscious state transiently, for a relative long period or permanently. Here we enrolled patients who had severe TBI and were in minimally conscious state from several days to years. Patients who had severe neurological, psychological, or heart and pulmonary disease before injury were excluded. Summary of characteristics in 65 patients were listed in Table 1.

According the timing of entering MCS, we divided the recruited patients into two groups. Patients who entered MCS within one month after injury went into the early MCS group. In contrast, the late MCS group consist patients of whom the MCS was detected later. Glasgow coma scale (GCS) and pupil reactivity were assessed and recorded on admission. The Glass outcome scale (GOS) was applied as a major parameter to compare the prognosis between the in two groups at the end of six-month follow-up.

Data were analyzed using the statistic software SPSS-16. t-tests were conducted to determine whether mean GOS differed significantly between early MCS and late MCS group. P values of $< 0.05$ were considered statistically significant.

## FINDINGS

Sixty-five patients were involved in this study, including 53 male sand 12 females, aging from 6 to 69 years (41.8 ± 13.5). All these patients suffered traumatic brain injury and loss of consciousness for several days to months. All of these patients were consistent with the diagnosis of MCS (3), according to behavioral criteria.

The GCS on admission were recorded from 3 to 15, but lowest GCS for these patients were all below 9 with the hematoma enlargement, edema deterioration, or whole brain swelling. Some patients even demonstrated enlarged pupils prior to surgery, implying brain herniation. After proper comprehensive treatment, the patients' condition became stable; gradually recovering partial consciousness and entry into a minimally conscious state. Within six months, some patients emerged from MCS but some did not. The early MCS group had 39 cases, including 29 males and 10 females, aging from 6 to 69(40.4 ± 15.1). Late MCS group had 26 cases, 24 males 2 females, aging from 18 to 61(43.9 ± 10.5).

The GOS of involved patients six months post-injury and are shown in Table 2. The mean GOS in the early MCS group was 4.31± 0.92, and 2.50 ± 0.91 and in the late MCS group (t value 7.798; $p < 0.001$), displaying significant differences between the two groups.

**Table 1. Summary of characteristics in 65 traumatic brain injury patients**

| Parameter | Early MCS patients(39) | Late MCS patients(26) |
|---|---|---|
| Age in years | | |
| Median | 40 | 44 |
| Range | | |
| 6-18 | 4 | 2 |
| 19-60 | 32 | 23 |
| 61-70 | 3 | 1 |
| Sex | | |
| Male | 29 | 24 |
| Female | 10 | 2 |
| GCS on admission | | |
| 3-5 | 3 | 4 |
| 6-8 | 17 | 19 |
| 9-12 | 16 | 3 |
| 13-15 | 3 | 0 |
| Hernia | 8 | 10 |

**Table 2. GOS difference six month later between early and late MCS group**

| GOS | Early MCS group (n=39) | Late MCS group (n=26) |
|---|---|---|
| 1 | 1 | 4 |
| 2 | 0 | 8 |
| 3 | 6 | 11 |
| 4 | 11 | 3 |
| 5 | 21 | 0 |

There were 32 patients who had GOS above four (suggesting good prognosis) at 6 months after injury, consisting 82.1% of patients in the early MCS group. In contrast, in the late MCS group, only three cases had GOS 4 and no one had GOS 5 at the end of 6-month follow-up. One patient died in the early MCS group, four in late MCS group for severe cardiopulmonary complication.

## DISCUSSION

The prognosis of severe brain injury patients was not only related to severity of injury, but also many other factors including patients' age, brain injury location, management, possible hypoxia or hypotension, and complications such as infections and heart failure. During rehabilitation, possible hydrocephalus and cardiopulmonary complication were the most important risk factors.

In the past few years, although great efforts have been made to explore new ways by which severely injured patients may to expedite recovery from minimally conscious state, there has been little effective treatment (4-6). Yet, the time point at which a patient recovers from coma and enters a MCS may indicate his/her final prognosis.

During the study, we divided patients with severe TBI and in MCS into two groups according to whether a MCS was detected within one month after injury. The reasons for adopting the "one-month" boundary mainly were that TBI edema usually disappears one month after injury, when structural deformity mostly becomes stable (7, 8).

From this study, we found that patients in the early MCS group displayed better prognosis than those in the late MCS group according to the GOS assessed at 6 months after injury. Since different prognosis may often induce dissimilar treatment decision, resource allocation, and even medicolegal judgment, we believed it would be meaningful to divide TBI patients into the early MCS and late MCS group to facilitate outcome predicting. Certainly further research was needed to testify the rationality for division to MCS patients.

## ACKNOWLEDGMENTS

The authors gratefully acknowledge financial support from grants (2010CB945500, 30870805, 90919002, 2007CB947902, 2009CB941100, 2010CB945500, 06dj14001, 08dj1400503, 075407070) from the National Nature Science Foundation, National Basic Research Program and Shanghai City Science Foundation.

## REFERENCES

[1] Schiff ND, Moreno R, Kamal A, Kim KHS, Giacino JT, Plum F, Hirsch J. fMRI reveals large-scale network activation in minimally conscious patients. Neurology 2005;64:514-23.

[2] Zhu J, Wu X, Gao L, Mao Y, Zhong P, Tang W, et al. Cortical activity after emotional visual stimulation in minimally conscious state patients. J Neurotrauma 2009;26(5):677-88.

[3] Giacino JT, Ashwa S, Childs N, Cranford R, Jennett B, Katz DI, et al. The minimally conscious state: Definition and diagnostic criteria. Neurology 2002;58(3):349-53.

[4] Bradley MM, Sabatinelli D, Lang PJ, Fitzsimmons JR, King W, Desai P. Activation of the visual cortex in motivated attention. Behav Neurosci 2003;117:369-80.

[5] D'Argembeau A, Van der Linden M. Influence of affective meaning on memory for contextual information. Emotion 2004;4:173–88.

[6] Di HB, Yu SM, Weng XC, Laureys S, Yu D, Li JQ, et al. Cerebral response to patient's own name in the vegetative and minimally conscious states. Neurology 2007;68:895-9.

[7] Wu XH, Zhu JH, Gao L, Zhong P, Tang WJ, Zhou LF. Functional magnetic imaging of brain cortical activities in minimally conscious patients stimulated by visual presentation. Chin Med J 2007;87:1894-9.

[8] Schiff ND, Rodriguez-Moreno D, Kamal A, Kim KH, Giacino JT, Plum F, et al. fMRI reveals large-scale network activation in minimally conscious patients. Neurology 2005;64:514-23.

In: Considering Consciousness Clinically
Editors: Gerry Leisman and Joav Merrick

ISBN: 978-1-63484-260-0


*Chapter 8*

# BRAIN DEAD: CLINICAL AND NEUROPATHOLOGICAL ASPECTS

***Jesús Perez-Nellar*, Calixto Machado, Claudio Scherle, Reynaldo Alvarez and Alejandro Areu***

Service of Neurology, Hermanos Ameijeiras Hospital, Havana and Institute of Neurology and Neurosurgery, Department of Clinical Neurophysiology, Havana, Cuba

## ABSTRACT

Brain death (BD) is caused by a catastrophic injury leading to irreversible coma, absent brainstem reflexes and apnea. Recent publications of autopsy studies in brain-dead patients have concluded that due to organ transplant protocols, the time to brain fixation has been abbreviated and consequently, no distinguishing BD neuropathologic features can be described. Nonetheless, as autopsies allow the most complete description of the disease leading to BD, the objective of this paper is to describe the clinical and pathologic features in a series of 26 brain-dead patients, from a tertiary hospital of Havana, Cuba, from 2006 to 2008. We concluded that although in transplant era it is not possible to find any distinctive neuropathologic feature in BD. Autopsy studies remain the best method to confirm the direct cause of death, leading to an irreversible destruction of the brain. Hence, we recommend performing neuropathologic and clinical studies in brain-dead patients.

## INTRODUCTION

Brain death (BD) is currently defined as a complete and irreversible loss of brain function. BD is caused by a catastrophic injury leading to irreversible coma, absent brainstem reflexes and apnea. This is a clinical diagnosis that requires a well-known cause and physician's

* Corresondence: Jesús Perez-Nellar, Hospital Hermanos Ameijeiras. Servicio de Neurologia. San Lazaro 701e/Belascoain. Centrohabana, Ciudad Habana, 10300, Cuba. E-mail: jesus.perez@infomed.sld.cu

certainty that the condition is potentially irreversible. In the great majority of patients neuroimages will show lesions explaining the loss of cerebral hemispheres and brainstem functions (1-15).

Wijdicks and Pfeifer have recently published an interesting series of autopsy studies in patients who were declared brain dead, concluding that due to organ transplant protocols, the time to brain fixation has been abbreviated and consequently, the so-called "respirator brain" is no longer found, and no distinguishing BD neuropathologic features can be described (16, 17) Nonetheless, autopsies allow the most complete description of the disease leading to BD, even though neuropathologic studies in patients who have been declared brain dead are rare (18-22).

The Hermanos Ameijeiras Hospital is the main tertiary referral center in Cuba. Patients with serious conditions, with the exception of traumatic brain injury, are admitted for complex medical and surgical treatments. The objective of this study is to describe the clinical and pathologic features in a series of 26 cases previously diagnosed as brain-dead, during a three-year period (2006-2008).

## OUR STUDY

We reviewed the medical records and autopsy protocols of 26 patients diagnosed as brain-dead from 2006 to 2008. We collected all data concerning demographics, cause of injury, time from admission to BD, time on ventilatory support, specialty of physician determining BD, findings on neurologic examination, ancillary tests, time from BD diagnosis to cardiac arrest, and all macroscopic and microscopic neurophatologic findings.

All cases were admitted in our intensive care unit, and hemodynamics and oxygenation were based on the use of vasopressors, vasopressin, and high positive end expiratory pressure mechanical ventilation.

A national protocol establishes that in BD cases family must be consulted about autopsy, and after informed consent, the pathologic study is performed. BD diagnosis was always performed by a neurologist and death was certified by the neurologist and two intensivists, based on the Cuban criteria for BD diagnosis (15, 23-27) The neurologist plays the fundamental role in this diagnosis, and without his/her presence, BD diagnosis can't be performed at our hospital.

Autopsy was performed by pathologist RA, without knowing any clinical detail related to BD diagnosis in all cases. The brains were fixed in 10% formalin before macroscopic neuropathology evaluation. Brain tissue from pathologic areas was selected for microscopic evaluation, in slides stained by hematoxylin and eosin.

Autopsy results were collected in a database according to the International Classification of Diseases, Ninth Revision (ICD-10), The following categories were established: direct cause of death (the condition that produces the death); basic cause of death (disease or condition that started the process that ends in death); contributing factors (pathologic conditions that affected the patient, but are not enough to cause the death) (28-30). Pathologist RA determined if the direct cause of death was either correlated with, destructive irreversible lesions of the cerebral hemispheres, or the brainstem, or both.

## FINDINGS

The relevant clinical and pathological data of the 26 cases are summarized in Table 1. Patients' age varied from 20 to 77 years (mean = 45,7 years). 18 were females (62,2%), and 8 men (30,8%); 15 whites (57,7%), 4 blacks (15,4%) and 7 black-white mestees (26,9%).

A total of 19 patients were supported by IV infusions of dobutamine (9 patients) or norepinephrine (10 patients). Patients were on ventilatory support from 17 to 288 hours (mean = 51,3 hours).

The clinical examination for BD diagnosis was performed by a neurologist in 25 cases, and by a neurosurgeon in one case. Most cases were examined by two of the authors, JP (10 cases), CS (9 cases).

**Table 1. Clinical and pathologic study of 26 consecutive brain-dead patients**

| | Age / sex / skin color | Direct cause of death | Observation period (Hrs) | Ventilatory Support (Hrs) | Ancillary tests | Time (Hrs) Brain Death to Cardiac Arrest | Donation |
|---|---|---|---|---|---|---|---|
| 1 | 26 / F / W | Hypoxic encephalopathy. Valvular heart surgery. | 5 | 148 | TCD | 22:00 | no |
| 2 | 57 / F / B | SAH. Cerebral aneurysms (surgery). | 6 | 32 | TCD | 2:20 | yes |
| 3 | 30 / F / M | ICH. Anticoagulation for valvular heart disease. | 24 | 100 | - | 0:30 | no |
| 4 | 77 / M /W | Cerebellar infarct. | 6 | 120 | - | 1:30 | no |
| 5 | 70 / F / W | Cerebellar astrocitoma. Intratumoral hemorrhage. | 6 | 52 | - | 2:00 | no |
| 6 | 20 / F / M | Intraventricular neurocitoma (surgery). | 4 | 88 | TCD | 2:20 | yes |
| 7 | 61 / F / W | ICH. Anticoagulation for valvular heart disease. | 7 | 44 | - | 1:30 | no |
| 8 | 47 / F / M | SAH. Basilar artery aneurysm. | 6 | 18 | - | 8:00 | yes |
| 9 | 55 / F / W | SAH. Internal carotid artery aneurysm. | 6 | 288 | TCD | 0:45 | yes |
| 10 | 22 / M /M | Herpes simplex encephalitis. | 7 | 29 | TCD | 0:18 | no |
| 11 | 39 / M /W | Glioblastoma multiforme. Intratumoral hemorrhage. | 0 | 24 | TCD | 1:10 | yes |
| 12 | 49 / F / W | SAH: malignant brain infarct. Acoa aneurysm. | 6 | 48 | TCD/EEG | 0:15 | yes |
| 13 | 42 / F / W | VIII nerve schwanoma. Surgical injury of brainstem. | 3 | 96 | TCD | 0:40 | yes |
| 14 | 44 / F / B | SAH: malignant brain infarct. Basilar artery aneurysm. | 0 | 48 | TCD | 2:20 | no |
| 15 | 41 / F / B | Hypertensive ICH. | 6 | 24 | TCD | 8:45 | yes |

**Table 1. (Continued)**

| | Age / sex / skin color | Direct cause of death | Observation period (Hrs) | Ventilatory Support (Hrs) | Ancillary tests | Time (Hrs) Brain Death to Cardiac Arrest | Donation |
|---|---|---|---|---|---|---|---|
| 16 | 70 / M /W | Brain stem infarct. | 4 | 41 | - | 18:00 | no |
| 17 | 34 / M /M | SAH. Acoa aneurysm. | 8 | 21 | - | 5:00 | yes |
| 18 | 53 / F / W | SAH. Acoa aneurysm. | 6 | 35 | - | 2:10 | yes |
| 19 | 41 / F / W | SAH: malignant brain infarct. PCoA aneurysm. | 5 | 23 | TCD | 1:00 | yes |
| 20 | 56 / F / W | Cranial Base meningioma. Surgical injury of brain. | 6 | 48 | - | 1:00 | yes |
| 21 | 29 / F / B | SAH. Basilar artery aneurysm. | 5 | 24 | TCD | 3:30 | yes |
| 22 | 42 / F / W | SAH. MCA aneurysm. | 0 | 48 | TCD | 2:50 | yes |
| 23 | 25 / M /M | ICH. Bone marrow aplasia. | 6 | 36 | - | 11:30 | no |
| 24 | 59 / F / M | SAH. Acoa aneurysm | 0 | 72 | TCD | 5:40 | yes |
| 25 | 53 / M /W | Cranial Base meningioma. Surgical injury of brain. | 0 | 17 | TCD/EEG | 0:30 | yes |
| 26 | 45 / M /W | SAH. Basilar artery aneurysm. | 0 | 18 | TCD/EEG | 0:30 | no |

SAH: Subarachnoid hemorrhage; ICH: Intracerebral hemorrhage; Hrs: Hours.
NE: Norepineprhine; DOB: Dobutamine; Skin color: W: White, B: Black, M: Mestee.

The majority of cases fulfilled all clinical criteria for BD diagnosis, but in one patient (case 12) apnea test was aborted because of an extreme bradycardia and BD was later confirmed using ancillary tests. The patient was a 49 years old woman complaining severe vasospasm associated to a subarachnoid hemorrhage due to a rupture of an aneurysm located at the top of the basilar artery.

Twenty patients required multiple examinations. The observation period varied from 3 to 24 hours (mean: 5,1 hours). Time from BD diagnosis to cardiac arrest, due to withdrawal of life support or after organ harvesting, varied from 15 minutes to 47 hours (mean = 305 minutes), although this time in most cases was less than 6 hours.

The most frequent etiology of BD was stroke: subarachnoid hemorrhage was diagnosed in 12, intracerebral hemorrhage in 4, and ischemic stroke in 2 patients. Other diagnoses were: malignant brain tumors in 4 cases, complications of brain surgery in 2, hypoxic encephalopathy in patient, and herpetic encephalitis in one patient.

Destructive lesions with cerebral edema, brain herniations and mass effect, were confirmed on macroscopic pathologic studies of patients. Microscopic evaluation revealed varying degrees of neuronal ischemic changes. hemispheres with a secondary involvement of the brainstem, in 21 cases; a primary compromise of the brainstem was found in 4 cases, and lesions involving the whole brain (cerebral hemispheres and brainstem) in 1 case. Neuropathologic examination confirmed a “respirator brain” in case 1 (Figure 1).

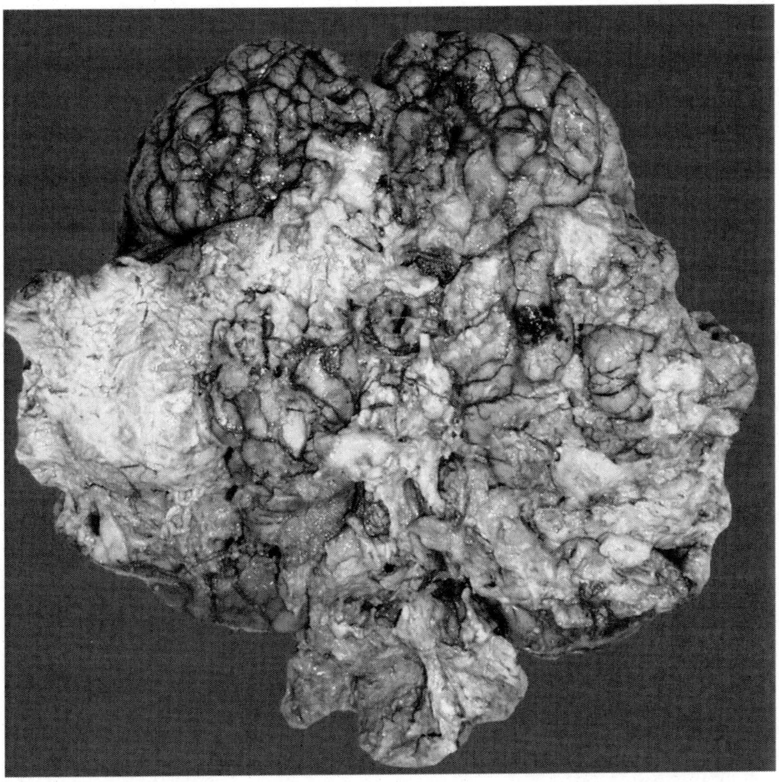

Figure 1. Respirator brain. The brain is fragmented, dusky congested and discolored, containing liquid portions. There are extensive destructive lesions with cerebral edema, brain herniation and mass effect.

The brain was fragmented, dusky congested and discolored, containing liquid portions. There were extensive destructive lesions with cerebral edema, brain herniation and mass effect. This patient had suffered a hypoxic encephalopathy during a heart surgery for valvular correction. She was under ventilatory support for 148 hours with a Glasgow Coma Scale scoring 3 point, but some brainstem reflexes still remained, until BD diagnosis was completed. Time since BD confirmation to cardiac arrest was 48 hours, because relatives denied life support withdrawal.

## DISCUSSION

Our hospital is a tertiary center with availability of neurologists on a 24-hour basis. Hence, BD determination is mainly performed by neurologists. Alternatively, this diagnosis in other institutions can be performed by intensivists, who are properly certified by the Cuban Commission for the Death Determination. By this way, it is not mandatory that a neurologist or a neurosurgeon must guide this diagnosis (15, 23-27).

According to the Cuba criteria for BD diagnosis in adults, ancillary tests are not mandatory. Confirmatory laboratory tests are only required when specific components of the clinical testing cannot reliably be evaluated (15, 15, 23-27, 31-37). In this study, only one patient did not fulfill all clinical BD criteria, requiring mandatory ancillary tests because the apnea test was aborted. Pfeifer and Wijdicks, in 228 patients pronounced brain dead at Mayo Clinic, found that the examiner decided not to proceed with the apnea test in 7% of the patients, and in 3% the apnea test was aborted because of hypotension or hypoxemia (16). However, we performed ancillary tests in 66% of cases, with the main objective of shortening the observation period to complete BD diagnosis. To demonstrate cerebral circulatory arrest we used transcranial Doppler (TCD) as ancillary test.

The AAN Therapeutics and Technology Assessment Subcommittee emphasized that the TCD sensitivity and specificity for detecting cerebral circulatory arrest were 91-100 and 97-100%, respectively (38-40).

In general, the principal advantages of TCD are: it is noninvasive, it can be carried out at the bedside, it can repeated as needed or in continuous monitoring, it is less expensive than other techniques, and dye contrast agents are not needed. Its main chief disadvantages are: it can only study CBF velocities in certain segments of large intracranial vessels, it is operator-dependent requiring training and experience to perform it and interpret results, and, up to 20% of studies may be unsuccessful because some patients have cranial vaults too thick impeding a proper visualization of intracranial arteries. In our service, all neurologists have been trained as TCD operators, easing the use of this technique in suspected brain-dead patients (35, 40-51) Nonetheless, we are now running a protocol to use CT angiography as a main ancillary test in detecting cerebral circulatory arrest, according to recent publications on this topic (47, 52-54). In the 1970´s neuropathologists coined the term "respirator brain" to describe particular characteristics in brain-dead cases kept on life support, and hence it was considered a BD pathologic hallmark (55) However, nowadays patients in BD are usually kept on the ventilator for shorter periods of time, and total brain necrosis is rarely observed (16, 17).

Time on the ventilator has been correlated with autopsy findings (17, 55-59). In the present study time since BD confirmation to cardiac arrest was less than 6 hours in most patients. We only found the so-called "respirator brain" in one case who was on ventilatory support for a long time period, and time since BD diagnosis to cardiac arrest was delayed up to 48 hours.

## Conclusion

As Widjicks and Pfeifer stated, "we found no prototypical examples of a respirator brain," and hence these authors affirmed that in the modern transplant era it is not possible to find any distinctive neuropathologic feature in BD (16). However, neuropathologic studies remain the best method to confirm the direct cause of death, leading to an irreversible destruction of the brain. Hence, it is recommended to perform neuropathologic studies correlated with clinical findings in all cases previously diagnosed as brain-dead.

## References

[1] Ingvar DH. Brain death--total brain infarction. Acta Anaesthesiol Scand Suppl 1971;45:129-140.
[2] Jennett B. Diagnosis of brain death. J Med Ethics 1977;3:4-5.
[3] Black PM. Brain death (first of two parts). N Engl J Med 1978 17;299:338-44.
[4] Pallis C. Brainstem death--the evolution of a concept. Med Leg J 1987;55(Pt 2):84-107.

[5] Bernat JL. The concept and practice of brain death. Prog Brain Res 2005;150:369-79.
[6] Lang CJ, Heckmann JG. Apnea testing for the diagnosis of brain death. Acta Neurol Scand 2005;112:358-69.
[7] Machado C. The first organ transplant from a brain-dead donor. Neurology 2005;64:1938-42.
[8] Shemie SD. Diagnosis of brain death in children-Technology and the inadequate lexicon of death. Lancet Neurology 2007;6:87-92.
[9] Wijdicks EFM. Determining Brain-Death in Adults. Neurology 1995;45:1003-11.
[10] Wijdicks EF. The diagnosis of brain death. N Engl J Med 2001;344:1215-21.
[11] Wijdicks EF. Brain death worldwide: accepted fact but no global consensus in diagnostic criteria. Neurology 2002;58:20-5.
[12] Wijdicks EF. The neurologist and Harvard criteria for brain death. Neurology 2003;61:970-6.
[13] Machado C, Korein J, Ferrer Y, Portela L, de la Garcia MC, Manero JM. The concept of brain death did not evolve to benefit organ transplants. J Med Ethics 2007;33:197-200.
[14] Machado C. The declaration of Sydney on death. he declaration of Sydney on human death. J Med Ethics 2007;33:699-703.
[15] Machado C. Brain death. A reappraisal. New York: Springer, 2007.
[16] Wijdicks EF, Pfeifer EA. Neuropathology of brain death in the modern transplant era. Neurology 2008;70:1234-7.
[17] Wijdicks EFM, Pfeifer EA. Neuropathology of brain death in the modern transplant era reply. Neurology 2009;72:1028.
[18] Alderete JF, Jeri FR, Richardson EP, Sament S, Schwab RS, Young RR. Irreversible coma: Aa clinical, electroencephalographic and neuropathological study. Trans Am Neurol Assoc 1968;93:16-20.
[19] Pearson J, Korein J, Harris JH, Wichter M, Braunstein P. Brain death: II. Neuropathological correlation with the radioisotopic bolus technique for evaluation of critical deficit of cerebral blood flow. Ann Neurol 1977;2:206-10.
[20] Schneider H, Matakas F. Pathological changes of the spinal cord after brain death. Acta Neuropathol (Berl) 1971;18:234-47.
[21] Cole G, Cowie VA. Long survival after cardiac arrest: case report and neuropathological findings. Clin Neuropathol 1987;6:104-9.
[22] Ujihira N, Hashizume Y, Takahashi A. A clinico-neuropathological study on brain death. Nagoya J Med Sci 1993;56:89-99.
[23] Machado-Curbelo C. (A new formulation of death: definition, criteria and diagnostic tests). Rev Neurol 1998;26:1040-7.
[24] Machado C, National Commission and Certification of Death. Resolution for the determination and certification of death in Cuba. Rev Neurol 2003;36:763-70.
[25] Machado C, Shewmon DL. Brain death and disorders of consciousness. New York: Kluwer Academics/Plenum Publishers, 2004.
[26] Machado C, Abeledo M, Alvarez C, Aroche RM, Barrios I, Lasanta AM, et al. Cuba has passed a law for the determination and certification of death. Brain Death Disorders Consciousness 2004;550:139-42.
[27] Machado C. Determination of death. Acta Anaesth Scand 2005;49:592-3.
[28] Joshi R, Lopez AD, MacMahon S, Reddy S, Dandona R, Dandona L, et al. Verbal autopsy coding: are multiple coders better than one? Bull World Health Organ 2009;87:51-7.
[29] Fillit HM. The pharmacoeconomics of Alzheimer's disease. Am J Manag Care 2000;6:S1139-44.
[30] Mony PK, Nagaraj C. Health information management: an introduction to disease classification and coding. Natl Med J India 2007;20:307-10.
[31] Machado C, Valdés P, Garcia-Tigera J, Virues T, Biscay R, Miranda J, et al. Brain-stem auditory evoked potentials and brain death. Electroencephalogr Clin Neurophysiol 1991;80(5):392-8.
[32] Machado C. Multimodality evoked potentials and electroretinography in a test battery for an early diagnosis of brain death. J Neurosurg Sci 1993;37:125-31.
[33] Machado C, Santiesteban R, Garcia O, Coutin P, Beurgo MA, Miranda J, et al. Visual evoked potentials and electroretinography in brain-dead patients. Doc Ophthalmol 1993;84(1):89-96.

[34] Machado C. An early approach to brain death diagnosis using multimodality evoked potentials and electroretinography. Minerva Anestesiol 1994;60:573-7.
[35] Machado C. Assessment: Transcranial Doppler ultrasonography: report of the Therapeutics and Technology Assessment Subcommittee of the American Academy of Neurology. Neurology 2004;63:2457-8.
[36] Machado C. Evoked potentials in brain death. Clin Neurophysiol 2004;115:238-9.
[37] Machado C, Garcia OD, Gutierrez J. Heart rate variability in comatose and brain-dead patients. Clin Neurophysiol 2005;116:2859-60.
[38] Sloan MA, Alexandrov AV, Tegeler CH, Spencer MP, Caplan LR, Feldmann E, et al. Assessment: Transcranial Doppler ultrasonography-Report of the Therapeutics and Technology Assessment Subcommittee of the American Academy of Neurology. Neurology 2004;62(9):1468-81.
[39] Ropper AH, Kehne SM, Wechsler L. Transcranial Doppler in brain death. Neurology 1987;37:1733-5.
[40] Previgliano IJ. Assessment: transcranial Doppler ultrasonography: report of the Therapeutics and Technology Assessment Subcommittee of the American Academy of Neurology. Neurology 2004;63:2457-8.
[41] Jonkman EJ, Mosmans PC. Doppler haematotachography: problems in interpretation and new applications. Clin Neurol Neurosurg 1977;80:33-45.
[42] Bode H, Sauer M, Pringsheim W. Diagnosis of brain death by transcranial Doppler sonography. Arch Dis Child 1988;63:1474-8.
[43] Lowe LH, Bulas DI. Transcranial Doppler imaging in children: sickle cell screening and beyond. Pediatr Radiol 2005;35:54-65.
[44] Schoning M, Scheel P, Holzer M, Fretschner R, Will BE. Volume measurement of cerebral blood flow: assessment of cerebral circulatory arrest. Transplantation 2005;80:326-31.
[45] de Freitas GR, Andre C. Sensitivity of transcranial Doppler for confirming brain death: a prospective study of 270 cases. Acta Neurologica Scand 2006;113:426-32.
[46] Molnar C, Rozsa L, Sarkany P, Horvath J, Fulesdi B, Szabo S. The role of transcranial Doppler sonography in diagnosis of brain death (a practical review). Orvosi Hetilap 2006;147:357-62.
[47] Young GB, Shemie SD, Doig CJ, Teitelbaum J. Brief review: the role of ancillary tests in the neurological determination of death. Can J Anaesth 2006;53:620-7.
[48] Saqqur M, Zygun D, Demchuk A. Role of transcranial Doppler in neurocritical care. Crit Care Med 2007;35:S216-23.
[49] Sardinha LAC, Araujo S, Boin IFSF. Brain death and transcranial Doppler ultrasound as exam for confirming test and its applicability in potential donors. Transplant Int 2007;20:346.
[50] Calderon CV, Portela PC. Recommendations of the transcranial Doppler in the diagnosis of brain death. Neurologia 2008;23:397-8.
[51] Conti A, Iacopino DG, Spada A, Cardali SM, Giusa M, La Torre D, et al. Transcranial Doppler Ultrasonography in the Assessment of Cerebral Circulation Arrest: Improving Sensitivity by Trancervical and Transorbital Carotid Insonation and Serial Examinations. Neurocrit Care 2009;10:326-35.
[52] Brock M, Schurmann K, Hadjidimos A. Cerebral blood flow and cerebral death. Acta Neurochir (Wien ) 1969;20:195-209.
[53] Escudero D, Otero J, Vega P, Gil A, Roger RL, Gonzalo JA, et al. Diagnosis of brain death by multislice CT scan: angioCT scan and brain perfusion. Med Intensiva 2007;31(6):335-41. (Spanish)
[54] Greer DM, Strozyk D, Schwamm LH. False positive CT angiography in brain death. Neurocrit Care 2009;11(2):272-5.
[55] Walker AE, Diamond EL, Moseley J. The neuropathological findings in irreversible coma. A critque of the "respirator." J Neuropathol Exp Neurol 1975;34:295-323.
[56] Walker AE. The death of a brain. Johns Hopkins Med J 1969;124:190-201.
[57] Moseley JI, Molinari GF, Walker AE. Respirator brain. Report of a survey and review of current concepts. Arch Pathol Lab Med 1976;100:61-4.
[58] Walker AE. Pathology of brain death. Ann NY Acad Sci 1978;315:272-80.
[59] Walker AE. Cerebral death, 3rd ed. Baltimore, MD: Urban Schwarzenberg, 1985.

In: Considering Consciousness Clinically
Editors: Gerry Leisman and Joav Merrick

ISBN: 978-1-63484-260-0


*Chapter 9*

# DIAGNOSIS OF DEATH IN MODERN HOSPITAL PRACTICE

***Dale Gardiner*[*], *Gemma Housley and Dominick Shaw***
Nottingham University Hospitals NHS Trust,
Nottingham, United Kingdom

## ABSTRACT

There is a potential for many death diagnoses in hospitals to not satisfy a philosopher's definition of irreversibility. It is estimated there are 360,000 deaths in UK hospitals each year. Our results of death diagnosis practices in a modern hospital indicates that in the UK over 133,000 patients each year would have to have the way their deaths were diagnosed to satisfy a 60 minutes standard and 300,000 (83% of all UK hospital deaths) to satisfy a three hour standard. The radicalness of an insistence on irreversibility as impossible to reverse has not been appreciated and is inconsistent with what is regarded as normal hospital practice. We note that physicians use permanence, being the chance that something will happen rather then could happen (impossible to reverse) to make their death declarations. This is a dignity-consistent approach to making a diagnosis of death, as it is both safe and timely. The five-minute observation standard, as first proposed by Eugene Bouchut in 1846, remains the most valid physiological and patient-centered criteria for modern doctors to employ when diagnosing death after cardio-respiratory arrest.

## INTRODUCTION

Concern has been expressed that the diagnosis of death, used in donation after circulatory death (DCD), will not satisfy the Dead Donor Rule (1). Since the USA Uniform Declaration of Death Act requires irreversible cessation of circulatory and respiratory functions, then the typical observation period before confirming death in DCD and organ donation commencing,

---

[*] Correspondence: Dale Gardiner, Nottingham University Hospitals NHS Trust, Nottingham, United Kingdom. E-mail: dalegardiner@doctors.net.uk.

of 2-10 minutes, would not appear to satisfy this criterion because were Cardio-Pulmonary Resuscitation (CPR) instituted, reversal of cardiac function may well be possible. This is to say that the standard of irreversibility required to meet this criterion should be 'impossible to reverse.' (1, 2). Others have argued that there is a distinction between irreversible and permanent 'will not reverse' and the Dead Donor Rule is satisfied (3-5).

How long doctors typically wait before confirming death after cardio-respiratory arrest is unknown. Most medical textbooks and curricula are silent on this matter and it was only in 2008 that in the UK the Academy of Medical Royal Colleges offered guidance suggesting a five-minute standard (6). The Lazarus phenomenon of auto-resuscitation described in the literature appears to occur only in the context of failed or inadvertent continued cardiopulmonary resuscitation (eg continuing mechanical ventilation in a patient declared 'dead') (7). A recent systematic review could identify no cases of spontaneous return of circulation not in the context of cardiopulmonary resuscitation (8). Following a decision to cease cardiopulmonary resuscitation, a longer observation period of seven minutes was inferred. In 2012 the UK National Patient Safety Agency (NPSA) issued an alert regarding five patients wrongly declared deceased after cardio-respiratory arrest and failed CPR (9). The recommendation from the NPSA was not that the UK observation time of five minutes to declare death after cardio-respiratory arrest was too short; it was that the doctors hadn't even waited this length of time.

It remains unclear if doctors, in modern hospital practice, routinely satisfy a criterion for death as impossible to reverse. If they do not then philosophical assertions for this standard may require a radical change in death determination practices and societal expectation. We sought to ascertain what the usual, ward based (non donation, non intensive care) time to diagnose death is in a modern hospital.

## Our Project

In our university tertiary referral hospital, after hours (between 1700-0800 Monday to Friday, and 1700 Friday to 0800 Monday), doctors use a Hospital at Night (H@N) electronic referral system that logs when a doctor accepts a job and when the doctor confirms the job complete.

All after hours 'tasks' are now logged via nurses onto a ward-based desktop Personal Computer (PC). The task is then sent wirelessly to a coordinator who carries a small tablet PC. This task can then be triaged and allocated wirelessly to junior doctors via a message to dedicated on-call mobile phones. The recipient accepts the task with a single button press and it is added to the freely accessible task list held on their phone. Once a task is passed to a junior doctor and accepted it stays active on both their and the co-ordinator's list until completion or reassignment to another individual.

This system was used to investigate all 'Certification of expected / unexpected death' category calls which would allow us to investigate the time from a nurse requesting a death certification to the completion of this task and the medical declaration of death by a junior doctor.

## FINDINGS

Between 01/11/12 - 30/04/13 (six months), 590 calls were logged into our Hospital at Night (H@N) electronic referral system for the 'Certification of expected / unexpected death' category. In 555 cases death was logged as expected. All calls were priority green meaning non-urgent attendance required. Median time from the nurse electronically requesting a death certification to the doctors' completion of the task was 83 minutes (40-148 minutes interquartile range). Within 30 minutes 17% of the deaths had been confirmed, within 60 minutes 37%, within 180 minutes 83% and within 240 minutes 91%. The spread of results can be seen in Figure 1 and the cumulative percentage in Figure 2.

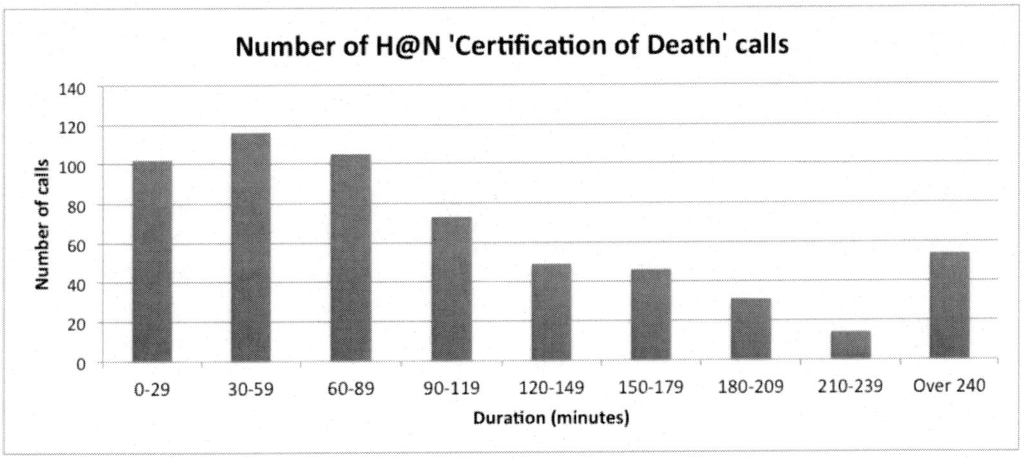


Figure 1.

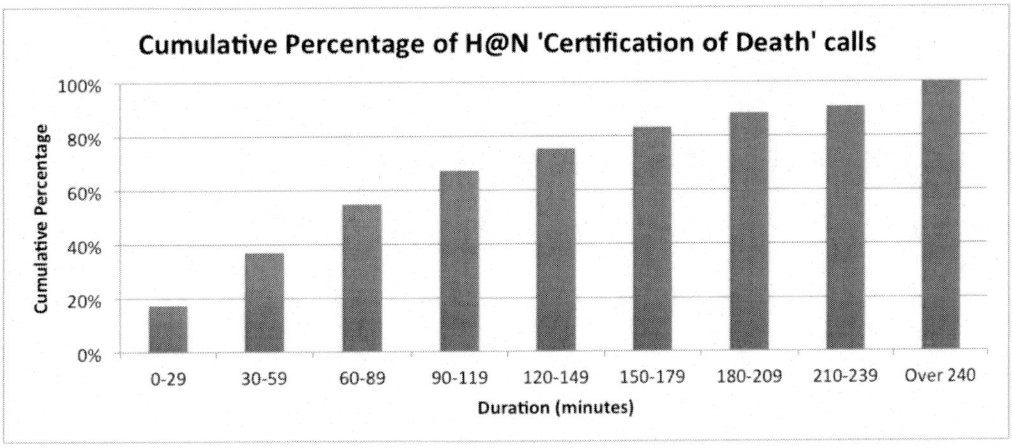


Figure 2.

## DISCUSSION

Until the re-introduction of DCD programs there was little guidance or debate about how doctors should diagnose death after cardio-respiratory arrest (10). Few critics of death diagnoses in DCD contexts have offered doctors guidance on how it might be possible for doctors to meet the impossible to reverse requirement of irreversibility or when this requirement might have occurred in an unconscious, apnoeic and asystolic patient.

Alan Shewmon however does offer, 'under normal circumstances (ie normal temperature), an educated guess is that twenty to thirty minutes probably suffice to surpass the point of no return." (11). This point according to Shewmon would satisfy a state of thermodynamically supracritical microstructural damage diffusely throughout the body. Unfortunately the time he suggests is too short for the state he desires to have developed.

In a case published in 2009 transplant surgeons in Cambridge restarted a heart inside the body under DCD conditions at 23 minutes using extra-corporeal membrane oxygenation (ECMO) and the heart function was considered good, almost transplantable (12). Since that time successful adult heart DCD has occurred in the UK and Australia. Given the current evidence from DCD transplantations, even after prolonged periods of organ warm ischemia, there is no evidence for the diffuse supra-critical microstructural damage that Shewmon speaks about, occurring within thirty minutes.

DeVita's review of both human and animal evidence dating back to the early 1900's suggests that 60 minutes is the shortest acceptable observation time for determination of death if the criterion is impossibility of restoring some brain activity because up until this point the brain may be stimulated and respond (13). If the chosen criterion is impossibility of restoring cardiac activity then an observation period, or as DeVita calls it a 'death watch' of many hours may be required, since the heart may still resume function in a laboratory or transplant setting.

It would seem that therefore that there is a potential for many death diagnoses in hospitals not to satisfy a philosophers definition of irreversibility. It is estimated there are 360,000 deaths in UK hospitals each year. Using DeVita's death watch criteria in order to satisfy a definition of irreversibility as 'impossible to reverse,' our results of death diagnosis practices in a modern hospital would suggest that in the UK over 133,000 patients each year would have to have the way their deaths were diagnosed to satisfy a 60 minutes standard and 300,000 (83% of all UK hospital deaths) to satisfy a three hour standard. The radicalness of an insistence on irreversibility as impossible to reverse has not been appreciated and is not consistent with what is regarded as normal hospital practice.

Limitations to our results are that the length of time from cardio-respiratory arrest to this being identified by a ward nurse and the request logged. Given the prolonged time frames suggested by DeVita to satisfy a concept of irreversibility as impossible to reverse, we do not believe this limits the interpretation of our findings that in modern hospitals doctors no not use a definition of irreversibility that philosophers might attest to. It would seem that doctors use permanence, being the chance that something will happen rather then could happen (impossible to reverse) to make their death declarations. This is a dignity-consistent approach to making a diagnosis of death, as it is both safe and timely. The five-minute observation standard, as first proposed by Eugene Bouchut in 1846 (14), remains the most valid physiological and patient centred criteria for modern doctors to employ when diagnosing death after cardio-respiratory arrest.

## REFERENCES


[1] Truog RD, Miller FG, Halpern SD. The dead-donor rule and the future of organ donation. N Engl J Med 2013;369(14):1287-9.

[2] Truog RD, Miller FG. The dead donor rule and organ transplantation. N Engl J Med 2008;359(7):674-5.

[3] Bernat JL. How the distinction between "irreversible" and "permanent" illuminates circulatory-respiratory death determination. J Med Philos 2010;35(3):242-55.

[4] Bernat JL, Capron AM, Bleck TP, Blosser S, Bratton SL, Childress JF, et al. The circulatory-respiratory determination of death in organ donation. Crit Care Med 2010;38(3):963-70.

[5] Bernat JL. Life or death for the dead-donor rule? N Engl J Med 2013;369(14):1289-91.

[6] Academy of Medical Royal Colleges. A code of practice for the diagnosis and confirmation of death, 2008. URL: http://www.aomrc.org.uk/publications/reports-guidance.html

[7] Maleck WH, Piper SN, Triem J, Boldt J, Zittel FU. Unexpected return of spontaneous circulation after cessation of resuscitation (Lazarus phenomenon). Resuscitation 1998;39(1-2):125-8.

[8] Hornby K, Hornby L, Shemie SD. A systematic review of autoresuscitation after cardiac arrest. Crit Care Med 2010;38(5):1246-53.

[9] National Patient Safety Agency (NPSA). Signal alert: Diagnosis of death after cessation of cardiopulmonary resuscitation. URL: http://www.nrls.npsa.nhs.uk/signals/?entryid45=132973

[10] Gardiner D, Shemie S, Manara A, Opdam H. International perspective on the diagnosis of death. Br J Anaesth 2012;108(Suppl 1):14-28.

[11] Shewmon DA. Chronic "brain death": meta-analysis and conceptual consequences. Neurology 1998;51(6):1538.

[12] Ali A, White P, Dhital K, Ryan M, Tsui S, Large S. Cardiac recovery in a human non-heart-beating donor after extracorporeal perfusion: source for human heart donation? J Heart Lung Transplant 2009;28(3):290-3.

[13] DeVita MA. The death watch: certifying death using cardiac criteria. Prog Transplant 2001;11(1):58-66.

[14] Bouchut E. Traité des signes de la mort et des moyens de prévenir les enterrements prématurés. Paris: JB Baillière, 1849. (French)


Conflicts of interest declaration

Dr Gardiner is deputy national clinical lead for organ donation in the UK for NHS Blood and Transplant.

In: Considering Consciousness Clinically
Editors: Gerry Leisman and Joav Merrick

ISBN: 978-1-63484-260-0


*Chapter 10*

# VEGETATIVE STATE AND THE OUTER WORLD

***Calixto Machado[1], Mario Estévez[1], Rafael Rodríguez[2], Maylén Carballo[2], Jesús Pérez-Nellar[3], Joel Gutiérrez[1], Marcia Fleitas[1] and Gerry Leisman[4,5*]***

[1]Institute of Neurology and Neurosurgery,
Department of Clinical Neurophysiology, Havana, Cuba
[2]International Center for Neurological Restoration Havana, Cuba
[3]Hermanos Ameijeiras Hospital, Service of Neurology, Havana, Cuba
[4]The National Institute for Brain and Rehabilitation Sciences, Nazareth, Israel
[5]Universidad de Ciencias Médicas de la Habana, Facultad Manuel Fajardo,
Havanna, Cuba

## ABSTRACT

Persistent vegetative state patients (PVS) cases reflect the only circumstance in which an apparent dissociation of both components of consciousness is found. The recent description of the MCS highlights the crucial role of unexpected and well documented recoveries of cognitive functions. Functional neuroimaging has provided new insights for assessing neuropathology and cerebral activity in these patients, providing information on the presence, degree, and location of any residual brain function in PVS or MCS cases. The main finding in PVS is preservation of wakefulness with apparent loss of awareness. Hence, by definition, subjects in PVS with no recognizable behavioral responses to external stimuli, are isolated from the outer world, and they cannot experience pain and suffering. Nonetheless, our results, suggest recognition of the mom's voice with an emotional content, indicating high-level residual linguistic processing, and brain activation after Zolpidem administration. These results differ with the current concept that by definition, subjects in PVS with no recognizable behavioral responses to external stimuli, are isolated from the outer world, and they cannot experience pain and suffering.

* Correspondence: Professor Gerry Leisman, Director, The National Institute for Brain and Rehabilitation Sciences, Biomechanics Laboratory, Department of Mechanical Engineering, ORT-Braude College of Engineering, Snunit 51 Street, POBox 78, IL-21982 Karmiel, Israel. E-mail: gerry.leisman@staff.nazareth.ac.il

These findings launch new medical, ethical and practical implications for the diagnosis and management of PVS and MCS patients.

## INTRODUCTION

Persistent vegetative state patients (PVS) cases reflect the only circumstance in which an apparent dissociation of both components of consciousness is found. The main finding in PVS is preservation of wakefulness with apparent loss of awareness (1-14). The recent description of the minimally conscious state (MCS) in some patients as a transitional phase towards the partial recovery of self awareness or environmental awareness while emerging from the PVA, highlights the crucial role of pathophysiological elucidation of consciousness generation in these cases (15-18).

The Schiavo case and other famous patients have made it necessary for neurologists and neuroscientists to propose reliable diagnostic guidelines for testing brain function in altered states of consciousness (19-27).

## TERMINOLOGY

Jennet and Plum first coined the term "persistent vegetative state" in 1972 to describe the condition of patients with severe brain damage in whom coma has progressed to a state of wakefulness without detectable awareness. Such patients have sleep-wake cycles but no ascertainable cerebral cortical function. Jennett and Plum thought that patients in a persistent vegetative state could be distinguished clinically from those with other conditions associated with disturbances of consciousness. These authors described a specific syndrome of reflex reactions without any meaningful response to the environment but in patients who have a sleep–awake pattern. They introduced the term because they were dissatisfied about the other terms used at the time. These terms referred to states, which were not true, e.g., prolonged *coma* or *coma* vigil (the patients, by definition, were not in coma), or described specific syndromes, e.g., decerebrate dementia, parasomnia, or akinetic mutism (28). This syndrome was originally termed *apallic syndrome* (29), because it was considered to be caused by the destruction of the "pallium, the cortical gray matter that covers the thelencephalon" (30). The term apallic syndrome, still used in some European countries, implies lack of the cortex (palium), but this is not the only pathologic pattern found in these cases (31-33).

After 35 years, The European Task Force on Disorders of Consciousness proposed a new term, *unresponsive wakefulness syndrome (UWS)*, to portray this syndrome for avoiding the depreciatory term *vegetative state* (34)˙ We fully agree that for physicians is very difficult to explain to anybody that his/her son or relative is in a vegetative state (VS). If we consider the translation to our mother tongue language (Spanish), the term "*estado vegetativo"* also represents a pejorative description for a patient who preserved sleep-wake cycles, respiration, digestion or thermoregulation, with an apparently loss of awareness of self and of the environment. In the Spanish language the term *"vegetal"* is relative to plants. Hence, when using the term "estado vegetativo" physicians are coining a PVS patient as a vegetable (35-39).

Giacino et al. first proposed to use the term MCS to describe patients showing a limited but clear evidence of awareness of themselves or their environment, based on a reproducible or sustained basis (15). We submitted a response to that paper, proposing the use of the term *minimally aware state* instead of *minimally conscious state,* because considering both components of consciousness, the main difference between a PVS and a MCS case, is a partial recovery of awareness (40). Hence, continuing in the direction of the new term, UWS, we could coin MCS as *minimally responsive wakefulness state* (MRWS), or *minimally aware wakefulness state (MAWS).*

As a conclusion, we agree with the new term proposed by the European Task Force on Disorders of Consciousness (34). In any way, physicians from all regions of the globe should find, according to their own respective languages, a term for avoiding a pejorative description of patients, that on the contrary, should mean a challenge for neuroscientists to offer them new hopes for neurorehabilitation.

## Clinical findings in PVS and MCS patients

### Persistent Vegetative State

Diagnostic criteria for PVS include: lack of evidence of awareness of self or environment, lack of interaction with others, and lack of comprehension or expression of language. By implication, external stimuli should not evoke purposeful or sustained and reproducible voluntary behavioral responses (41-45). The accurate diagnosis of PVS requires the skills of a multidisciplinary team experienced in the management of people with complex disabilities and consciousness disorders. Accurate clinical assessments of patients in these conditions must be obtained before they undergo neuroimaging (1, 6,42, 46-52).

The Multi-Society Task Force on PVS has classified the causes of PVS in 3 main groups: *Acute injuries*, where the most common causes are traumatic and hypoxic-ischemic encephalopathy; *degenerative and metabolic disorders*, including dementia*; developmental malformations*, where the most important is anencephaly (44, 45). These causes have been taken as models to describe the three main patterns of the neuropathological damage in PVS cases (53, 54). The Multi-Society Task Force on PVS has defined the precise use of the terms *"persistent"* and *"permanent."* "Persistent refers only to a condition of past and continuing disability with an uncertain future, whereas permanent implies irreversibility." This Task Force likewise addressed that "a patient in a persistent vegetative state becomes permanently vegetative when the diagnosis of irreversibility can be established with a high degree of clinical certainty." According to the etiology, a period of observation has been proposed to define when a *persistent vegetative state*, has become a *permanent vegetative state* (44, 45).

PVS state can be diagnosed considering the following criteria: lack of awareness of self or environment and the inability to interact with other; lack of sustained, reproducible, purposeful or voluntary behavioral responses to visual auditory, tactile or noxious stimuli, and a lack of evidence of language comprehension or expression. There is intermittent wakefulness manifested by the presence of sleep-wake cycles, a sufficient hypothalamic and brain-stem autonomic function for survival with medical and nursing care, bowel and bladder incontinence, and finally there are variably preserved cranial-nerve reflexes and spinal reflexes (1, 41-45, 52). The crux of the problem lies in the determination of a person's internal mental state using external proofs (5, 35, 55-59).

Eye tracking and emotional responses are the most common ways of determining whether a patient is responding and therefore no longer in a vegetative state. The first sign of a patient emerging from PVS is the localizing of the eyes on a visual stimulus. This can be observed because persons in a vegetative state are unable to track moving objects or fixate their vision on an object, and as a patient recovers they regain this ability (60-63). Several authors have reported that recovery of visual pursuit may presage recuperation of other signs of consciousness (64, 65). Giacino and Kalmar reported a significantly higher incidence of visual pursuit among MCS patients admitted for inpatient rehabilitation, independent of time post-injury. Additionally, among the 20% of VS patients who exhibited visual pursuit, 73% showed clear-cut signs of consciousness by 12 months post-injury, while only half of the VS patients without pursuit movements emerged from VS (17).

However, Andrews et al. have emphasized that many patients who are misdiagnosed as being in the vegetative state are blind or have severe visual handicap, and then lack of eye blink to threat or absence of visual tracking might be not reliable signs for diagnosing the vegetative state (60).

Giacino et al., have developed the JFK Coma Recovery Scale (CRS-R) to follow up the clinical evolution in these patients and their potential recovery. If trained examiners apply the CRS-R by repeated measurements, it could yield stable estimates of patient status. This scale contains 6 subscale scores: Auditory function, visual function, motor function, oromotor/verbal function, communication, and arousal scales (66-68).

Misdiagnoses of vegetative state, minimally conscious state, and locked-in syndrome are common. Unexpected and well-documented recoveries of cognitive functions have been described in patients diagnosed by neurologists experienced and skilled in the diagnosis of this condition (33, 69-74). Childs et al. reported that 37% of 49 cases admitted to a special unit for rehabilitation were incorrectly diagnosed, according to the American Medical Association guidelines on PVS and the decision to withdraw support. Although imaging techniques have the potential to improve both diagnostic and prognostic accuracy, careful and repeated neurological assessment by a trained examiner remains best practice (72).

## Minimally Conscious State (MCS)

MCS patients have to shows a limited but clear evidence of awareness of themselves or their environment, based on a reproducible or sustained basis, by at least one of the next behaviors: gestural or verbal yes/no response (regardless of accuracy), following simple commands, intelligible speech, purposeful behavior (including movements or affective behavior that happen in response to stimuli in the environment and are not due to reflexive activity) (18, 55, 56, 75-78).

The Aspen group proposed the criteria for MCS to categorize patients who are not in a vegetative state but are unable to communicate consistently (15). MCS in some patients is a transitional phase towards the partial recovery of self-awareness or environmental awareness while emerging from the vegetative state (17, 51, 79). Emergence from the minimally conscious state is defined by the ability to communicate or use objects functionally. Further improvement is more likely than in patients in a vegetative state, although some cases remain in a MCS permanently (15, 80, 81).

## ANATOMICAL AND FUNCTIONAL CONNECTIVITY IN PVS AND MCS

According to Kinney et al. (53, 54), PVS denotes a "locked-out-syndrome" because "the cerebral cortex is disconnected from the external world, and all awareness of the external world is lost." They suggested that the loss of awareness in the PVS is caused by three main patterns: widespread and bilateral lesions of the cerebral cortex, diffuse damage of intra- and subcortical connections in the cerebral hemispheres white matter, and necrosis of the thalamus.

In widespread and bilateral lesions of the cerebral cortex, hypoxic-ischemic encephalopathy is the main etiology. It could be the consequence of acute hypoxic-ischemic insults after cardio-respiratory arrest, strangulation, suffocation, near-drawing, prolonged hypotension, and perinatal asphyxia in neonates (53, 55, 82-89). Other damages, such as neuronal loss and small infarcts, are also typically found in the cerebellum, basal ganglia, thalamus and hippocampus; the latter being particularly sensitive. Other anatomical structures of the brain are relatively undamaged: brainstem, hypothalamus, basal forebrain and amygdala. This distribution of brain damage reflects the differential vulnerability of brain regions to hypoxia-ischemia (53, 56, 84-86, 90-94).

The second pattern, characterized by diffuse damage subcortical connections in the cerebral hemispheres white matter, could be explained in head trauma and hypoxic-ischemic injury. After head trauma, a widespread damage of axons in the cerebral hemispheres white matter occurs, known as diffuse axonal injury (DAI). The DAI is probably caused by the acceleration suffered by the head immediate after the injury (88, 95-102).

Diffuse damage of intra- and subcortical connections in the cerebral hemispheres white matter could be also occurred after hypoxic-ischemic accidents in a pathological pattern known as *leukoencephalopathy* (103-106). It is characterized by "extensive symmetrical necrotic lesions in the central white matter of the cerebral hemispheres, with minimal or no damage to gray matter structures" (53). These patients yield antecedents of prolonged periods of hypotension, hypoxemia and increased venous pressure (53, 54, 84).

The third pattern is characterized by a selective necrosis of the thalamus and, although the cortex is not totally spared, the lesions are focal and restricted (53, 54, 84, 88, 95, 102, 107-112). It has been explained by several possible factors, such as: partial or immediately reversed transtentorial herniation, cerebral edema causing hypoxia-ischemia, and intrinsic metabolic vulnerability of the thalamus (53, 84).

Nonetheless, in many PVS patients the lesions are mixed of the above mentioned neuropathological findings. Hence, it is important to describe in detail the location of lesions in these cases. Undoubtedly, magnetic resonance imaging (MRI) is the most powerful technique to describe neuropathological findings in alive PVS patients' brains (86, 114, 115).

One of the main obstacles for detailed morphometric evaluation in these cases is that the common very abnormal anatomy hampers the use of software for automatic segmentation to separate brains' gray and white matter. Hence, it is necessary to apply manual segmentation of brains, which is just a time consuming task (35, 116-118). For assessment of regional atrophy, a morphometric analysis is necessary applying the method of voxel-based morphometry (VBM), as described elsewhere. Since the patients' brain morphologies vary due to various degrees of atrophy as identifiable by visual assessment, the standard SPM MRI is not appropriate for VBM analysis and for the co-registration with other functional imaging (119-122).

We are running protocols to evaluate neuropathology in all PVS and MCS cases, studying patients with T1 MRI technique, with slices of I 1mm, and 3D reconstruction of brain images (56, 86) We studied a 21 years old female patient (YOR), who suffered a stroke causing a top of the basilar artery syndrome, and who had been in PVS for 5 years (Figure 1).

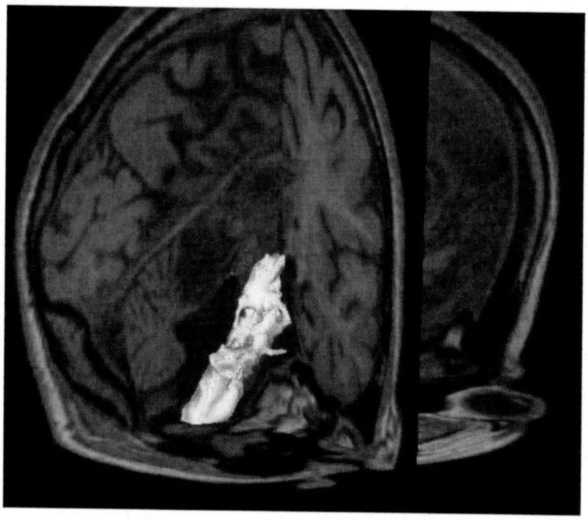

Figure 1. A 3D MRI reconstruction of the brainstem is shown inserted on the three axial planes: sagittal, coronal, and axial. A destruction of the rostral part of the pons, the mesencephalon, and both thalami is demonstrated.

## Anatomical Connectivity

We used MRI diffusion tensor imaging (DTI) technique to study anatomical connectivity by assessing fractional anisotropy (FA) in a 15-year-old girl complaining sickle cell disease, who developed important cognitive impairment, due to multiple strokes, and who had been diagnosed as a PVS. Nonetheless, when she was later admitted to our Institute, accordingly with the presence of inconsistent, but clearly demonstrable behavioral evidence of consciousness awareness, we changed our diagnosis to MCS. Co-registration of FA and MRI showed preservation of anatomical connectivity among posterior brain regions, which were also connected with the frontal remaining cortex islands. These remaining cortical regions were also connected with the thalami (Figure 2). We concluded that white matter connectivity among posterior and frontal cortical regions and the thalami, and CBF preservation in the cortical areas, might explain the recovery of minimum awareness despite huge anatomical brain lesions (86). A possible axonal rewiring mechanism could explain late recoveries in these cases, as reported by other authors (86, 123).

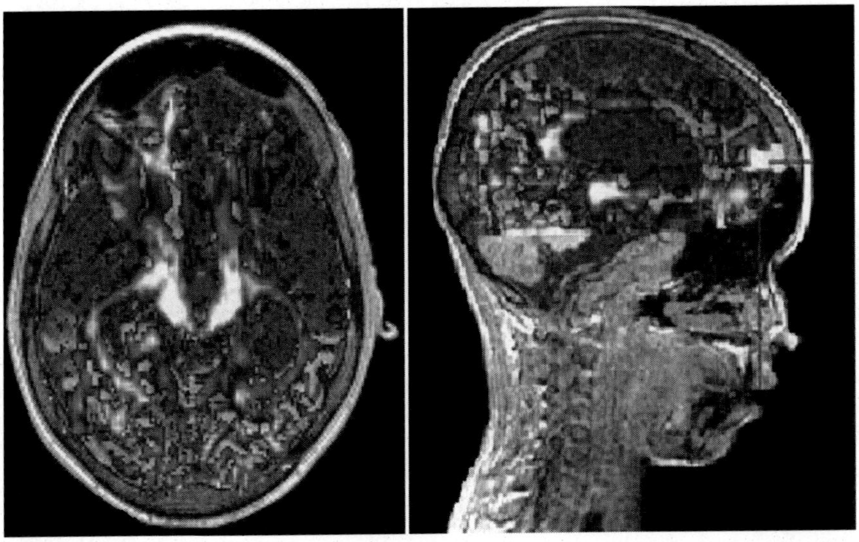

Figure 2. Co-registration of FA and MRI in axial (left) and sagittal (right) planes demonstrates relative preservation of anatomical connectivity within the posterior brain regions which are also connected with the frontal tissue islands. These remaining cortical regions are also connected with the thalamus.

## CEREBRAL BLOOD FLOW (CBF) IN PVS PATIENTS

Compared to controls, positron emission tomography (PET) and single photon emission tomography (SPECT) have shown a substantial reduction of global brain cerebral glucose metabolism and perfusion in PVS (39, 56, 63, 115, 124-127).

SPECT is a powerful technique to demonstrate cerebral blood flow changes in disorders of consciousness. In Figure 3 we present A 3D MRI of the brain reconstruction with SPECT co-registered from the same patient shown in Figure 2, who suffered a stroke causing a top of the basilar artery syndrome (Figure 3). 3D MRI image reveals marked atrophy consistent with progressive cerebral cell loss in the parietal, temporal and frontal lobes of both hemispheres, associated with dilated ventricles and wide cerebral sulci. Brain structures are mainly preserved in the posterior areas of both cerebral hemispheres. Small tissue islands are present in both frontal lobes, mainly preserved in the right one. Co-registration of SPECT and MRI shows maintenance of CBF in the posterior brain regions and cerebellum and in those frontal tissue islands, primarily in the right frontal lobe.

On the other hand, transcranial Doppler ultrasonography (TCD) assesses local blood flow velocity and direction in the proximal portions of large intracranial arteries. Moreover, it is a noninvasive technique, it can be carried out at the bedside, and it is a cost effective method (128-132). Nonetheless, few studies have applied TCD to study intracranial circulation in PVS. Shan et al. used this technique concluded that this technique is a valuable tool in distinguishing PVS, locked-in syndrome and brain death patients according to the differences in velocities and patterns of anterior and posterior cerebral arteries (133-134). Shiogai et al. evaluated cerebrovascular reserve capacity in relation to cerebral cognitive impairments between PVS and vascular dementia, assessing TCD acetazolamide vasoreactivity (133).

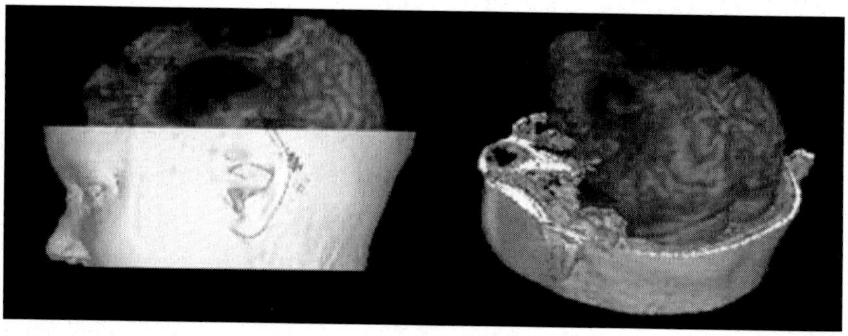

Figure 3. A 3D MRI of the brain reconstruction with SPECT co-registered is shown. 3D MRI image reveals marked atrophy in the parietal, temporal and frontal lobes of both hemispheres, associated with dilated ventricles and wide cerebral sulci. Brain structures are mainly preserved in the posterior areas of both cerebral hemispheres. Small tissue islands are present in both frontal lobes, mainly preserved in the right one. Co-registration of SPECT and MRI shows maintenance of CBF in the posterior brain regions and cerebellum and in those frontal tissue islands, primarily in the right frontal lobe.

We assessed intracranial circulation by TCD in 5 PVS patients. The cause of brain insult was hypoxic encephalopathy in 4 cases, and the other suffered an embolic cerebral infarct causing a top of the basilar artery syndrome. Two experienced operators performed TCD studies. The sample volume was set at 12 mm; power output and gain settings were maximized as needed. The temporal bone acoustic window was not suitable for intracranial vessel insonation in all patients. As an alternative, the internal carotid artery siphon was assessed by orbital insonation between 55-70 mm. Systolic velocity was within a normal range, between 44 and 62 cm/second in all cases. However, the diastolic flow curve amplitude was reduced, as well as the end diastolic velocity, and the pulsatility Index was increased in all patients (Figure 4). We conclude that TCD diastolic velocity decrement and PI augmentation in our cases might be related to uncoupling of CBF and cerebral metabolic rate, arising from reduced cerebral glucose consumption and oxygen uptake, after extensive brain injury (128).

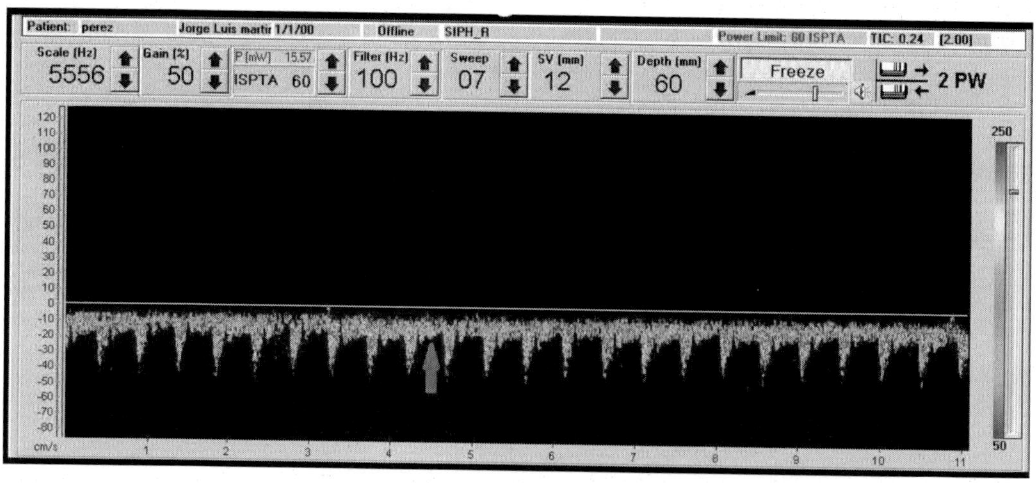


Figure 4. A TCD study of the right internal carotid artery siphon reveals a decreased diastolic flow, as well as the end diastolic velocity (arrow).

## PROTON MRS STUDIES IN PVS AND MCS PATIENTS

Proton magnetic resonance spectroscopy ($^{1}$H-MRS) is useful in monitoring biochemical changes in metabolic, traumatic, infectious, and oncologic disorders of the brain. N-acetyl aspartate (NAA) content is a measure of neuronal integrity, choline (Cho) content mirrors membrane turnover, and creatine (Cre) relates to energy dependent systems. A decrement of NAA concentration has been interpreted as a sign of neuronal loss or dysfunction (87, 135-138).

We recently described the metabolic changes assessed by MRS comparing 2 patients who evolved from PVS to MCS and 2 others who remained in PVS (87). We believe the most important finding in our studies was the increment of the NAA/Cre ratio in the cortex in the two cases of transition of from PVS to MCS, while the pair who remained in PVS showed lower values of this MRS measure (Figure 5). Of course, due to our small sample of patients we were not able to apply a valid statistical analysis, but we consider that it is important to report cognitive recovery assessment in PVS cases, even in single or few cases, as other authors have done (73, 139-142). Hence, MRS seems to be a useful technique as a neurobiological marker to follow up cognitive recovery in PVS patients transiting to MCS (39, 56, 87).

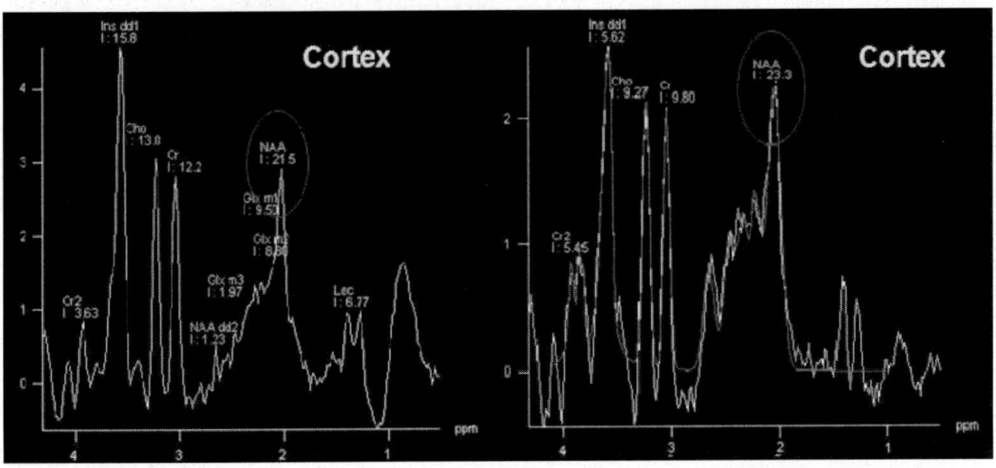


Figure 5. MRS spectra were obtained from 2 x 2 x 2 cm volumes of interest (VOI) placed in cerebral cortex at the left frontal hemisphere. The VOI was localized in three dimensions using T1- and T2-weighted, multisection, spin-echo images. It is shown an increment of NAA when a PVS patient improved to a MCS state.

## RECOGNITION OF THE MOM'S VOICE WITH AN EMOTIONAL CONTENT IN A PVS PATIENT

We recently reported an 8-year-old boy who after a near-drowning remained in a PVS for 4 years before the study (35, 143). We investigated whether there was significant differential brain activation in response to hearing his mother's voice (mom's voice), compared with the voices of unknown women (sham voice). The data were assessed using quantitative electric tomography (QEEGt), a technique that combines anatomical information of the brain by MRI with EEG patterns to estimate the sources of the EEG within the brain. We found an activation for EEG frequencies from 14-58 Hz, with a peak at 33.2 Hz (gamma band), localized in the lateral and posterior regions of the left hemisphere (Figure 6) (35). These results suggested recognition of the mom's voice, indicating a high-level residual linguistic processing in a patient meeting clinical criteria for PVS.

It is important to consider the time and space resolutions in assessing brain function comparing neurophysiologic with other neuroimaging methods. EEG, ERP, and other neurophysiologic techniques, have a high time resolution, which allows assessing early brain functional changes, in the time dominium of milliseconds, contrary to CBF measurements achieved my fMRI, PET and SPECT, which express metabolic and functional changes of the brain in seconds and minutes. Furthermore, QEEGt solves the low spatial resolution of the EEG and ERP estimating the sources of bioelectric generators inside the anatomical voxels of the patient's MRI (116, 118, 144, 145).

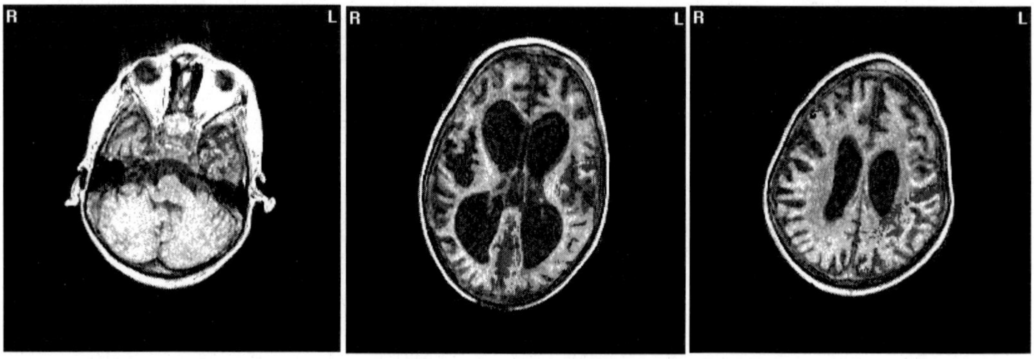


Figure 6. QEEGt calculated in three axial planes illustrate localization of activation in the left lateral and posterior region of the left hemisphere when his mother talks to the patient.

We also assessed autonomic responses to mom's voice, by heart rate variability (HRV) technique (143). We processed HRV using a time-varying spectral analysis applied to sequential series of electrocardiogram (ECG) R-R normal. We found that during the sham voice experimental condition there was significant increase in the HRV very low frequency (VLF) band, and a significant decrease in the HRV high frequency (HF) band, indicating sympathetic triggering and a reduction of parasympathetic activity. Nonetheless, during the mom's voice condition, there was again increase in the VLF band, but a significant recovery of the HF band also occurred, revealing both sympathetic and parasympathetic activation (Figure 7). This can be explained on the basis that the sham voice induces an arousal characterized by the sympathetic activation, while the mom's voice induced arousal, but it also prompted parasympathetic activity, probably related to a shift to a positive emotion during this experimental condition (146, 147).

We also had studied a group of four patients, comparing three diagnosed as PVS, and one as MCS, demonstrating that auditory stimulation can induce recordable changes in HRV, in some patients fulfilling the clinical diagnosis of PVS (148).

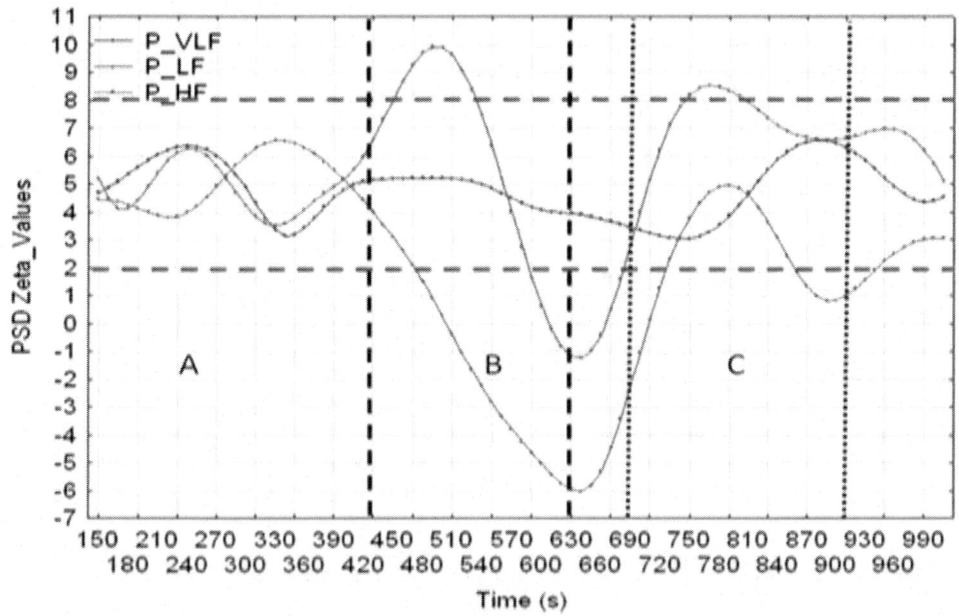


Figure 7. A time-varying spectral analysis applied to sequential series of electrocardiogram (ECG) R-R normal intervals in patient OC is shown in three experimental conditions:(A) Basal;(B) Sham voice;(C) Mother voice. During the sham voice experimental condition there was significant increase in the HRV very low frequency (VLF) band, and a significant decrease in the HRV high frequency (HF) band, indicating sympathetic triggering and a reduction of parasympathetic activity. Nonetheless, during the mom's voice condition, there was again increase in the VLF band, but a significant recovery of the HF band also occurred, revealing both sympathetic and parasympathetic activation (Modified from (143)).

The main finding in PVS is preservation of wakefulness with apparent loss of awareness. Hence, by definition, subjects in PVS with no recognizable behavioral responses to external stimuli, are isolated from the outer world, and they "cannot experience pain and suffering" (44, 45). Nonetheless, our results, combined with the EEG data previously published, suggest recognition of the mom's voice with an emotional content, indicating high-level residual linguistic processing, connected with neural network controlling emotion (35, 143, 148). This entails new medical and ethical discussion on the management of PVS cases.

## PHARMACOLOGICAL INTERVENTION IN PVS CASES: ZOLPIDEM

Several reports have been published over recent years about the paradoxical "arousing" effect of Zolpidem, a highly selective nonbenzodiazepine gamma aminobutyric acid (GABA) agonist acting on the (omega)-1 site of the GABA A receptor (149), in PVS, (150, 151)in MCS (152), in ischemic stroke cases (153, 154), and in patients suffering hypoxic encephalopathy (155).

We studied a 21 years old female patient (YOR), who suffered a stroke causing a top of the basilar artery syndrome, and who had been in PVS for 5 years. MRI showed destruction of the rostral part of the pons, the mesencephalon, and both thalami. YOR showed circadian wakefulness, although she maintained longer periods of time with her eyes closed. With informed written consent of her parents, 10 mg of Zolpidem were administered through a percutaneous endoscopic gastrostomy (156).

After the administration of Zolpidem, and for some 15-20 minutes, patient YOR began to open and close her eyes, until her eyes remained opened. Later, yawns appeared spontaneously at minutes 27, 28, 29, 31, 37 and 39. Usual respiratory and facial muscular movements accompanied inspiratory and expiratory phases of yawns. Her eyes remained opened after minute 25 to minute 46.

The main feature in both experimental phases was the dominance of slow delta waves in all EEG leads. The relative PSD in the delta band constituted 89 - 96% of the whole power density for the EEG spectra in the different EEG-leads, and the mean frequency was near to 1.34 Hz. Over higher frequency ranges (theta, alpha, and beta) the EEG activity was negligible. So, the quantitative analysis was focused on possible changes in the lower frequencies of the EEG (0.146-2 Hz). During the post-Zolpidem period some modulation was observed in the amplitude and morphology of delta waves, coinciding with spontaneous eye movements, and yawning, but the quantitative analysis did not result in significant differences compared to the control EEG. Post-yawning averaged EEG spectra showed a significant ($p < 0.05$) increment of delta PSD considered in normalized units (%) in all EEG leads in comparison with the pre-yawning EEG segments of the same duration of 40.96 seconds, and a corresponding reciprocal significant decrease of the PSD of EEG activity in the infra-slow EEG frequency band in the post-yawning averaged spectra (Figure 8).

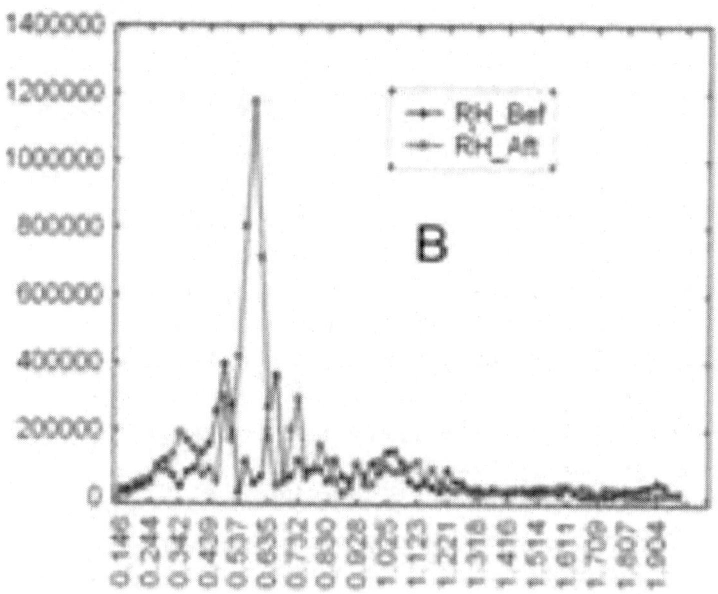


Figure 8. In this figure EEG comparisons are confined to the 0.146 to 2.0 Hz frequency range in F4 lead. Post-yawning averaged EEG spectra (red line) showed a significant ($p < 0.05$) increment of delta PSD, and, and a corresponding reciprocal significant decrement of the PSD of EEG activity in the infra-slow EEG frequency band, compared with the pre-yawning EEG segments (blue line) (Modified from (156)).

The effect of Zolpidem on autonomic function was also assessed by HRV methodology. Dynamics of low frequency (LF), high frequency (HF), and very low frequency (VLF), bands considering normalized units (%) showed from minutes 6 to 16 a definitive increase of HF power and a corresponding reciprocal reduction behavior of the LF band power. Similar changes were observed from minute 20 to 23, 28 to 30, 53 to 54, and finally from 58 to 60. From minute 24 to minute 27, there was observed a reversal of the previously described situation, characterized by increased power in the LF band with reciprocal reduction in the HF band. This pattern reappeared from minutes 37 to 43. Power values in the VLF band markedly increased its control values from minutes 25 to 35, and later, although not as a peak, remained significantly increased until minute 47.

Autonomic dynamics after Zolpidem in patient YOR, as described earlier, clearly showed periods of parasympathetic and of sympathetic cardiovascular predominance. The most interesting findings showed as sympathetic cardiovascular predominance coincided with yawns and behavioral signs of arousal.

Although this is report of a single case, our findings showing a clear relationship between arousal behavioral signs and specific changes of the autonomic cardiovascular regulation, as well as the minimal but significant shift to faster frequencies of the EEG spectrum, demonstrate the importance to assess the so-called brain-heart connections to explain the paradoxical effect of Zolpidem in PVS and MCS patients, reported by other authors (151-153, 155-160).

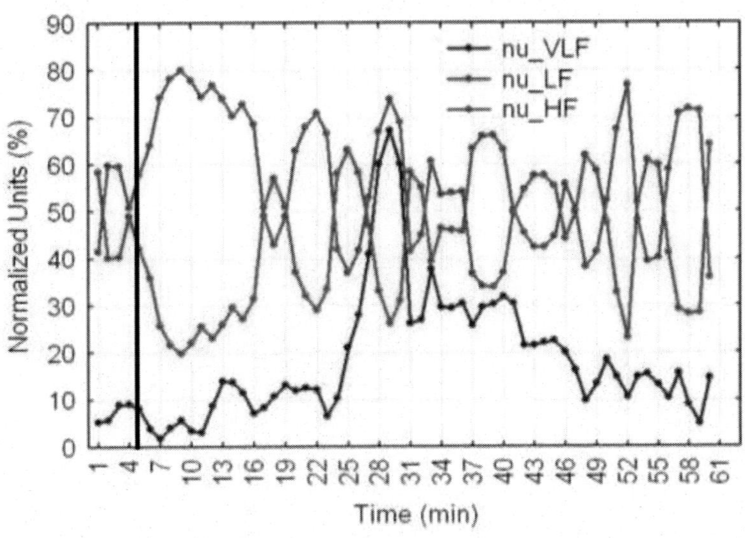


Figure 9. The effect of Zolpidem on autonomic function was assessed by HRV methodology, comparing basal record (vertical line). Dynamics of low frequency (LF), high frequency (HF), and very low frequency (VLF), bands considering normalized units (%) showed from minutes 6 to 16 a definitive increase of HF power and a corresponding reciprocal reduction behavior of the LF band power. Similar changes were observed from minute 20 to 23, 28 to 30, 53 to 54, and finally from 58 to 60. From minute 24 to minute 27, there was observed a reversal of the previously described situation, characterized by increased power in the LF band with reciprocal reduction in the HF band. This pattern reappeared from minutes 37 to 43. Power values in the VLF band markedly increased its control values from minutes 25 to 35, and later, although not as a peak, remained significantly increased until minute 47 (Modified from (156)).

## METABOLIC CHANGES PREDICT VARIATION IN BOLD AND MRS SIGNALS AFTER ADMINISTRATION OF ZOLPIDEM IN A PVS PATIENT

We also studied Patient YOR using $^{1}$H-MRS and BOLD signal, before and after Zolpidem administration. Significantly increased BOLD signal were localized in left frontal superior cortex, bilateral cingulated areas, left thalamus and right head of the caudate nucleus (Figure 10). A transient activation was observed in frontal cortex, comprising portions of anterior cingulate, medial, and orbito-frontal cortices. Additionally, significant pharmacological activation in sensory-motor cortex 1 hour after Zolpidem intake. Significant linear correlations of BOLD signal changes were found with primary concentrations Glutamate at the right frontal cortex. We discussed that when Zolpidem attaches to the modified GABA receptors of the neurodormant cells, dormancy is switched off, inducing brain activation. This might explain the significant correlations of BOLD signal changes and $^{1}$H-MRS metabolites in our patient. We concluded that $^{1}$H-MRS and BOLD signal assessment might contribute to study neurovascular coupling in PVS cases after Zolpidem administration. Although this is report of a single case, considering our results we recommend to apply this methodology in series of PVS and MCS patients.

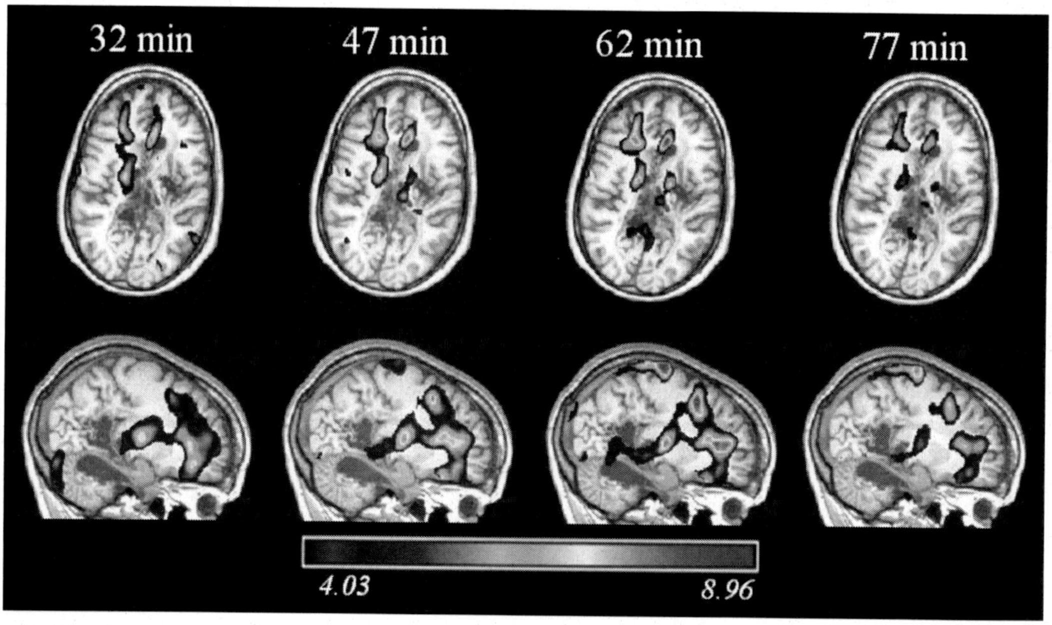


Figure 10. Statistically thresholded Zolpidem-induced BOLD activation in four time points (32, 47, 62, and 77 minutes), rendered on the patient'sT1-weighted axial and sagittal views. Results are thresholded for display at whole brain family wise error corrected (P<0.05). Colour scale represents t-values BOLD signal shows a transient activation in right frontal cortex, comprising portions of anterior cingulate, medial, and orbito-frontal cortices, after Zolpidem intake.

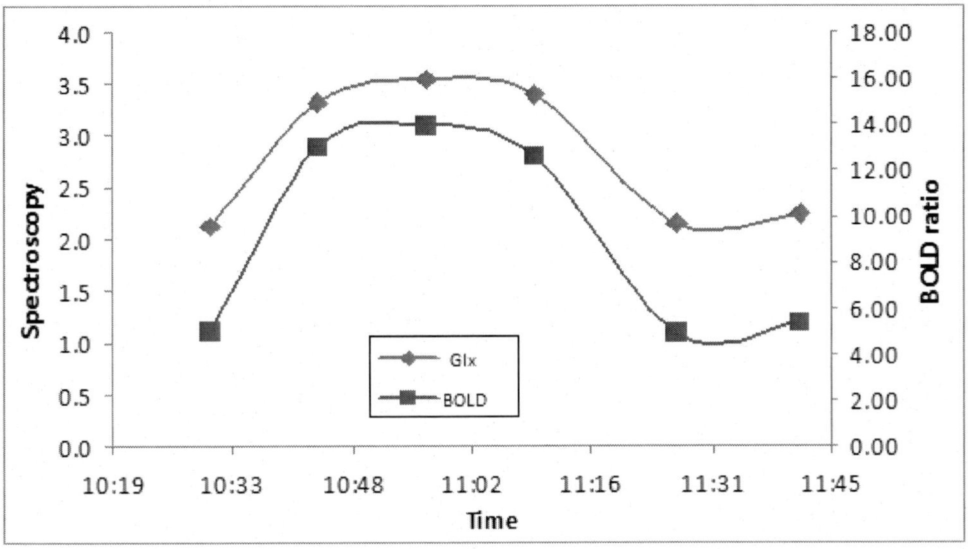


Figure 11. The voxel in right frontal cortex BOLD activated voxel was selected to MRS acquisition in four time points (32, 47, 62, and 77 is shown.. Time dependent behaviour of BOLD time course and metabolites concentrations were compared. Significant linear correlations ($p<0.05$) of BOLD signal changes were found with primary concentrations glutamate (Glx).

We conclude that $^{1}$H-MRS and BOLD signal assessment might contribute to study neurovascular coupling in PVS cases after Zolpidem administration. Although this is report of a single case, considering our results we recommend to apply this methodology in series of PVS and MCS patients.

## CONCLUSION

The diagnosis and management of PVS and MCS cases entail powerful medical, ethical and legal debates. The recent description of the MCS highlights the crucial role of unexpected and well documented recoveries of cognitive functions. Anatomic and functional neuroimaging has provided new insights for assessing neuropathology and cerebral activity in these patients, providing information on the presence, degree, and location of any residual brain and autonomic functions in PVS or MCS cases.

The main finding in PVS is preservation of wakefulness with apparent loss of awareness. Hence, by definition, subjects in PVS with no recognizable behavioral responses to external stimuli, are isolated from the outer world, and they “cannot experience pain and suffering” (44, 45). Nonetheless, our results, suggest recognition of the mom’s voice with an emotional content, and indicating high-level residual linguistic processing, and brain activation after Zolpidem administration (35, 143, 148). These results differ with the current concept that by definition, subjects in PVS with no recognizable behavioral responses to external stimuli, are isolated from the outer world, and they “cannot experience pain and suffering” (44, 45). These findings launch new medical, ethical and practical implications for the diagnosis and management of PVS and MCS patients.

## REFERENCES


[1] Bernat JL. Current controversies in states of chronic unconsciousness. Neurology 2010;75:S33-8.

[2] Byrne S, Hardiman O. Willful modulation of brain activity in disorders of consciousness. N Engl J Med 2010;362:1936-8.

[3] Carelli F. Persistent vegetative state. Br J Gen Pract 2010;60:132.

[4] Cruse D, Owen AM. Consciousness revealed:New insights into the vegetative and minimally conscious states. Curr Opin Neurol 2010;23:656-60.

[5] Fernandez-Espejo D, Bekinschtein T, Monti MM, et al. Diffusion weighted imaging distinguishes the vegetative state from the minimally conscious state. Neuroimage 2011;54:103-12.

[6] Laureys S, Owen AM, Schiff, ND. Brain function in coma, vegetative state, and related disorders. Lancet Neurol 2004;3:537-46.

[7] Machado C. Consciousness as a definition of death:Its appeal and complexity. Clin Electroenceph 1999;30:156-64.

[8] Machado C, Korein, J. Persistent vegetative and minimally conscious states. Rev Neurosci 2009;20:203-20.

[9] Machado C, Leisman, G. Towards an effective definition of death and disorders of consciousness. Rev Neurosci 2009;20:147-50.

[10] Machado C, Rodriguez R, Carballo M, Korein J, Sanchez-Catasus C, Perez J, et al. Brain anatomy, cerebral blood flow, and connectivity in the transition from PVS to MCS. Rev Neurosci 2009;20:177-80.

[11] Machado C, Rodriguez R, Carballo M, Perez J, Korein J. Results of proton MRS studies in PVS and MCS patients. Can J Neurol Sci 2009;36(3):365-9.

[12] Machado C, Perez-Nellar J, Rodriguez R. Emergence from minimally conscious state:insights from evaluation of posttraumatic confusion. Neurology 2010;74:1156-7.

[13] Machado C, Estevez M, Rodriguez R. Wakefulness and loss of awareness:Brain and brainstem interaction in the vegetative state. Neurology 2010;75:751.

[14] Machado C, Perez-Nellar J, Rodriguez R. Emergence from minimally conscious state:insights from evaluation of posttraumatic confusion. Neurology 2010;74:1156-7.

[15] Giacino JT, Ashwal S, Childs N, Cranford R, Jennett B, Katz DI, et al. The minimally conscious state: Definition and diagnostic criteria. Neurology 2002;58:349-53.

[16] Giacino JT. The vegetative and minimally conscious states:consensus-based criteria for establishing diagnosis and prognosis. NeuroRehabil 2004;19:293-8.

[17] Giacino JT, Kalmar K. Diagnostic and prognostic guidelines for the vegetative and minimally conscious states. Neuropsychol Rehabil 2005;15:166-74.

[18] Giacino JT, Malone R. The vegetative and minimally conscious States. Handb Clin Neurol 2008;90:99-111.

[19] Whelan CM. Karen Ann Quinlan: Patient or prisoner? America (NY) 1975;133:346-7.

[20] Becker-Schwarze K. Terri Schiavo:the assessment of the persistent vegetative state in accordance with German law. Eur J Health Law 2005;12:321-34.

[21] Blendon RJ, Benson JM, Herrmann MJ. The American public and the Terri Schiavo case. Arch Intern Med 2005;165:2580-4.

[22] Goodnough A. U.S. judge denies feeding-tube bid in Schiavo's case;parents quickly appeal;family cites urgency as woman enters 5th day without nutrition. NY Times 2005:A1,A14.

[23] Silverman HJ. Withdrawal of feeding-tubes from incompetent patients:the Terri Schiavo case raises new issues regarding who decides in end-of-life decision making. Intensive Care Med 2005;31:480-1.

[24] Dyer C. Tony Bland awaits final hearing. BMJ 1993;306:11-2.

[25] McCormick RA. The Nancy Cruzan case. Midwest Med Ethics 1989;5:2-31.

[26] Attorney for Cruzans discusses legal 'odyssey.' Iowa Med 1991;81:249-50.

[27] Keyser PK. After Cruzan:the "values base" to advance directives. Orthop Nurs 1992;11:37-40.

[28] Jennett,B, Plum, F. Persistent vegetative state after brain damage. A syndrome in search of a name. Lancet 1972;1:734-7.

[29] Kretschmer E. Das apallische syndrom. Z Ges Neurol Psychiat 1940;169:576-9.

[30] Ingvar DH, Brun A, Johansson L, Sammuelsson SM. Survival after severe cerebral anoxia with destruction of the cerebral cortex:the apallic syndrome. In: Korein J, ed. Brain death: Interrelated medical and social issues. New York: Ann NY Acad Sci 1977:184-214.
[31] Hassler R, Ore GD, Dieckmann G, Bricolo A, Dolce G. Behavioural and EEG arousal induced by stimulation of unspecific projection systems in a patient with post-traumatic apallic syndrome. Electroenceph Clin Neurophysiol 1969;27:306-10.
[32] Bergamasco B, Bergamini L, Bricolo A, Dolce G. Studies on sleep during the apallic syndrome. Monogr Gesamtgeb Psychiatr Psychiatry Ser 1977;14:155-9.
[33] Kotchoubey B. Apallic syndrome is not apallic:is vegetative state vegetative? Neuropsychol Rehabil. 2005;15:333-56.
[34] Laureys S, Celesia GG, Cohadon F, Lavrijsen J, Leon-Carrion J, Sannita WG, et al. Unresponsive wakefulness syndrome:a new name for the vegetative state or apallic syndrome. BMC Med 2010;8:68.
[35] Machado C, Korein J, Aubert E, Bosch J, Alvarez MA, Rodgiguez R, et al. Recognizing a mother's voice in the persistent vegetative state. Clin EEG Neurosci 2007;38(3):124-6.
[36] Machado C. Terminating artificial nutrition and hydration in persistent vegetative state patients:current and proposed state laws. Neurology 2007;68:312-3.
[37] Machado C. Cerebral response to patient's own name in the vegetative and minimally conscious states. Neurology 2007;69:708-9.
[38] Machado C. Cerebral response to patient's own name in the vegetative and minimally conscious states. Neurology 2007;69:708-9.
[39] Macahdo C. Brain death: A reappraisal. New York: Springer, 2007, 121-26.
[40] Machado C. The minimally conscious state:definition and diagnostic criteria. Neurology 2002;59:1473-4.
[41] Danze F, Brule JF, Haddad, K. Chronic vegetative state after severe head injury:clinical study;electrophysiological investigations and CT scan in 15 cases. Neurosurg Rev 1989;12(1):477-99.
[42] Giacino J, Whyte, J. The vegetative and minimally conscious states:current knowledge and remaining questions. J Head Trauma Rehabil 2005;20:30-50.
[43] Wijdicks EF, Cranford RE. Clinical diagnosis of prolonged states of impaired consciousness in adults. Mayo Clin Proc 2005;80:1037-46.
[44] The Multi-Society Task Force on PVS. Medical aspects of the persistent vegetative state (2). N Engl J Med 1994;330:1572-9.
[45] The Multi-Society Task Force on PVS. Medical aspects of the persistent vegetative state (1). N Engl J Med 1994;330:1499-1508.
[46] Shah SA, Schiff ND. Central thalamic deep brain stimulation for cognitive neuromodulation - a review of proposed mechanisms and investigational studies. Eur J Neurosci 2010;32:1135-44.
[47] Laureys S, Giacino JT, Schiff ND, Schabus M, Owen AM. How should functional imaging of patients with disorders of consciousness contribute to their clinical rehabilitation needs? Curr Opin Neurol 2006;19:520-7.
[48] Schiff ND, Plum, F. Cortical function in the persistent vegetative state. Trends Cogn Sci 1999;3:43-4.
[49] Schiff ND. Commentary:neurobiology, suffering, and unconscious brain states. J Pain Symptom Manage 1999;17:303-4.
[50] Racine E, Rodrigue C, Bernat JL, Riopelle R, Shemie SD. Observations on the ethical and social aspects of disorders of consciousness. Can J Neurol Sci 2010;37:758-68.
[51] Bernat JL. Questions remaining about the minimally conscious state. Neurology 2002;58:337-8.
[52] Bernat JL. The boundaries of the persistent vegetative state. J Clin Ethics 1992;3:176-80.
[53] Kinney HC, Samuels MA. Neuropathology of the persistent vegetative state. A review. J Neuropathol Exp Neurol 1994;53:548-58.
[54] Kinney HC, Korein J, Panigrahy A, Dikkes P, Goode R. Neuropathological findings in the brain of Karen Ann Quinlan. The role of the thalamus in the persistent vegetative state. N Engl J Med 1994;330:1469-75.
[55] Machado C, Perez-Nellar J, Rodriguez R. Emergence from minimally conscious state:insights from evaluation of posttraumatic confusion. Neurology 2010;74:1156-7.

[56] Machado C, Korein, J. Persistent vegetative and minimally conscious states. Rev Neurosci 2009;20:203-20.
[57] Monti MM, Laureys S, Owen AM. The vegetative state. BMJ 2010;341:c3765.
[58] Monti MM, Vanhaudenhuyse A, Coleman MR, Boly M, Pickard JD, Tshibanda L, et al. Willful modulation of brain activity in disorders of consciousness. N Engl J Med 2010;362(7):579-89.
[59] Owen AM, Coleman MR. Detecting awareness in the vegetative state. Ann N Y Acad Sci 2008;1129:130-8.
[60] Andrews K. Recovery of patients after four months or more in the persistent vegetative state. BMJ 1993;306:1597-1600.
[61] Andrews K, Murphy L, Munday R, Littlewood C. Misdiagnosis of the vegetative state:retrospective study in a rehabilitation unit. BMJ 1996;313:13-6.
[62] Ng YS, Chua KS. States of severely altered consciousness:Clinical characteristics, medical complications and functional outcome after rehabilitation. NeuroRehabil 2005;20:97-105.
[63] Bruno MA, Vanhaudenhuyse A, Schnakers C, Boly M, Gosseries O, Demertzi A, et al. Visual fixation in the vegetative state:an observational case series PET study. BMC Neurol 2010;10:35.
[64] Ansell BJ, Keenan JE. The Western Neuro Sensory Stimulation Profile:a tool for assessing slow-to-recover head-injured patients. Arch Phys Med Rehabil 1989;70:104-8.
[65] Shiel A, Horn SA, Wilson BA, Watson MJ, Cambell MJ, McLellan DL. The Wessex Head Injury Matrix (WHIM) main scale:a preliminary report on a scale to assess and monitor patient recovery after severe head injury. Clin Rehabil 2000;14:408-16.
[66] Løvstad M, Froslie KF, Giacino JT, Skandsen T, Anke A, Schanke AK. Reliability and diagnostic characteristics of the JFK coma recovery scale-revised:exploring the influence of rater's level of experience. J Head Trauma Rehabil 2010;25:349-56.
[67] Kalmar, K and Giacino, JT. The JFK Coma Recovery Scale--Revised. Neuropsychol Rehabil 2005;15:454-60.
[68] Giacino JT, Kalmar K, Whyte, J. The JFK Coma Recovery Scale-Revised:measurement characteristics and diagnostic utility. Arch Phys Med Rehabil 2004;85:2020-9.
[69] Childs N. Differences in vegetative states. Tex Med 1999;95:6.
[70] Childs NL, Mercer, WN. Misdiagnosing the persistent vegetative state. Misdiagnosis certainly occurs. BMJ 1996;313:944.
[71] Childs NL, Mercer, WN. Brief report:late improvement in consciousness after post-traumatic vegetative state. N Engl J Med 1996;334:24-5.
[72] Childs NL, Mercer, WN, Childs, HW. Accuracy of diagnosis of persistent vegetative state. Neurology 1993;43:1465-7.
[73] Kotchoubey B, Jetter U, Lang S, Semmler A, Mezger G, Schmalohr D, et al. Evidence of cortical learning in vegetative state. J Neurol 2006;253:1374-6.
[74] Kotchoubey B. Event-related potential measures of consciousness:two equations with three unknowns. Prog Brain Res 2005;150:427-44.
[75] Boly M, Faymonville ME, Schnakers C, Peigneux P, Lambermont B, Phillips C, et al. Perception of pain in the minimally conscious state with PET activation:an observational study. Lancet Neurology 2008;7:1013-20.
[76] Machado C. Cerebral response to patient's own name in the vegetative and minimally conscious states. Neurology 2007;69:708-9.
[77] Giacino JT. The minimally conscious state:defining the borders of consciousness. Prog Brain Res 2005;150:381-95.
[78] Giacino JT, Kalmar, K. Diagnostic and prognostic guidelines for the vegetative and minimally conscious states. Neuropsychol Rehabil 2005;15:166-74.
[79] Leong B. The vegetative and minimally conscious states in children:spasticity, muscle contracture and issues for physiotherapy treatment. Brain Inj 2002;16:217-30.
[80] Cicerone KD, Dahlberg C, Malec JF, Langenbahn DM, Felicetti T, Kneipp S, et al. Evidence-based cognitive rehabilitation:updated review of the literature from 1998 through 2002. Arch Phys Med Rehabil 2005;86:1681-92.

[81] Schiff ND, Ribary U, Moreno DR, Beattie B, Kronberg E, Blasberg R, et al. Residual cerebral activity and behavioural fragments can remain in the persistently vegetative brain. Brain 2002;125:1210-34.

[82] Ingvar DH. The pathophysiology of cerebral anoxia. Acta Anaesthesiol Scand Suppl 1968;29:47-59.

[83] Rothstein TL. Recovery from near death following cerebral anoxia:A case report demonstrating superiority of median somatosensory evoked potentials over EEG in predicting a favorable outcome after cardiopulmonary resuscitation. Resuscitation 2004;60:335-41.

[84] McKinney JS, Giacino JT. Diagnostic accuracy in disorders of consciousness. Neurologist 2008;14:340.

[85] Machado C, Estevez M, Redriguez R. Wakefulness and loss of awareness:brain and brainstem interaction in the vegetative state. Neurology 2010;75:751-2.

[86] Machado C, Rodriguez R, Carballo M. Brain anatomy, cerebral blood flow, and connectivity in the transition from PVS to MCS. Rev Neurosci 2009;20:177-80.

[87] Machado C, Rodriguez R, Carballo M, Perez J, Korein J. Results of proton MRS studies in PVS and MCS patients. Can J Neurol Sci 2009;36:365-9.

[88] Graham, DI, Adams JH, Murray LS, Jennett B. Neuropathology of the vegetative state after head injury. Neuropsychol Rehabil 2005;15:198-213.

[89] Stevens RD, Bhardwaj A. Approach to the comatose patient. Crit Care Med 2006;34:31-41.

[90] Machado C. Can vegetative state patients retain cortical processing? Clin Neurophysiol 2005;116:2253-4.

[91] Ingvar DH. EEG and cerebral circulation in the apallic syndrome and akinetic mutism. Electroencephalogr Clin Neurophysiol 1971;30:272-3.

[92] Rap ZM. Influence of damage of hypothalamo-hypophysial neurosecretory system and adrenalectomy on the blood-brain barrier alteration during intracranial hypertension. Acta Neuropathol Suppl (Berl) 1981;7:10-2.

[93] Geocadin RG, Muthuswamy J, Sherman DL, et al. Early electrophysiological and histologic changes after global cerebral ischemia in rats. Mov Disord 2000;15(1):14-21.

[94] McDonald JW, Althomsons SP, Hyrc KL, Choi DW, Goldberg MP. Oligodendrocytes from forebrain are highly vulnerable to AMPA/kainate receptor-mediated excitotoxicity. Nature Med 1998;4:291-7.

[95] Jennett B, Adams JH, Murray LS, Graham DI. Neuropathology in vegetative and severely disabled patients after head injury. Neurology 2001;56:486-90.

[96] Chiaretti A, Visocchi M, Viola L, De Benedictis R, Langer A, Tortorolo L, et al. (Diffuse axonal lesions in childhood). Pediatr Med Chir 1998;20:393-7. (Italian)

[97] Vuilleumier P, Assal, G. (Lesions of the corpus callosum and syndromes of interhemispheric disconnection of traumatic origin). Neurochirurgie 1995;41:98-107.

[98] Cordobes F, Lobato RD, Rivas JJ, Cabrera A, Sarabia M, Castro S, et al. Post-traumatic diffuse axonal brain injury. Analysis of 78 patients studied with computed tomography. Acta Neurochir (Wien) 1986;81:27-35.

[99] Graham DI, McLellan D, Adams JH, Doyle D, Kerr A, Murray LS. The neuropathology of the vegetative state and severe disability after non-missile head injury. Acta Neurochir Suppl (Wien) 1983;32:65-7.

[100] Gentleman SM, McKenzie JE, Royston MC, McIntosh TK, Graham DI. A comparison of manual and semi-automated methods in the assessment of axonal injury. Neuropathol Appl Neurobiol 1999;25:41-7.

[101] Tong KA, Ashwal S, Holshouser BA, Nickerson JP, Wall CJ, Shutter LA, et al. Diffuse axonal injury in children:clinical correlation with hemorrhagic lesions. Ann Neurol 2004;56:36-50.

[102] Graham DI, Maxwell WL, Adams JH, Jennett B. Novel aspects of the neuropathology of the vegetative state after blunt head injury. Prog Brain Res 2005;150:445-55.

[103] Heye N, Terstegge K, Gosztonyi, G. Vasculitic, hypoxic-ischemic leukoencepha-lopathy. Clin Neurol Neurosurg 1994;96:156-60.

[104] Mahler ME, Cummings JL, Tomiyasu U. Atypical dementia syndrome in an elderly man. J Am Geriatr Soc 1987;35:1116-26.

[105] Ginsberg MD, Hedley-Whyte ET, Richardson, EP Jr. Hypoxic-ischemic leukoencephalopathy in man. Trans Am Neurol Assoc 1974;99:213-6.

[106] Roman GC. Vascular dementia today. Rev Neurol (Paris) 1999;155 Suppl 4:S64-S72.
[107] Villablanca J, Salinas-Zeballos ME. Sleep-wakefulness, EEG and behavioral studies of chronic cats without the thalamus:the 'athalamic' cat. Arch Ital Biol 1972;110:383-411.
[108] Tsubokawa T, Yamamoto T, Katayama Y, Hirayama T, Maejima S, Moriya T. Deep-brain stimulation in a persistent vegetative state:follow-up results and criteria for selection of candidates. Brain Inj 1990;4:315-27.
[109] Zhou J, Liu X, Song W, Yang Y, Zhao Z, Ling F, et al. Specific and nonspecific thalamocortical functional connectivity in normal and vegetative states. Conscious Cogn 2011;20(2):257-68.
[110] Lull N, Noe E, Lull JJ, Garcia-Panach J, Garcia-Marti G, Chirivella J, et al. (Thalamic metabolism and neurological outcome after traumatic brain injury. A voxel-based morphometric FDG-PET study). Neurologia 2010;25:174-80.
[111] Laureys S, Faymonville ME, Peigneux P, Damas P, Lambermont B, Del Fiore G, et al. Cortical processing of noxious somatosensory stimuli in the persistent vegetative state. Neuroimage 2002;17:732-41.
[112] Jellinger KA. The brain of Karen Ann Quinlan. N Engl J Med 1994;331:1378-9.
[113] Adams JH, Graham DI, Jennett, B. The neuropathology of the vegetative state after an acute brain insult. Brain 2000;123(7):1327-38.
[114] Ropper AH. Cogito ergo sum by MRI. N Engl J Med 2010;362:648-9.
[115] Juengling FD, Kassubek J, Huppertz HJ, Krause T, Els T. Separating functional and structural damage in persistent vegetative state using combined voxel-based analysis of 3-D MRI and FDG-PET. J Neurol Sci 2005;228:179-84.
[116] Machado C, Cuspineda E, Valdes P, Virues T, Llopis F, Bosch J, et al. Assessing acute middle cerebral artery ischemic stroke by quantitative electric tomography. Clin EEG Neurosci 2004;35:116-24.
[117] Fernandez-Bouzas A, Harmony T, Fernandez T, Silva-Pereyra J, Valdes P, et al. Sources of abnormal EEG activity in brain infarctions. Clin Electroencephalogr 2000;31:165-9.
[118] Bosch-Bayard J, Valdes-Sosa P, Virues-Alba T, Aubert-Vazquez E, John ER, et al. 3D statistical parametric mapping of EEG source spectra by means of variable resolution electromagnetic tomography (VARETA). Clin Electroencephalogr 2001;32:47-61.
[119] Hutton C, Draganski B, Ashburner J, Weiskopf N. A comparison between voxel-based cortical thickness and voxel-based morphometry in normal aging. Neuroimage 2009;48:371-80.
[120] Good CD, Scahill RI, Fox NC, Ashburner J, Friston KJ, Chan D, et al. Automatic differentiation of anatomical patterns in the human brain:validation with studies of degenerative dementias. Neuroimage 2002;17:29-46.
[121] Salmond CH, Ashburner J, Vargha-Khadem F, Connelly A, Gadian DG, Friston KJ. Distributional assumptions in voxel-based morphometry. Neuroimage 2002;17:1027-30.
[122] Ashburner J, Friston KJ. Voxel-based morphometry--the methods. Neuroimage 2000;11:805-21.
[123] Voss HU, Uluc AM, Dyke JP, Watts R, Kobylarz EJ, McCandliss BD, et al. Possible axonal regrowth in late recovery from the minimally conscious state. J Clin Invest 2006;116:2005-11.
[124] Kremer S, Nicolas-Ong C, Schunck T, Schenck M, Collange O, Mutschler V, et al. Usefulness of functional MRI associated with PET scan and evoked potentials in the evaluation of brain functions after severe brain injury:preliminary results. J Neuroradiol 2010;37:159-66.
[125] Owen AM, Coleman MR, Menon DK, Johnrude IS, Rodd JM, Davis MH, et al. Residual auditory function in persistent vegetative state:a combined PET and fMRI study. Neuropsychol Rehabil 2005;15:290-306.
[126] Beuthien-Baumann B, Holthoff VA, Rudolf, J. Functional imaging of vegetative state applying single photon emission tomography and positron emission tomography. Neuropsychol Rehabil 2005;15:276-82.
[127] Estraneo A, Moretta P, Loreto V, Lanzillo B, Santoro L, Trojano L. Late recovery after traumatic, anoxic, or hemorrhagic long-lasting vegetative state. Neurology 2010;75(3):239-45.
[128] Perez-Nellar J, Machado C, Scherle CE, Chinchilla M. TCD diastolic velocity decay and pulsatility index increment in PVS cases. Can J Neurol Sci 2010;37:831-6.

[129] Conti A, Iacopino DG, Spada A, Cardali SM, Giusa M, La Torre D, et al. Transcranial Doppler ultrasonography in the assessment of cerebral circulation arrest:improving sensitivity by transcervical and transorbital carotid insonation and serial examinations. Neurocrit Care 2009;10:326-35.

[130] Dosemeci L, Dora B, Yilmaz M, Cenqiz M, Balkan S, Ramazanoglu A. Utility of transcranial doppler ultrasonography for confirmatory diagnosis of brain death:two sides of the coin. Transplantation 2004;77:71-5.

[131] Machado C. Assessment:transcranial Doppler ultrasonography:report of the Therapeutics and Technology Assessment Subcommittee of the American Academy of Neurology. Neurology 2004;63:2457-8.

[132] Sadik JC, Riquier V, Koskas P, Zylberberg F, Beyloune-Mainardi C, Szmaraqd V, et al. (Transcranial Doppler imaging:state of the art). J Radiol 2001;82:821-31.

[133] Shiogai T, Koshimura M, Uebo C, Makino M, Mizuno T, Nakajima K. Acetazolamide vasoreactivity in persistent vegetative state and vascular dementia evaluated by transcranial harmonic perfusion imaging and Doppler sonography. Acta Neurochir Suppl 2003;87:63-9.

[134] Shan G, Yining H, Xia H, Yicheng Z, Bo W, Shunwei L. Transcranial Doppler characteristics in persistent vegetative status, locked-in syndrome and brain death. Chin Med Sci J 1999;14:211-14.

[135] Tshibanda L, Vanhaudenhuyse A, Boly M, Soddu A, Bruno MA, Moonen G, et al. Neuroimaging after coma. Neuroradiology 2010;52:15-24.

[136] Wartenberg KE, Patsalides A, Yepes MS. Is magnetic resonance spectroscopy superior to conventional diagnostic tools in hypoxic-ischemic encephalopathy? J Neuroimaging 2004;14:180-6.

[137] Aubert A, Costalat R, Duffau H, Benali H. Modeling of pathophysiological coupling between brain electrical activation, energy metabolism and hemodynamics:insights for the interpretation of intracerebral tumor imaging. Acta Biotheor 2002;50:281-95.

[138] Morales-Chacon L. Magnetic resonance spectroscopy and functional magnetic resonance images:Non-invasive alternatives for identification of the zone. Revista de Neurologia 2001;32:234-6.

[139] Kotchoubey B, Schneck M, Lang S, Birbaumer N. Event-related brain potentials in a patient with akinetic mutism. Neurophysiol Clin 2003;33:23-30.

[140] Kotchoubey B, Lang S, Bostanov V, Birbaumer N. Is there a mind? Electrophysiology of unconscious patients. News Physiol Sci 2002;17:38-42.

[141] Schiff ND, Plum F, Rezai AR. Developing prosthetics to treat cognitive disabilities resulting from acquired brain injuries. Neurol Res 2002;24:116-24.

[142] Berstad J, Undseth S, Kunz R, Schanke AK, Christensen S, Andersson S. (Severely injured patients after the initial phase--vegetative state or remaining cognitive functions?). Tidsskr Nor Laegeforen 2001;121:794-6. (Norwegian)

[143] Machado C, Estevez M, Gutierrez J, Beltran C, Machado Y, Machado Y, et al. Recognition of the mom's voice with an emotional content in a PVS patient. Clin Neurophysiol 2011;122(5):1059-60.

[144] Cuspineda Bravo ER, Iturria Y, Praderes JC, Melie L, Valdes PA, Virues T, et al. Noninvasive multimodal neuroimaging for Rasmussen encephalopathy surgery:simultaneous EEG-fMRI recording. Clin EEG Neurosci 2010;41:159-65.

[145] Cuspineda ER, Machado C, Virues T, Martinez-Montes E, Ojeda A, Valdes PA, et al. Source analysis of alpha rhythm reactivity using LORETA imaging with 64-channel EEG and individual MRI. Clin EEG Neurosci 2009;40:150-6.

[146] Riganello F, Candelieri A, Dolce G, Sannita WG. Residual emotional processing in the vegetative state:A scientific issue? Clin Neurophysiol 2011;122(5):1061-2.

[147] Riganello F, Candelieri A, Quintieri M, Conforti D, Dolce G. Heart rate variability:an index of brain processing in vegetative state? An artificial intelligence, data mining study. Clin Neurophysiol 2010;121:2024-34.

[148] Gutierrez J, Machado C, Estevez M, Olivares A, Hernandez H, Perez J, et al. Heart rate variability changes induced by auditory stimulation in persistent vegetative state. Int J Disabil Hum Dev 2010;9(4):357-62.

[149] Chen L, Xie JX, Fung KS, Yung WH. Zolpidem modulates GABA(A) receptor function in subthalamic nucleus. Neurosci Res 2007;58:77-85.

[150] Clauss RP, van der Merwe CE, Nel HW. Arousal from a semi-comatose state on zolpidem. S Afr Med J 2001;91:788-9.

[151] Clauss RP, Guldenpfennig WM, Nel HW, Sathekge MM, Vankannagari RR. Extraordinary arousal from semi-comatose state on zolpidem. A case report. S Afr Med J 2000;90:68-72.

[152] Singh R, McDonald C, Dawson K, Lewis S, Pringle AM, Smith S, et al. Zolpidem in a minimally conscious state. Brain Inj 2008;22:103-6.

[153] Clauss RP, Nel WH. Effect of zolpidem on brain injury and diaschisis as detected by 99mTc HMPAO brain SPECT in humans. Arzneimittelforschung 2004;54:641-6.

[154] Cohen L, Chaaban B, Habert MO. Transient improvement of aphasia with zolpidem. N Engl J Med 2004;350:949-50.

[155] Cohen SI, Duong, TT. Increased arousal in a patient with anoxic brain injury after administration of zolpidem. Am J Phys Med Rehabil 2008;87:229-31.

[156] Machado C, Estevez M, Perez-Nellar J, Gutierrez J, Rodriguez R, Carballo M, et al. Autonomic, EEG, and behavioral arousal signs in a PVS case after Zolpidem intake. Can J Neurol Sci 2011;38(2):341-4.

[157] Chen YY, Sy HN, Wu, SL. Zolpidem improves akinesia, dystonia and dyskinesia in advanced Parkinson's disease. J Clin Neurosci 2008;15:955-6.

[158] Du B, Shan AJ, Yang D. Induced arousal following zolpidem treatment in a vegetative state after brain injury in 7 cases - Analysis using visual single photon emission computerized tomography and digitized cerebral state monitor. Neural Regener Res. 2008;3:94-6.

[159] Brefel-Courbon C, Payoux P, Ory F, Sommet A, Slaqui T, Raboyeau G, et al. Clinical and imaging evidence of zolpidem effect in hypoxic encephalopathy. Ann Neurol 2007;62:102-5.

[160] Clauss R, Sathekge M, Nel W. Transient improvement of spinocerebellar ataxia with zolpidem. N Engl J Med 2004;351:511-12.

In: Considering Consciousness Clinically
Editors: Gerry Leisman and Joav Merrick

ISBN: 978-1-63484-260-0


*Chapter 11*

# PERSISTENT VEGETATIVE STATE: VENTRICULAR CSF PULSATION ARTIFACT

***Jesús Perez-Nellar*[1], *Calixto Machado*[2], *Claudio Scherle*[1], *Rafael Rodríguez*[3], *Maylen Carballo*[3], *Gerry Leisman*[4,5,*] *and Robert Melillo*[4]**

[1]Institute of Neurology and Neurosurgery, Department of Clinical Neurophysiology, Havana, Cuba
[2]Hermanos Ameijeiras Hospital, Stroke Unit, Havana, Cuba
[3]International Center for Neurological Restoration, Havana, Cuba
[4]The National Institute for Brain and Rehabilitation Sciences, Karmiel, Israel
[5]Universidad de Ciencias Médicas de la Habana, Facultad Manuel Fajardo, Havana, Cuba

## ABSTRACT

One of the major limitations of FLAIR imaging is the ventricular CSF pulsation artifact (VCSFA). This artifact could compromise the study of ventricular abnormalities by leading to false-negative or false-positive interpretations. We report 4 young persistent vegetative state (PVS) patients with severe ventriculomegaly and brain atrophy who showed VCSFA on FLAIR MR imaging. FLAIR axial images showed the presence of a hyperintensity. occupying the fourth, third, lateral ventricles, and the aqueduct of Sylvius. VCSFA was more prominent in the third and fourth ventricles, compared with the lateral ventricles. In PVS, both severe ventriculomegaly and brain atrophy might induce non-appropriate CSF circulation nulling, which remains hyperintense on axial FLAIR images, leading to VCSFA coming out. This is the first report in literature about the presence of VCSFA in PVS patients.

[*] Correspondence: Professor Gerry Leisman, Director, The National Institute for Brain and Rehabilitation Sciences, Biomechanics Laboratory, Department of Mechanical Engineering, ORT-Braude College of Engineering, Snunit 51 Street, POBox 78, IL-21982 Karmiel, Israel. E-mail: gerry.leisman@staff.nazareth.ac.il/

## INTRODUCTION

Fast fluid-attenuated inversion recovery (FLAIR) magnetic resonance imaging (MRI) technique were first reported by Hajnal et al. (1-3) FLAIR technique is based on a pulse sequence with an inversion time that nulls the signal from cerebrospinal fluid (CSF), providing heavy T2 weighting, due to its very long echo time (4-6). This technique increases MRI sensitivity in depicting lesions when causing T2 prolongation against a suppressed CSF background (5-8).

A major limitation of FLAIR MRI is the ventricular CSF pulsation artifact (VCSFA). This artifact might compromise the study of ventricular abnormalities by leading to false-negative or false-positive interpretations (9, 10).

We report 4 young persistent vegetative state (PVS) patients with marked ventriculomegaly and brain atrophy who showed the VCSFA on FLAIR MRI. This is the first report in literature about the presence of the VCSFA in PVS patients.

## FOUR PATIENTS

We studied four patients (ranging from 12 to 31 years old) who suffered hypoxic-ischemic insult resulting in PVS of long-term clinical evolution (4-8 years). The patients fulfilled current diagnostic criteria for PVS: no evidence of awareness of self or environment, no interaction with others, and no comprehension or expression of language. Noxious stimuli frequently resulted in massive stretching or startle reactions, without habituation, sometimes with massive flexor responses. Occasionally grimacing followed stimulation. Nonetheless, external stimuli did not evoke purposeful or sustained and reproducible voluntary behavioral responses (11, 12). Patients were assessed by the JFK Scale (13, 14). Patients' demographic features are summarized in Table 1.

Patients were studied by a 1.5T MR scanner (Symphony, Siemens). FLAIR technique description is found elsewhere (15, 17). MRI were reviewed by two independent observers to detect the VCSFA in the aqueduct of Sylvius, and the lateral, third, and fourth ventricles. VCSFA intensity was classified as slight, moderate, and high, by the two independent observers.

**Table 1. Demographic features of patients**

| PVS patients | OC | JM | RH | AG |
|---|---|---|---|---|
| Age | 12 | 18 | 18 | 31 |
| Sex | Male | male | male | male |
| Skin color | Mestee | black | mestee | black |
| Etiology | Near drown | Near drown | Near drown | Anesthetic accident |
| PVS duration | 6 years | 8 years | 4 years | 6 years |
| JFK scale | 6 points | 4 points | 3 points | 4 points |

JFK Scale from Giacino et al. (13, 14).

**Table 2. VCSFA intensity in cerebral ventricles and aqueduct of Sylvius.**

| PVS patients | OC | JM | RH | AG |
|---|---|---|---|---|
| Lateral ventricles | + | + | + | + |
| III ventricle | +++ | +++ | ++ | +++ |
| Aqueduct | ++ | +++ | + | + |
| IV ventricle | +++ | ++ | ++ | ++ |

+ Slight VCSFA intensity, ++ Moderate VCSFA intensity, +++ High VCSFA intensity.

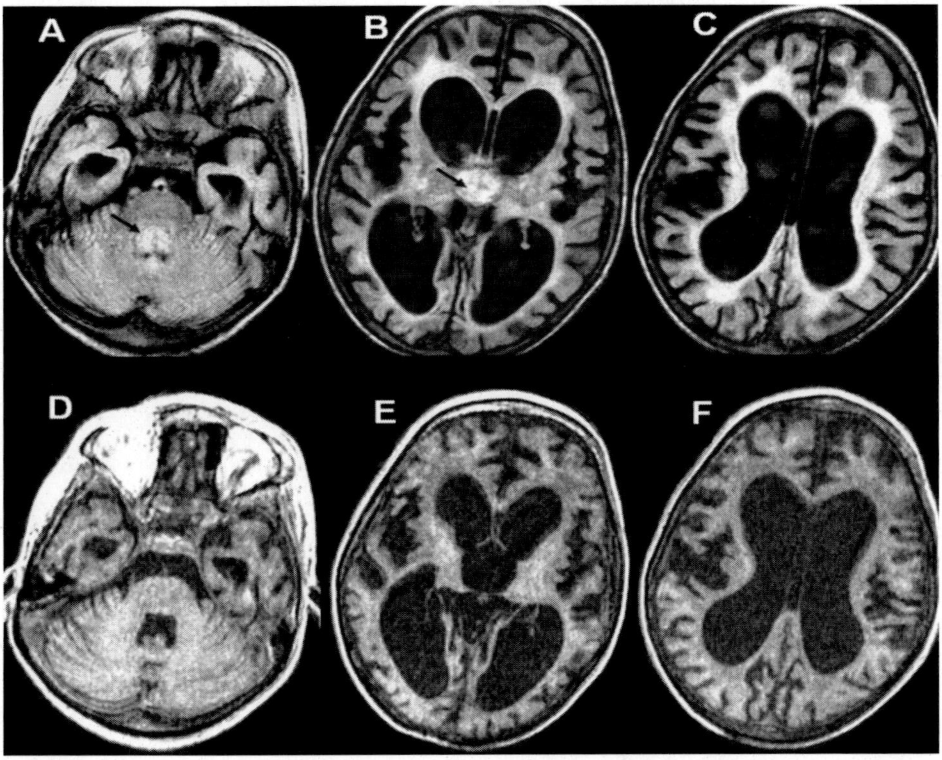


Figure 1. MRI data set in axial views from patient OC are presented (A to F images).
A–C: MRI FLAIR axial images show the VCSFA in the fourth (A) and in the third (B) ventricles the VCSFA (arrows), meanwhile this artifact is comparatively less pronounced, visualized as small white spots. There is also parenchymal atrophy and white matter hyperintensity.
D-F: MRI-T1 images in axial views revealed marked atrophy in both cerebral hemispheres, associated with dilated ventricles and wide cerebral sulci, but no intraventricular abnormalities are present (Figure 1 D-F).

## FINDINGS

The VCSFA was found in all patients, and it was more prominent in the third and fourth ventricles, compared with the lateral ventricles (Table 2). In Figure 1, MRI data sets on axial views from patient OC are presented (A to F images). MRI FLAIR axial images showed the VCSFA in the fourth, and in the third ventricles, meanwhile this artifact was comparatively less pronounced in the lateral ventricles, visualized as small white spots. There was also parenchymal atrophy and white matter hyperintensity. MR T1 axial images of the same patient (D to F) revealed severe brain atrophy in both cerebral hemispheres, associated with dilated ventricles and wide cerebral sulci, but no intraventricular abnormalities were found. In one patient the VCSFA was found on axial images but it was not detected on sagittal planes.

## DISCUSSION

The prominent hyperintensity occupying the cerebral ventricles in our patients most probably represents the VCSFA, due to an inversion delay and ghosting effects (4, 18-22).

Several mechanisms have been proposed to explain the VCSFA. When CSF goes into the brain sections between the inversion pulse and the commencement of signal sampling, it is not appropriately nulled, and remains hyperintense on axial FLAIR images. Hence, the causes of VCSFA seem to be multifactorial (4, 18, 19, 21-24).

Bakshi et al. (29) reported that increasing ventricular size and, to a lesser extent increasing age, were significantly associated with VCSFA. In PVS cases is frequent to find marked brain atrophy and ventriculomegaly. These morphological put forth their maximal force on the CSF circulation. Ventriculomegaly may induce an increment of CSF flow velocity through the third and fourth ventricles (19, 23).

Other possible mechanism could be the reflux of spinal CSF into the fourth and third ventricles from the cisterna magna. Some authors have shown increased passage of subarachnoid dye into the fourth ventricle from the cisterna magna in cases ventriculomegaly, due to brain volume loss, as occurs in hydrocephalus (25, 26). This reflux may be also enhanced in normal-pressure (27, 28), and pyogenic meningitis (29, 30).

Brain atrophy might produce a decrement in the compliance of periventricular tissues that may allow for more vigorous transmission of systolic and diastolic pulsations to the ventricles, further increasing CSF velocity. These strong CSF pulsations that occur in synchrony with the systole and diastole put forth their maximal force at the base of the brain through the third ventricle, where CSF velocities are also maximal (30).

Hence, marked ventriculomegaly and brain atrophy might explain the presence of the VCSFA in PVS cases, because CSF circulation might not be appropriately nulled, remaining hyperintense on MR axial images (19).

In one case the VCSFA was found on axial images but it was not detected on sagittal planes. This is most likely because sagittal imaging induces the required nulling of in-plane midline brain and cervical spinal CSF, before the fluid arrives at the third and fourth ventricles during readout (19, 23).

Several authors have proposed technical variations to reduce this artifact, such as, using a wider slice-selective inversion to increase the inversion of CSF outside the imaging section, to use other section-selective inversion pulses, to utilize cardiac synchronization during MRI acquisition (19, 22, 23).

Other authors have recommended using a nonslice-selective inversion pulse to eliminate the VCSFA using the K-space Reordered by Inversion-time for each Slice Position (KRISP) technique, in order to achieve constant contrast in a multislice acquisition (18, 31-33).

We conclude that it is extremely important to consider the possible presence of the VCSFA in PVS patients, because it may induce false-negative or false-positive diagnosis of intraventricular abnormalities.

## References


[1] Bydder GM, Rutherford MA, Hajnal JV. How to perform diffusion-weighted imaging. Childs Nerv Syst 2001;17:195-201.

[2] Hajnal JV, Collins AG, White SJ, Pennock JM, Oatridge A, Baudouin CJ, et al. Imaging of human brain activity at 0.15 T using fluid attenuated inversion recovery (FLAIR) pulse sequences. Magn Reson Med 1993;30:650-3.

[3] Hajnal JV, Bryant DJ, Kasuboski L, Pattany PM, De Coene B, Lewis PD, et al. Use of fluid attenuated inversion recovery (FLAIR) pulse sequences in MRI of the brain. J Comput Assist Tomogr 1992;16:841-4.

[4] Tanaka N, Abe T, Kojima K, Nishimura H, Hayabuchi N. Applicability and advantages of flow artifact-insensitive fluid-attenuated inversion-recovery MR sequences for imaging the posterior fossa. AJNR Am J Neuroradiol 2000;21:1095-8.

[5] Alibek S, Adamietz B, Cavallaro A, Stemmer A, Anders K, Kramer M, et al. Contrast-enhanced T1-weighted fluid-attenuated inversion-recovery BLADE magnetic resonance imaging of the brain: an alternative to spin-echo technique for detection of brain lesions in the unsedated pediatric patient? Acad Radiol 2008;15:986-95.

[6] Alkan O, Kizilkiliç O, Yildirim T, Alibek S. Comparison of contrast-enhanced T1-weighted FLAIR with BLADE, and spin-echo T1-weighted sequences in intracranial MRI. Diagn Interv Radiol 2009;15:75-80.

[7] Okuda T, Korogi Y, Shigematsu Y, Sugahara T, Hirai T, Ikushima I, et al. Brain lesions: when should fluid-attenuated inversion-recovery sequences be used in MR evaluation? Radiology 1999;212:793-8.

[8] Sun J, Zhang S, Jiang D, Zhang D, Xu X. Application of turbo fluid-attenuated inversion-recovery MRI in evaluation of intraspinal tumors. Clin Imaging 2008;32:103-8.

[9] Bakshi R, Caruthers SD, Janardhan V, Wasay M. Intraventricular CSF pulsation artifact on fast fluid-attenuated inversion-recovery MR images: analysis of 100 consecutive normal studies. Am J Neuroradiol 2000; 21:503-8.

[10] Bakshi R, Kamran S, Kinkel PR, Bates VE, Mechtler LL, Janardhan V, et al. Fluid-attenuated inversion-recovery MR imaging in acute and subacute cerebral intraventricular hemorrhage. AJNR Am J Neuroradiol 1999; 20:629-36.

[11] Giacino JT, Malone R. The vegetative and minimally conscious States. Handb Clin Neurol 2008;90:99-111.

[12] Andrews K. International working party on the management of the vegetative state: Summary report. Brain Injury 1996;10:797-806.

[13] Giacino JT, Kalmar K, Whyte J. The JFK Coma Recovery Scale-Revised: measurement characteristics and diagnostic utility. Arch Phys Med Rehabil 2004;85:2020-9.

[14] Kalmar K, Giacino JT. The JFK Coma Recovery Scale--Revised. Neuropsychol Rehabil 2005;15:454-60.

[15] Cabrera-Gómez J, Saiz-Hinarejos A, Graus F, González-Quevedo A, Rodríguez-Rojas R, Quevedo-Sotolongo L, et al. Brain magnetic resonance imaging findings in acute relapses of neuromyelitis optica spectrum disorders. Mult Scler 2008;14:248-51.

[16] Canales-Rodríguez EJ, Lin CP, Iturria-Medina Y, Yeh CH, Cho KH, Melie-García L. Diffusion orientation transform revisited. Neuroimage 2010; 49:1326-39.

[17] Iturria-Medina Y, Canales-Rodríguez EJ, Melie-García L, Valdés-Hernández PA, Martínez-Montes E, Alemán-Gómez Y, et al. Characterizing brain anatomical connections using diffusion weighted MRI and graph theory. Neuroimage 2007;36:645-60.

[18] Oatridge A, Curati WL, Herlihy AH, Hajnal JV, Virji N, Puri BK, et al. Evaluation of a FLAIR sequence designed to reduce CSF and blood flow artifacts by use of k-space reordered by inversion time at each slice position (KRISP) in high grade gliomas of the brain. J Comput Assist Tomogr 2001; 25:251-6.
[19] Tha KK, Terae S, Kudo K, Miyasaka K. Differential diagnosis of hyperintense cerebrospinal fluid on fluid-attenuated inversion recovery images of the brain. Part II: non-pathological conditions. Br J Radiol 2009;82(979):610-4.
[20] Neema M, Guss ZD, Stankiewicz JM, Arora A, Healy BC, Bakshi R. Normal findings on brain fluid-attenuated inversion recovery MR images at 3T. Am J Neuroradiol 2009;30:911-6.
[21] Kallmes DF, Hui FK, Mugler JP III. Suppression of cerebrospinal fluid and blood flow artifacts in FLAIR MR imaging with a single-slab three-dimensional pulse sequence: initial experience. Radiology 2001;221:251-5.
[22] Cianfoni A, Martin MG, Du J, Hesselink JR, Imbesi SG, Bradley WG, et al. Artifact simulating subarachnoid and intraventricular hemorrhage on single-shot, fast spin-echo fluid-attenuated inversion recovery images caused by head movement: A trap for the unwary. Am J Neuroradiol 2006; 27:843-9.
[23] Chagla GH, Busse RF, Sydnor R, Rowley HA, Turski PA. Three-dimensional fluid attenuated inversion recovery imaging with isotropic resolution and nonselective adiabatic inversion provides improved three-dimensional visualization and cerebrospinal fluid suppression compared to two-dimensional flair at 3 tesla. Invest Radiol 2008;43(8):547-51.
[24] Maeda M, Yagishita A, Yamamoto T, Sakuma H, Takeda K. Abnormal hyperintensity within the subarachnoid space evaluated by fluid-attenuated inversion-recovery MR imaging: a spectrum of central nervous system diseases. Eur Radiol 2003;13(Suppl 4):L192-L201.
[25] Phuenpathom N, Ratanalert S, Saeheng S, Sripairojkul B. Post-traumatic hydrocephalus: experience in 17 consecutive cases. J Med Assoc Thai 1999; 82:46-53.
[26] Appenzeller O, Salmon JH, Blatt E. Effect of ventriculoatrial shunts on postoperative pneumoencephalograms in patients with hydrocephalus ex-vacuo. Trans Am Neurol Assoc 1968;93:163-5.
[27] Mahler ME, Cummings JL, Tomiyasu U. Atypical dementia syndrome in an elderly man. J Am Geriatr Soc 1987;35:1116-26.
[28] Hurley RA, Bradley WG Jr, Latifi HT, Taber KH. Normal pressure hydrocephalus: significance of MRI in a potentially treatable dementia. J Neuropsychiatry Clin Neurosci 1999;11:297-300.
[29] Bakshi R, Kinkel PR, Mechtler LL, Bates VE. Cerebral ventricular empyema associated with severe adult pyogenic meningitis: computed tomography findings. Clin Neurol Neurosurg 1997;99:252-55.
[30] Sherman JL, Citrin CM, Gangarosa RE, Bowen BJ. The MR appearance of CSF flow in patients with ventriculomegaly. Am J Roentgenol 1987; 148:193-9.
[31] Curati WL, Oatridge A, Herlihy AH, Hajnal JV, Puri BK, Bydder GM. Contributions of an adiabatic initial inversion pulse and K-space re-ordered by inversion-time at each slice position (KRISP) to control of CSF artifacts anti visualization of the brain in FLAIR magnetic resonance imaging. Clin Radiology. 2001;56:375-84.
[32] Herlihy AH, Hajnal JV, Curati WL, Virji N, Oatridge A, Puri BK, et al. Reduction of CSF and blood flow artifacts on FLAIR images of the brain with k-space reordered by inversion time at each slice position (KRISP). Am J Neuroradiology 2001;22:896-904.
[33] Herlihy AH, Oatridge A, Curati WL, Puri BK, Bydder GM, Hajnal JV. FLAIR imaging using nonselective inversion pulses combined with slice excitation order cycling and k-space reordering to reduce flow artifacts. Magn Reson Med 2001;46:354-64.

In: Considering Consciousness Clinically
Editors: Gerry Leisman and Joav Merrick

ISBN: 978-1-63484-260-0


*Chapter 12*

# SOMATOSENSORY EVOKED POTENTIALS (SSEP) IN ANOXIC COMA AND THE INFLUENCE OF HYPOTHERMIA

***Ted L Rothstein****

Department of Neurology, George Washington University, Washington, DC, United States of America

## ABSTRACT

The early recognition of those comatose patients with a hopeless prognosis—regardless of how aggressively they are managed—is critical to rational medical management. Median somatosensory evoked potentials (SSEP) have been used to supplement and enhance neurologic examination findings in anoxic–ischemic coma following cardiac arrest and have been useful as an early guide in predicting unfavorable outcome. The bilateral absence of the $N_{20}$ component of cortical evoked potentials has reliably predicted death or persistent vegetative state in patients who remain comatose after cardiac arrest. Two randomized trials have demonstrated that mild therapeutic hypothermia (TH) if provided immediately in the management of comatose patients after cardiac arrest improves neurologic outcomes. There have been 8 recent studies in which SSEP have been used as a predictor of outcome in comatose patients following cardiac arrest in whom TH was administered.

These studies are reviewed. At issue is whether the rules for using SSEP to predict unfavorable outcome in those who have received TH still apply.

## INTRODUCTION

The most common cause of anoxic brain injury is cardiac arrest, which affects approximately 450,000 Americans every year, and accounts for about half the deaths due to cardiovascular

* Correspondence: Ted L. Rothstein MD, Department of Neurology, George Washington University, Washington, DC, United States. E-mail: trothstein@mfa.gwu.edu.

disease. Modern resuscitation techniques applied directly to victims of cardiac arrest from automatic external defibrillators as well as the use of therapeutic hypothermia (TH) have resulted in increased rates of survival (1-6). However, less than 1/3 of patients comatose survivors of cardiac arrest awaken within the first week, and those who do awaken are often left with persistent motor or cognitive deficits (7, 8).

When cerebral anoxia occurs after cardiac arrest, the duration and severity of the interruption of cerebral blood flow determines the potential for recovery. These factors are usually unknown, or may be difficult to estimate in any given patient. The extent of brain injury is usually evaluated indirectly by performing a detailed neurological examination and assessing cortical and brainstem function and whether there is evidence of recovery or deterioration over time. The degree of eventual recovery is dependent on the localization and extent of permanently damaged brain structures.

Cerebral neurons cannot tolerate complete normothermic ischemic anoxia for more than 5 minutes (9-10). After this period of time the cerebrum and brainstem are destroyed, and brain death eventually ensues. It is more difficult to predict outcome for patients with severe anoxic brain damage than to diagnose brain death, which is based on widely accepted criteria (11, 12). Using criteria based on physical examination findings alone, only 1.5% of patients in coma after cardiac arrest present with brain death (13).

The adult cerebral cortex is more vulnerable to the effects of anoxia than the more primitive brainstem parenchyma (10, 14). If the brainstem is damaged by an anoxic insult, the cerebral cortex is likely to have sustained an even worse injury and may be completely destroyed (10, 13). It is common for patients to sustain a critical measure of anoxia sufficient to damage or destroy the cerebral cortex while preserving some or all brainstem function. Therefore, those prognostic scales that rely to great extent on preserved brainstem function such as the Glasgow Coma Scale (GCS) may be seriously flawed (15, 16).

There remains an urgent need to develop reliable criteria for the early prediction of outcome in comatose patients following cardiac arrest. An initial step is to identify those patients whose prognosis is hopeless regardless of how aggressively they are managed. Conversely, it is of paramount importance for physicians to recognize those patients with the potential to recover. Accurate prognostication allows physicians to channel resources to those who could benefit, counsel family members with realistic expectations, allow for earlier identification of potential organ donors, and aid in the selection of patients for TH and other innovative or experimental therapies.

Hypothermia has been used as a therapeutic technique to protect the brain from anoxic injury as in cardiac surgery with cardiopulmonary bypass. In 2002, two randomized trials utilizing TH were performed on post cardiac arrest patients, lowering their body temperature to 33 degrees Centigrade, which resulted in significant improvement in survival (4,5). To prevent one unfavorable neurologic outcome, the need to treat with TH was only 6 patients. Moreover, many of those randomized to the TH group made a meaningful neurologic recovery. The mechanism whereby TH produces benefit is not established, but may cause a reduction in cerebral oxygen requirements. TH is now recommended as the standard of care in the management of patients with out of hospital cardiac arrest (17). However, recent articles have raised concerns that the evidence for benefit was unclear given the studies small sample size (18). Indeed, a study of 939 patients who were unconscious survivors after cardiac arrest showed no improvement in mortality between patients with targeted temperatures of 33 and 36 degrees Centigrade (19).

Practice parameters for predicting outcome after cardiac arrest were developed by the Quality Standards Subcommittee of the American Academy of Neurology (AAN) and were based on evidence-based reviews of studies between 1966 and 2006 (20). Taken into consideration were a variety of clinical and electrophysiologic variables, but have not been revised to address whether TH had modified outcome prediction. At issue, then, is whether the rules for using SSEP in predicting unfavorable outcome in post arrest patients who have received TH still apply.

The EEG has been the key test for evaluating coma over the past 30 years (20). However, SSEP has proved to be more reliable than EEG in predicting neurologic outcome (15, 16, 21,22).

Zandbergen and colleagues reviewed the relevant literature to assess the prognostic value of early neurologic and electrophysiologic studies in anoxic coma (23). They compared the results of clinical findings, EEG, and SSEP in 563 patients, and concluded that the absence of cortical evoked potentials (CEP) was the most discriminating predictor of unfavorable outcome. It has been established that the EEG becomes isoelectric during circulatory arrest which can persist for several hours after restoration of the cerebral circulation (24). Further, I reported a post arrest patient with an isoelectric EEG but normal SSEP, both obtained 5 hours after arrest and resuscitation, who achieved full neurologic recovery after 4 days (22). Another study described two patients with burst suppression patterns on EEG who recovered with minimal or no neurologic sequelae (25). Two additional patients with burst suppression on EEG have been reported to recover from their cardiac arrest (26, 27).

SSEPs are a relatively simple, convenient, non-invasive, and inexpensive bedside technique for assessing the integrity of transmission within the central nervous system, and are commonly used to assess both brainstem and cortical function (Figure 1). The SSEP has been studied extensively in anoxic coma, but its potential for predicting outcome accurately remains mostly neglected in clinical practice (28) or controversial (29).

SSEPs provide information limited to the somatosensory pathways and primary sensory cortex, and must be interpreted with caution. Patients with focal brain disease involving the sensory pathways may have SSEPs that are misleading. For example, I have found bilateral absence of CEP in patients with advanced multiple sclerosis, brainstem hemorrhage and basilar artery occlusion causing bilateral thalamic infarcts. Metabolic factors can also distort the interpretation of SSEP. Kaplan (2004) described a patient found pulseless as a result of a heroin overdose, with absent CEP, who eventually regained cortical potentials and fully recovered (30).

Numerous studies confirm that the absence of short-latency CEP is associated with a uniformly unfavorable prognosis (14-16, 22, 27-46). Robinson and associates performed a meta-analysis of 336 normothermic patients with absent cortical SSEP after day one and all died or became vegetative (44). However, Young et al. (2002) identified a single patient with bilateral absence of N20 who recovered (47). Young attributed this unique case to watershed ischemia with selective damage (personal communication, 2010). However, in a subsequent paper Young makes no mention of this case, and identifies the lack of an N20 response as "the most accurate predictor of poor outcome in patients with anoxic-ischemic encephalopathy" (48). There is single case report of a 16 year old student who had a cardiac arrest while playing soccer and received resuscitation within 3 minutes. Hypothermia was not administered. The N20 response was bilaterally absent at 72 hours and on day 9. He experienced constant improvement in his neurologic status and eventually recovered with only residual dysarthria and impaired fine motor control (49).

The N20 peak represents the earliest cortical response, and its delay or loss signifies an interruption of the connecting pathway between the cervico-medullary junction and the sensory cortex (50). A neuropathologic study of 7 comatose patients with bilateral absent N20 revealed diffuse cortical necrosis in each instance (15,16) suggesting there were no functioning neurons left to respond to an afferent stimulus. Does the bilateral absence of the N20 peak in TH patients have the same significance as in almost all normothermic patients, i.e., does it reliably predict an unfavorable outcome leading to death or persistent vegetative state?

SSEP in post-arrest patients treated with TH have now been reported in 8 recent studies (51-58).

Tiainen and colleagues identified three patients following cardiac arrest treated with hypothermia with absent N20 responses, and 8 normothermic controls with absent N20, all of whom died without awakening (51). Bouwes and associates described 13 patients with absent N20 who died without awakening (52). Cronberg et al. reported on 14 patients with similar SSEP results with a similar outcome (53). Rossetti et al. studied 3 clinical variables, EEG and SSEP in 111 post arrest patients, and found that the bilateral absence of N20 on SSEP in 33 patients was significantly associated with death at the time of hospital discharge (54). Fugate et al. had 2 hypothermic patients with absent cortical potentials who did not survive (55). Samaniego et al. reported upon 24 additional patients with absent cortical potentials none of whom survived (56). Bisschops and colleagues found no survivors among 18 post anoxic patients with absent SSEP treated with TH (57). In sum, a total of 331 post cardiac arrest patients were studied in these 7 reports of whom 104 had absent N20 potentials and there were no survivors.

Leithner and associates retrospectively assessed SSEP in 112 patients treated with hypothermia and identified 36 with bilateral absent N20, 35 of whom died without awakening or entered a persistent vegetative state (58). However, a single patient with bilateral absence of N20 at day 3 eventually regained consciousness and recovered normal cognitive function. The authors drew the conclusion that bilateral absence of N20 as an outcome predictor in hypothermic patients needs to be re-evaluated and not used as a decision to stop therapy. There is sparse data on their sole survivor. The patient is a 43 year old man with alcoholism who developed sepsis and had asystole for 10 minutes. SSEP was not repeated until 18 months later, when the N20 responses were intact.

Are Leithner and colleagues justified in refuting the role of SSEP as a negative outcome predictor on the basis of a single patient? Could there have been technical factors which might have contributed to this case? Could the patient have had metabolic confounders or "watershed ischemia" which resulted in the elimination of the N20. Other factors such as brain trauma with hemorrhage could abolish evoked responses which might eventually result in clinical and electrical recovery in 10.2% of patients with severe head injury (16). Neuroimaging is not described in Leithner's report nor in their subsequent correspondence under "Reply from the Authors" (58-60). However, Blondin and Greer went on to assert that in the setting of TH, "owing to this isolated case of recovery, a bilateral absent N20 at 72 h may not predict poor prognosis with absolute certainty" (61).

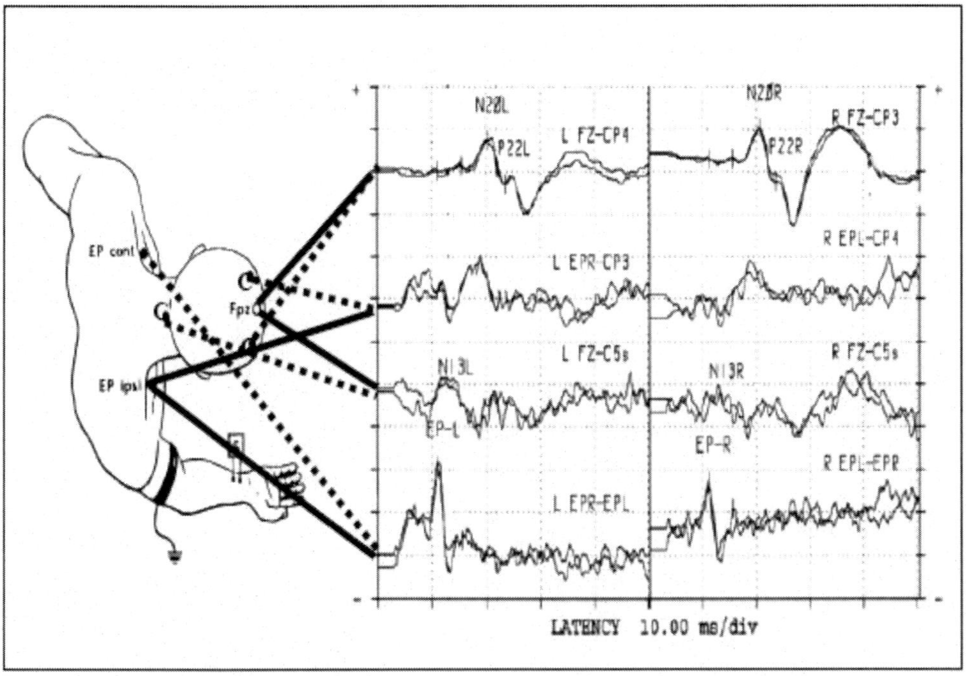


Figure 1. Technique used in recording median nerve somatosensory evoked potential (SSEP), which defines Erb's point (EP), the N13 peak, the N13–N20 interpeak latency, and the N20/P23 cortical evoked potential.

## Discussion

Clinical and neurologic evaluation alone of patients comatose after cardiac arrest does not establish ultimate neurologic outcome reliably. Accurate prognostication has been supplemented and enhanced by the use of SSEP. The bilateral absence of N20 has been used to identify those normothermic patients who will not survive anoxic–ischemic coma no matter how aggressively they are managed. Only one of the 8 recent studies in which Therapeutic Hypothermia has been used to improve outcome raises concern that SSEP may no longer be unfailingly predictive of unfavorable outcome and that report has significant flaws (58- 60).

There are now 3 case reports of recovery following cardiac arrest when SSEP has documented the bilateral absence of N20. These reports provide the basis for the false positive rate of 0.7% (CI 95%) for poor outcome using the absence of N20 as a predictor (47, 62).

As Sir William Osler instructed "medicine is a science of uncertainty and an art of probability" (63). In accord with this aphorism, SSEP remains the most reliable predictor of unfavorable outcome and the bilateral absence of N20 indicates, with the highest probability, that the patient will not recover (16, 20).

In conclusion, SSEP remains the most valuable, non invasive bedside test for determining prognosis in patients who are comatose following cardiac arrest, whether or not they have received Therapeutic Hypothermia. With very rare exceptions, SSEP should be used to identify those patients with a hopeless prognosis who will not respond to aggressive therapy no matter how skillfully applied.

## REFERENCES

[1] Thompson RG, Hallstrom AP, Cobb LA. Bystander-initiated cardio pulmonary resuscitation in the management of ventricular fibrillation. Ann Intern Med 1979;90:737–40.
[2] Hicks SD, DeFranco DB, Calloway CW. Hypothermia during reperfusion after asphyxial cardiac arrest improves functional recovery and selectively alters stress-induced protein expression. J Cereb Blood Flow Metab 2000; 20:520-30.
[3] Safar P, Kochanek P. Therapeutic hypothermia after cardiac arrest. N Engl J Med 2002;346:612-3.
[4] Bernard SA, Gray TW, Buist MD, Jones BM, Silvester W, Gutteridge G, et al. Treatment of comatose survivors of out of hospital cardiac arrest with induced hypothermia. N Engl J Med 2002;346:557-63.
[5] The Hypothermia after Cardiac Arrest Study Group. Mild therapeutic hypothermia to improve the Neurologic Outcome after cardiac arrest. N Engl J Med 2002;346:549-56.
[6] Sterz F, Holzer M, Roine R. Hypothermia after cardiac arrest: a treatment that works. Curr Opin Crit Care 2003;9(3):205-10.
[7] Longstreth WT Jr, Diehr P, Inui TS. Prediction of awakening after out-of-hospital cardiac arrest. N Engl J Med 1983;308:1378–82.
[8] Curfman GD. Hypothermia to protect the brain. N Engl J Med 2002;346: 546.
[9] Heymans C. Survival and revival of nervous tissue after prolonged cerebral ischemia. Physiol Rev 1950;30:375–92.
[10] Mullie A, van Hoeyweghen R, Quets A. Influence of time intervals on outcome of CPR. The Cerebral Resuscitation Study Group. Resuscitation 1989;17(suppl):S23–33.
[11] Plum F, Posner JB. Prognosis in coma. In: Plum F, Posner JB, eds. The Diagnosis of Stupor and Coma. 3rd edition. Contemporary Neurology Series. Philadelphia, PA: FA Davis, 1982:846-69.
[12] Bernat JL. A defense of the whole-brain concept of death. Hastings Cent Rep 1998;28:14–23.
[13] Longstreth WT Jr. Neurological complications of cardiac arrest. In: Aminoff MJ, ed. Neurology and general medicine. New York: Churchill Livingstone, 1994:166-82.
[14] Brierly JB. Cerebral hypoxia. In: Blackwood W, Corsellis JAN, eds. Greenfield's neuropathology. Edinburgh: Edward Arnold, 1976:43-85.
[15] Rothstein TL, Thomas EM, Sumi SM. Predicting outcome in hypoxic–ischemic coma. A prospective clinical and electrophysiologic study. Electroencephalogr Clin Neurophysiol 1991;79:101–7.
[16] Rothstein TL. The role of evoked potentials in anoxic-ischemic coma and severe brain trauma. J Clin Neurophysiol 2000;17:486-97.
[17] American Heart Association guidelines for cardiopulmonary resuscitation and emergency cardiovascular care. Circulation 2005;112(IV):1-203.
[18] Gibson A, Andrews PJ. Therapeuric hypothermia still "too cool to be true" F1000Prime Rep 2013;5:26-9.
[19] Nielsen N, Wetterslev J, Cronberg T, Erlinge D, Gasche Y et al. Targeted Temperature Management at 33 and 36 degrees Centigrade after Cardiac Arrest. N Engl J Med 2013;369:2197-2205.
[20] Wijdicks EFM, Hijdra A, Young GB, Bassetti CL, Wiebe S. Practice Parameter: Prediction of outcome in comatose survivors after cardiopulmonary resuscitation (an evidence-based review). Neurology 2006; 67:203-10.
[21] Kaplan PW. Electrophysiological prognostication and brain injury from cardiac arrest. Semin Neurol 2006;26:403-12.
[22] Rothstein TL. Recovery from near death following cerebral anoxia: A case report demonstrating superiority of median somatosensory evoked potentials over EEG in predicting a favorable outcome after cardiopulmonary resuscitation. Resuscitation 2004;60:335-41
[23] Zandbergen EGJ, deHaan RJ, Stoutenbeek CP, Koelman CP, Johannes HTM, et al. Systematic review of early prediction of poor outcome in anoxic–ischemic coma. Lancet 1998;352:1808–12

[24] Jørgenson EO, Malchow-Møller A. Natural history of global and critical brain ischemia. Resuscitation 1981;9:133-8.
[25] Chen R, Bolton CF, Young GB. Prediction of outcome in patients with anoxic coma: a clinical and electrophysiologic study. Crit Care Med 1996; 24:672–5.
[26] Crepeau AZ, Rabinstein AA, Fugete JE, Mandrekar J, Wijdicks EF et al. Continuous EEG in therapeutic hypothermia after cardiac arrest: prognostic and clinical value. Neurology 2013: 80: 339-44.
[27] Lucas JM, Cocchi MN, Salciccioli JA, Geocardin R, Romergryko GH, et al. Neurologic recovery aftertherapeutic hypothermia in patients with post-cardiac arrest. Resuscitation 2012; 83:265-9.
[28] Attia J, Cook DJ. Prognosis in anoxic and traumatic coma. Crit Care Med 1998;14:497–511.
[29] Kreiger D. Evoked potentials not just to confirm hopelessness in anoxic brain injury. Lancet 1998;352:1796–7.
[30] Kaplan PW. Stupor and coma: metabolic encephalopathies. Clin Neurophyiol 2004;57(Suppl):667-80.
[31] Ahmed I. Use of somatosensory evoked responses in the prediction of outcome from coma. Clin Electroencephalogr 1988;19:78–86.
[32] Bassetti C, Bomio F, Mathis J, Hess CW. Early prognosis in coma after cardiac arrest: a prospective clinical, electrophysiological, and biochemical study of 60 patients. J Neurol Neurosurg Psychiatry 1996;61:610–5.
[33] Berek K, Jeschow M, Aichner F. The prognostication of cerebral hypoxia after out-of hospital cardiac arrest in adults. Eur Neurol 1997;37:135–45.
[34] Berek K, Taferner E, Jeschow M, Voller B, Saltuari L. Euthanasia, physician-assisted suicide, and persistent vegetative state. Lancet 1996;348(9026):549.
[35] Brierly JB, Graham DI, Adams JH, Simpson JA. Neocortical death after cardiac arrest: a clinical, neurophysiological and neuropathological report of two cases. Lancet 1971;2:560–5.
[36] Brunko E, and Zegers de Beyl D. Prognostic value of early cortical somatosensory evoked potentials after resuscitation from cardiac arrest. Electroencephalogr Clin Neurophysiol 1987;66:15–24.
[37] Cheliout–Héraut F, Durand MC, Clair B, Gajdos P, Raphaël JC. Intérêt des potentiels évoqués dans le pronostic évolutif des comas par anoxie cérébrale chez l'adulte. Neurophysiol Clin 1992;22:269–80. (French)
[38] Fischer C, Luaute J, Nemoz C. Improved prediction of awakening or nonawakening from severe anoxic coma using tree-based classification analysis. Crit Care Med 2006;34:1520-4.
[39] Ganji S, Peters G, Frazier E. Somatosensory and brainstem auditory evoked potential studies in non-traumatic coma. Clin Electroencephalogr 1988;19: 55–66.
[40] Kano T, Shimoda O, Morioka T, Yagashita Y, Hashiguchi A. Evaluation of the central nervous function in resuscitated comatose patients by multilevel evoked potentials. Resuscitation 1992;23:235–48.
[41] Madl C, Grimm G, Kramer al. Early prediction of individual outcome after cardiopulmonary resuscitation. Lancet 1993;341:855-8.
[42] Marcus EM, Stone B. Short-latency median nerve somatosensory evoked potentials in coma: relationship to BAEP, etiology, age, and outcome. In: Nodar RH, Barber C, eds. Evoked potentials. Vol. II. The Second International Evoked Potentials Symposium. Stoneham: Butterworth, 1984: 609-23.
[43] Ragazzoni A, Cincotta M, Chiaramonti R. Electrophysiological early predictors of outcome in patients with anoxic coma: EEG and SEPs. Clin Neurophysiol 1999;110:S245–6.
[44] Robinson LR, Micklesen PJ, Tirschwell DL, Lew HL. Predictive value of somatosensory evoked potentials for awakening from coma. Crit Care Med 2003;31:960-7.
[45] Walser H, Mattle H, Keller HM, Janzer R. Early cortical median nerve somatosensory evoked potentials. Prognostic value in anoxic coma. Arch Neurol 1986;42:32–8.
[46] Ying Z, Schmid UD, Schmid J, Hess CW. Motor and somatosensory evoked potentials in coma: analysis and relation to clinical status and outcome. J Neurol Neurosurg Psychiatry 1992;55:470-4.
[47] Young GB, Doig G, Ragazzoni A. Anoxic-ischemic encephalopathy and electrophysiological associations with outcome. Neurocrit Care 2002;2:5-10. ).
[48] Young GB. Neurologic prognosis after cardiac arrest. N Engl J Med 2009: 361(6): 605-11.
[49] Bender A, Howell F, Frey M, Berlis A, Naumann M et al. Bilateral loss of cortical SSEP responses is compatible with good outcome after cardiac arrest. J Neurol 2012: 259:2481-3.

[50] Nuwer MR, Aminoff M, Desmedt J. IFCN recommended standards for short latency somatosensory evoked potentials. Report of an IFCN committee. International federation of clinical neurophysiology. Electroencephalogr. Clin Neurophysiol 1994;9:6–11.
[51] Tiainen M, Kovala TT, Takkunen OS, Roine RO. Somatosensory and brainstem auditory evoked potentials in cardiac arrest patients treated with hypothermia. Crit Care Med 2005;33:1736-40.
[52] Bouwes A, Binnekade JM, Zandstra DF, Koelman JHTM, van Schaik IN, Hijdra A, Horn J. Somatosensory evoked potentials during mild hypothermia after cardiopulmonary resuscitation. Neurology 2009;73:1457-61.
[53] Cronberg T, Lilja G, Rudgren M, Friberg H, Widdner H. Long term neurological outcome after cardiac arrest and therapeutic hypothermia. Resuscitation 2009; 80: 1119-23.
[54] Rossetti AO, Oddo M, Logroscino F, Kaplan PW. Prognostication after cardiac arrest and hypothermia. A prospective study. Ann Neuro 2010; 67:301-7.
[55] Fugate JE, Wijdicks EF, Mandrekar J, Classen DO, White RD et al. Predictors of neurologic outcome after cardiac arrest and therapeutic hypothermia. Resuscitation 2009; 80:1119-23.
[56] Samaniego EA, Mlynash M, Caulfield AF, Eyngorn I, Wijman CA. Sedation confounds outcome prediction in cardiac arrest survivors treated with hypothermia. Neurocritical Care 2011; 15: 113-9.
[57] Bisschops LLA, van Alfen M, Bons S, vander Hoeven JG, Hoedemakers CWE. Predictors of poor neurologic outcome in pateints after cardiac arrest threated with hypothermia: a retrospective study. Resuscitation 2011; 82: 696-701.
[58] Leithner C, Ploner CJ, Hasper D, Storm C. Does hypothermia influence the predictive value of bilateral absent N20 after cardiac arrest? Neurology 2010;74:965-9.
[59] Leithner C, Ploner CJ, Hasper D, Storm C. Does hypothermia influence the predictive value of bilateral absent N20 after cardiac arrest. Reply from the Authors. Neurology 2010;75:575-6.
[60] Rothstein TL Does hypothermia influence the predictive value of bilateral absent N20 after cardiac arrest? Letter to the Editor. Neurology 2010;75: 575.
[61] Blondin NA, Greer DM. Neurologic Prognosis in Cardiac Arrest Patients Treated with Therapeutic Hypothermia. The Neurologist 2011; 17:241-8.
[62] Wijdicks EFM, Young GB, Wang JT, Connolly J. Prognostic Determination in Anoxic-Ischemic and Traumatic Encephalopathies. J Clin Neurophys 2004;21:379-90.
[63] Bean RB, Aphorisms of Sir William Osler: From his bedside teachings and writings. New York: Schuman, 1950.

In: Considering Consciousness Clinically
Editors: Gerry Leisman and Joav Merrick
ISBN: 978-1-63484-260-0


*Chapter 13*

# AUTONOMIC ASSESSMENT DURING RECOGNITION OF THE MOTHER'S VOICE IN A PERSISTENT VEGETATIVE STATE PATIENT

***Calixto Machado*[1,*], *Mario Estévez*[1], *Mauricio Chinchilla*[2], *Jesús Pérez-Nellar*[2], *Joel Gutiérrez*[1], *Ana Olivares*[1], *Carlos Beltrán*[1], *Yazmina Machado*[1] *and Yanín Machado*[2]**

[1]Institute of Neurology and Neurosurgery, Department of Clinical Neurophysiology, Havana, Cuba and [2]Hermanos Ameijeiras Hospital, Service of Neurology, Havana, Cuba

By definition, persistent vegetative state (PVS) cases should be isolated from the outer world. Consequently, one of the most essential challenges in patients with severe brain damage is to assess their residual conscious perception of the environment. Moreover, other key point is to evaluate whether these responses also endow autonomic changes with possible emotional content. Heart rate variability (HRV) is considered a major index of the sympathetic/parasympathetic balance acting on the heart, and a powerful objective descriptor of individual differences in controlling the emotional conditions or responses to external and internal stimuli. We report an 8-year-old boy who after a near drowning remained in a PVS for 4 years before the study. We investigated whether there was significant differential brain activation in response to hearing his mother's voice (mom's voice), compared with the voices of unknown women (sham voice). During the sham voice experimental condition there was a significant increase in the HRV very low frequency (VLF) band, and a significant decrease in the HRV high frequency (HF) band, indicating sympathetic triggering and a reduction of parasympathetic activity. Nonetheless, during the mom's voice condition, there was again an increase in the VLF band, but a significant recovery of the HF band also occurred, revealing both a sympathetic and parasympathetic activation. We conclude that our results here suggest recognition of the mom's voice with an emotional content, indicating high-level residual linguistic processing, connected with neural network controlling emotion.

---

[*] Correspondence: Calixto Machado, MD, PhD, FAAN Institute of Neurology and Neurosurgery Department of Clinical Neurophysiology, 29 y D, Vedado La Habana 10400, Havana, Cuba. E-mail: braind@infomed.sld.cu.

## INTRODUCTION

Diagnostic criteria for persistent vegetative state (PVS) include: lack of evidence of awareness of self or environment, lack of interaction with others, and lack of comprehension or expression of language (1-5). Hence, by definition PVS cases should be isolated from the outer world. Consequently, one of the most essential challenges in patients with severe brain damage is to assess their residual conscious perception of the environment (6, 7). Different methods have been applied to evaluate the preservation of responses in the ascending sensory systems, such as event related potentials and EEG, fMRI and PET (8-11).

Nonetheless, other key point is to evaluate whether these responses also endow autonomic changes with possible emotional content, taking in consideration that PVS, by definition, should not present any recognizable behavioral responses to external stimuli (6-7). Emotions require wide cortical–subcortical interaction to occur, with involvement of limbic and paralimbic structures mediating in both emotional and autonomic response, which might be damaged due to massive brain injury which could be present in PVS cases (12).

Heart rate variability (HRV) allows measuring of autonomic and intrinsic influences on heart rate, and thus, it is considered a major index of the sympathetic/parasympathetic balance acting on the heart (13-15). This method can reflect complex patterns of brain activation and it is considered as an objective descriptor of individual differences in controlling the emotional conditions or responses to external and internal stimuli (15-17).

Riganello et al. assessed persistent vegetative state (PVS) patients using heart rate variability (HRV) and concluded that emotional brain processing can be preserved in these cases when they are passively listening to symphonic music pieces, which prompt known emotional responses. These authors also assessed the effect of music on emotion in PVS cases, using compressed power density values, obtained with a time-varying spectral analysis method (12).

We report here a PVS case assessed by HRV methodology to investigate whether there was significant differential brain activation with emotion content in response to hearing his mother's voice (mom's voice), compared with the voices of unknown women (sham voice).

### Our case story

We report an 8-year-old boy who after a near drowning remained in a PVS for 4 years before the study. We investigated whether there was significant differential brain activation in response to hearing his mother's voice (mom's voice), compared with the voices of unknown women (sham voice).

Electrocardiogram (ECG) was continually digitally recorded in precordial V5 lead during all the experimental session, with the MEDICID-05 system (Neuronic S. A.), using the following technical parameters: gain 5,000, filters pass-band 0.1-30 Hz, 60 Hz "notch" filter, level of noise 2μv RMS, sampling period of 5 ms, and environmental temperature of approximately 23°C.

ECG was exported in ASCII format to a custom-tailored software tool, developed by our staff, for visual inspection and detection of the "R" wave peaks. Accurate "R" peak detections were visually controlled and properly corrected when it was necessary.

The obtained RR interval sequence (RRI) was submitted to a previous preprocessing including: (i) application of a median filter; (ii) resampling of the sequence with an interpolation method (piecewise cubic Hermite) to obtain a sampling period of approximately 146 ms; (iii) removing of the mean value of the sequence; (iv) standard lineal detrending; (v) high-pass filtering at 0.01 Hz. A dynamic time-frequency spectral was then applied to the RRI sequence.(18) The sliding window was 300 seconds duration, and the sliding step was 10 seconds. The obtained spectral matrix comprised 87 sequential spectra for the whole experimental session.

For each spectrogram were calculated usual absolute and relative spectral indices in the frequency range: very low frequency band (0.02-0.04 Hz), low frequency band (0.4-0.15 Hz), high frequency band (0.15-0.40 Hz), and for the total frequency spectral range from 0.02 to 0.4 Hz. To provide an easier visual assessment of the whole compressed spectral matrix there were also calculated the independent compressed matrices for the three spectral ranges.

For calculations and diagrams, custom routines written in MATLAB (Mathworks, Natick, MA) were used.

## RESULTS

In Figure 1 we present the main results of the time-varying spectral analysis applied to the sequential RRI series of the ECG in patient OC. During the sham voice experimental condition there was a significant increase in the HRV very low frequency (VLF) band, and a significant decrease in the HRV high frequency (HF) band, indicating sympathetic triggering and a reduction of parasympathetic activity. Nonetheless, during the mom's voice condition, there was again an increase in the VLF band, but a significant recovery of the HF band also occurred, revealing both a sympathetic and parasympathetic activation. In Figure 2 the above described dynamics are more clearly shown.

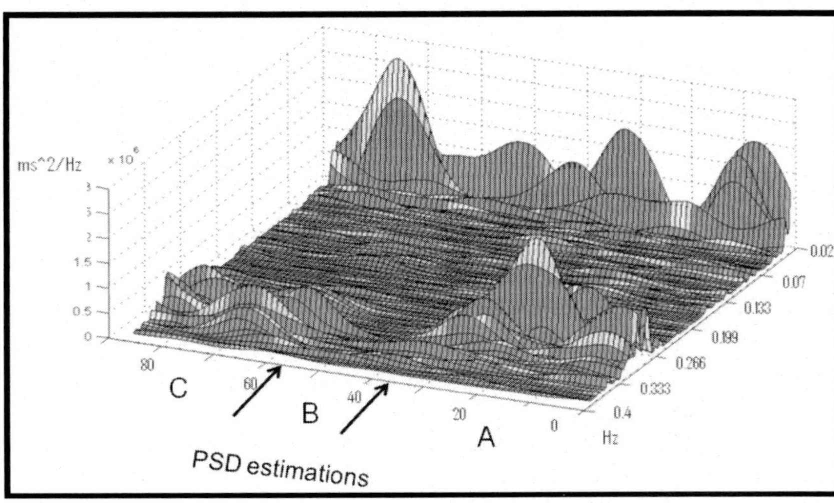


Figure 1. The whole compressed spectral matrix of patient O. calculated with a time-varying spectral analysis, applied to the sequential series of ECG R-R normal intervals in patient OC during the control basal condition, labeled as "A," and during the "sham voice" (B), and "mother talks" (C) experimental conditions.

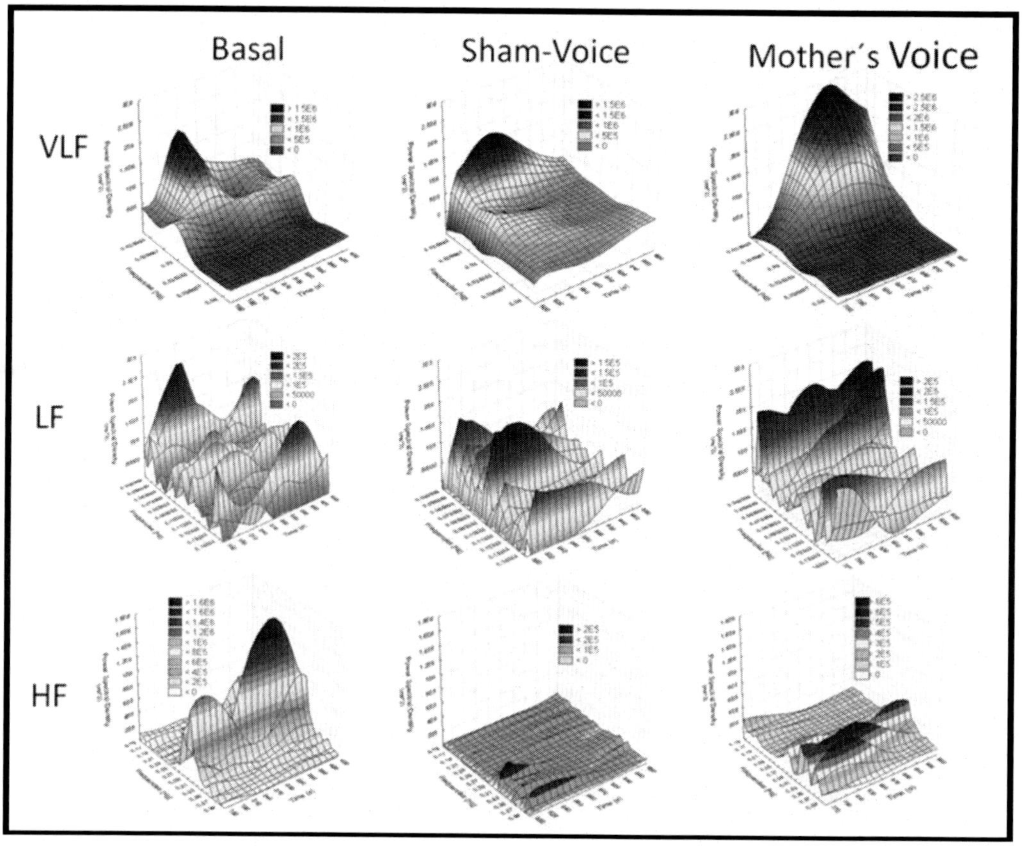


Figure 2. Compressed spectral matrices calculated for the three main HRV spectral ranges: VLF: very low frequency band (0.02-0.04 Hz); LF: low frequency band (0.04-0.15 Hz); HF: high frequency band (0.15-0.4 Hz) during the different experimental conditions.

## DISCUSSION

Mom's voice is probably one of the strongest stimuli inducing emotive and affective response in nature (19). Hence, using mom's voice as stimulus might be a suitable experimental condition to evaluate residual emotive responses in brain-injured patients (19-22).

We had studied the case reported here in the same experimental conditions, but assessing the patient using quantitative electric tomography, a technique that combines anatomical information of the brain by MRI with EEG patterns to estimate the sources of the EEG within the brain. We found an activation for EEG frequencies from 14-58 Hz, with a peak at 33.2 Hz (gamma band), localized in the lateral and posterior regions of the left hemisphere. These results suggested recognition of the mom's voice, indicating a high-level residual linguistic processing in a patient meeting clinical criteria for PVS (19). Although we only published the EEG data in that time, this patient was also simultaneously assessed by HRV.

Nonetheless, our results here suggest recognition of the mom's voice with an emotional content, indicating high-level residual linguistic processing, connected with neural network controlling emotion (12, 19). It was also interesting that HRV spectral analysis allowed us to decompose sympathetic/parasympathetic balance acting on the heart (13). In our case the sham voice induced an autonomic arousal characterized by the sympathetic activation, while the mom's voice induced arousal, but it also prompted parasympathetic high frequency activity, probably related to a shift to a "positive" emotion during this experimental condition (12, 23).

Riganello et al., using a data mining classification model in PVS cases, found that nu_LF changes clustered patients into classes comparable to normal subjects. According to their results, passively listening to music induced only sympathetic emotional changes in PVS cases, similar to normal controls (12).

Nonetheless, our results, combined with the EEG data previously published (19), suggests that autonomic changes with possible emotional content can be induced in PVS cases by complex stimuli, like voices and music (19).

Emotions entail cortical-subcortical interactions and involve limbic and paralimbic structures in mediating both emotional and autonomic responses (12, 24). Therefore, these results suggest that PVS cases can retain partial connectivity and functional integrity in networks involved in emotion processing.

Hence, HRV, which is a non-invasive and easy to assess technique even at bedside, is a powerful tool to study functional responses in these non-collaborative patients, providing additional information after emotional and affective stimuli (12, 19, 23).

Moreover, we conclude that these findings will promote discussion about conceptual, ethical and practical implications for the diagnosis and management of PVS and minimally conscious state patients.

## REFERENCES

[1] Machado C, Perez-Nellar J, Rodriguez R, Scherle.C, Korein J. Emergence from minimally conscious state: insights from evaluation of posttraumatic confusion. Neurology 2010;74:1156-7.

[2] Monti MM, Laureys S, Owen AM. The vegetative state. BMJ 2010;341:c3765.

[3] Machado C, Korein J. Persistent vegetative and minimally conscious states. Rev Neurosci 2009;20:203-20.

[4] Giacino JT, Malone R. The vegetative and minimally conscious States. Handb Clin Neurol 2008;90:99-111.

[5] Owen AM, Coleman MR. Detecting awareness in the vegetative state. Ann NY Acad Sci 2008;1129:130-8.

[6] Medical aspects of the persistent vegetative state (2). The Multi-Society Task Force on PVS. N Engl J Med 1994;330:1572-9.

[7] Medical aspects of the persistent vegetative state (1). The Multi-Society Task Force on PVS. N Engl J Med 1994;330:1499-1508.

[8] Laureys S, Giacino JT, Schiff ND, Schabus M, Owen AM. How should functional imaging of patients with disorders of consciousness contribute to their clinical rehabilitation needs? Curr Opin Neurol 2006;19:520-7.

[9] Kobylarz EJ, Schiff ND. Neurophysiological correlates of persistent vegetative and minimally conscious states. Neuropsychol Rehabil 2005;15:323-32.

[10] Schiff ND, Rodriguez-Moreno D, Kamal A, Kim KHS, Giacino JT, Plum F, Hirsch J. fMRI reveals large-scale network activation in minimally conscious patients. Neurology 2005;64:514-23.

[11] Laureys S, Owen AM, Schiff ND. Brain function in coma, vegetative state, and related disorders. Lancet Neurol 2004;3:537-46.

[12] Riganello F, Candelieri A, Dolce G, Sannita W. Residual emotional processing in the vegetative state: A scientific issue? Clin Neurophysiol 2010 Sep 30. Doi:10.1016/j.clinph.2010.05.010.

[13] Su CF, Kuo TB, Kuo JS, Lai HY, Chen HI. Sympathetic and parasympathetic activities evaluated by heart-rate variability in head injury of various severities. Clin Neurophysiol 2005;116:1273-9.
[14] Machado C, Garcia OD, Gutierrez J. Heart rate variability in comatose and brain-dead patients. Clin Neurophysiol 2005;116:2859-60.
[15] Baillard C, Vivien B, Mansier P, Mangin L, Jasson S, Riou B, et al. Brain death assessment using instant spectral analysis of heart rate variability. Crit Care Med 2002;30:306-10.
[16] Machado C, Garcia OD, Gutierrez J, Portela L, Garcia MC. Heart rate variability in comatose and brain-dead patients. Clin Neurophysiol 2005;116:2859-60.
[17] Neumann T, Post H, Ganz RE, Walz MK, Skyschally A, Schulz R, et al. Linear and non-linear dynamics of heart rate variability in brain dead organ donors. Z Kardiol 2001;90:484-91.
[18] de Souza Neto EP, Abry P, Loiseau P, Cejka JC, Custaud MA, Frutoso J, et al. Empirical mode decomposition to assess cardiovascular autonomic control in rats. Fundam Clin Pharmacol 2007;21:481-96.
[19] Machado C, Korein J, Aubert E, Bosch J, Alvarez MA, Rodríguez R, et al. Recognizing a mother's voice in the persistent vegetative state. Clin EEG Neurosci 2007;38:124-6.
[20] Chleboun S, Hux K, Snell J. Changes in responsiveness when brain injury survivors with impaired consciousness hear different voices. Brain Injury 2009;23(2):101-10.
[21] Di HB, Yu SM, Weng XC, Laureys S, Yu D, Li JQ, et al. Cerebral response to patient's own name in the vegetative and minimally conscious states. Neurology 2007;68:895-9.
[22] Purhonen M, Kilpelainen-Lees R, Valkonen-Korhonen M, Karhu J, Lehtonen J. Cerebral processing of mother's voice compared to unfamiliar voice in 4-month-old infants. Int J Psychophysiol 2004;52:257-66.
[23] Montano N, Porta A, Cogliati C, Costantino G, Tobaldini E, Casali KR, et al. Heart rate variability explored in the frequency domain: a tool to investigate the link between heart and behavior. Neurosci Biobehav Rev 2009;33:71-80.
[24] Kotchoubey B. Event-related potentials, cognition, and behavior: a biological approach. Neurosci Biobehav Rev 2006;30:42-65.

In: Considering Consciousness Clinically
Editors: Gerry Leisman and Joav Merrick

ISBN: 978-1-63484-260-0


*Chapter 14*

# A MODEL TO EXPLAIN DISORDERS OF CONSCIOUSNESS AND COGNITION IN THE BRAIN AND NERVOUS SYSTEM

***Gerry Leisman* and Robert Melillo***
The National Institute for Brain and Rehabilitation Sciences, Israel and Institute for Neurology and Neurosurgery, Universidad de Ciencias Médicas de la Habana, Facultad Manuel Fajardo, Havana, Cuba

## ABSTRACT

We will explain why despite children with autistic Spectrum disorder (ASD) having a possible common neurological basis, differing symptoms present from one child to another. The explanation is that a primary problem relates to the failure to achieve equal activity and resonance in both right and left cerebral hemispheres, in general and in local brain interconnectivities in particular. There exists an asymmetric distribution of almost all human functions within the cerebral cortex including cognitive, motor, sensory, neurohormonal, immune, autonomic, and endocrine. Failure to develop and achieve temporal coherence between brain regions will result in a form of functional independence of brain regions, resulting in dysfunction in the adaptive functioning of the brain and its control properties. This may sometime result in high degrees of functioning in specific tasks, and dysfunction in others. An example is the savant syndrome, but the same process is seen throughout all disorders in the spectrum and may even be a basis for individual differences in cognitive style. We will discuss the ramifications of viewing many of the cognitive and motor effects of developmental disabilities as based on a functional disconnection syndrome. Additionally, it will be noted that in these children, global functions are not affected, but many specific functions are decreased while others are enhanced, demonstrating region specific brain effects. We will also attempt to explain how the process of functional disconnection may inform altered and disordered states of consciousness.

* Correspondence: Professor Gerry Leisman, Director, The National Institute for Brain and Rehabilitation Sciences, Biomechanics Laboratory, Department of Mechanical Engineering, ORT-Braude College of Engineering, Snunit 51 Street, PO Box 78, IL-21982 Karmiel, Israel. E-mail: gerry.leisman@staff.nazareth.ac.il.

## INTRODUCTION

Traditionally clinicians have looked at various disorders like attention deficit hyperactive disorder, Tourette's, and obsessive-compulsive disorder as separate and distinct clinical entities. However, recently many of these disorders have been shown to have significant overlap and many children that have one disorder will often be diagnosed with at least one other. Neurobiological research and functional imaging tests have given science a new way of examining the brain in its functional and dysfunctioning states. These new tests have also revealed striking similarities in the brains of children and adults with various cognitive and behavioral disorders. As a result, we are arriving at the view that rather than consisting of separate processes, most of the common cognitive and behavioral disorders of childhood rest along a continuum all with a similar underlying mechanism. At one end of the spectrum is attention deficit disorder, then attention deficit hyperactive disorder, learning disability, pervasive developmental disorders, autism, obsessive-compulsive disorder, Tourette's, and the schizophrenias. From an anatomical and functional perspective, we find many of the same areas of the brain are affected. Some regions are smaller or appear atrophied, other regions appear to be functionally hyperactive, and some are hypoactive (1).

What seems to disturb and confuse many clinicians is the wide variety of symptoms that a child may express. Most of these children do not present solely with behavioral or learning problems although these may be of greatest concern or the most obvious. These children usually exhibit a combination of emotional, behavioral, cognitive, sensory, motor and autonomic symptoms. The broad range of symptoms causes even more anxiety and confusion to parents and professionals and leads them to think that the problem is overwhelming and insurmountable. Guiding principles in understanding these conditions and in fomenting intervention strategies starts with the caveat that the greater the number of symptoms, the more likely the problem is centered in the brain where all bodily and behavioral systems are controlled. If one can isolate specific dysfunctioning regions, one can then better understand the nature of the problem making treatment more specific and effective.

While many of the same pathways are involved in disorders within the continuum, their involvement appears restricted to either right-sided or left-sided hemispheric and subcortical areas. Elsewhere (2, 3) we have reported on how the brain functions, including the existence of a baseline arousal level of subcortical and cortical structures, appears to make up the contextual aspect of cognition, emotion, and perception. Superimposed on this baseline arousal level we have described specific pathways that convey content specific information to areas of the brain (1). Normal functions can be disrupted if the contextual information, which is arousal dependent, or the context specific information is disrupted in is progression through the nervous system.

From a functional perspective, we can examine by brain imaging techniques underactive or overactive brain regions that in turn relate to ineffectiveness of the arousal non-specific system or the specific content pathways. We have discussed how if neurons are active they will maintain a normal metabolic resting level. If not effectively stimulated they will be underactive, but eventually more active and relatively unstable. The result is that these neurons will fatigue more quickly and may even fire spontaneously as in the case of seizures or hyperkinetic disorders.

From an anatomic perspective, we see that certain areas of the brain are physically smaller and different from normal in children with these disorders (4-14). When an area is abnormally smaller, it either is usually due to failure to develop properly or is a result of disease. As with most areas of our body, when we use a structure it becomes larger with use, when we do not use it, we will often see atrophy of that area. Even with lack of development, we see that a region will fail to develop due to lack of exposure to stimuli, which will promote a developmental delay of the growth of the understimulated region.

In most of the cognitive and behavioral disorders that we will discuss we will see that there is a combination of alteration of function usually underactivity or hypoactive states, as well as atrophy or smaller physical size of neural structures. We also will recognize a common link between hypoactivity and atrophy of many of the same areas in all of these disorders. The only difference is usually if they are restricted to left or right side of the subcortical and cortical structures resulting in different symptoms. Many of the symptoms result from lack of inhibition of one area resulting in that region's functional hyperactivity; this in turn we hypothesize to be due to the hypoactivity of a region that would normally inhibit that function. In behavioral disorders, we know that the limbic system, especially on the right, is responsible for the production of many primitive or survival-driven emotions, such as fear, rage, anger, or approach and avoidance behaviors.

These brain regions in humans are normally modulated or inhibited by higher centers in the neocortex, especially the prefrontal cortex. Decreased stimulation or hypoactivity of the prefrontal cortex will reduce inhibitory control over the limbic system which can result in abnormal behavior, uncontrollable emotions especially aggression, increase in either avoidance or withdrawal behavior, perseveration, inability to focus attention and hypo or hyperactivity in a way not unlike that seen in the early Klüver-Bucy preparations in chimpanzees. The type of symptoms will depend on which hemisphere is dysfunctional. Autonomic systems can be affected or imbalanced due to dysfunction of the cortex and failure to modulate the limbic system and the hypothalamus. Neurotransmitter systems, especially serotonin, norepinephrine and dopamine systems can be dysfunctional, which system is affected is usually the result of the side of the brain affected as there exists an asymmetric distribution of neurotransmitters in the brain.

Finally, most of the development and normal function of the cerebrum is dependent on subcortical structures especially the cerebellum, thalamus, and basal ganglia. A failure to develop and or a dysfunction in these areas can affect both the nonspecific arousal system as well as specific transfer of information in the brain. Dysfunction in these areas will usually result in specific motor and sensory symptoms that are commonly seen in children with cognitive or behavioral disorders. These brain regions are often seen to be underactive or atrophied as well in these children. These cortical loci have been shown to be connected with the prefrontal cortex, which have also often been noted to be underactive or atrophied in children with the neurobehavioral developmental disorders. The underactivity and or atrophy is usually either restricted to the right or left side of the sub-cortex and cortex.

An imbalance of activity or arousal of one side of the cortex or the other can result in a functional disconnection syndrome similar to what is seen in split-brain patients, this could be an underlying source of many if not all of the symptoms that we see with children with behavioral and cognitive disorders.

For example, post-mortem examinations have indicated structural differences between the brains of good and impaired readers. High concentrations of micro-dysgenesis are noted in the left temporoparietal regions of dyslexic brains. The concentration is most evidenced in the planum temporale region (15-17). These micro-dysgeneses seriously impair the normal pattern of architecture of dyslexics and remove the asymmetry normally observed between the enlarged language areas of the left temporoparietal region and the smaller homologous areas of the right hemisphere (14, 17). The capacity for language is generally correlated with a significant development in the magnitude of the left temporoparietal region and an attrition of neurons in the right hemisphere. These neuronal casualties may produce the observed asymmetry between corresponding areas in the left and right hemispheres (14, 18). The relative symmetry in the dyslexics' brains might reflect their impaired linguistic development.

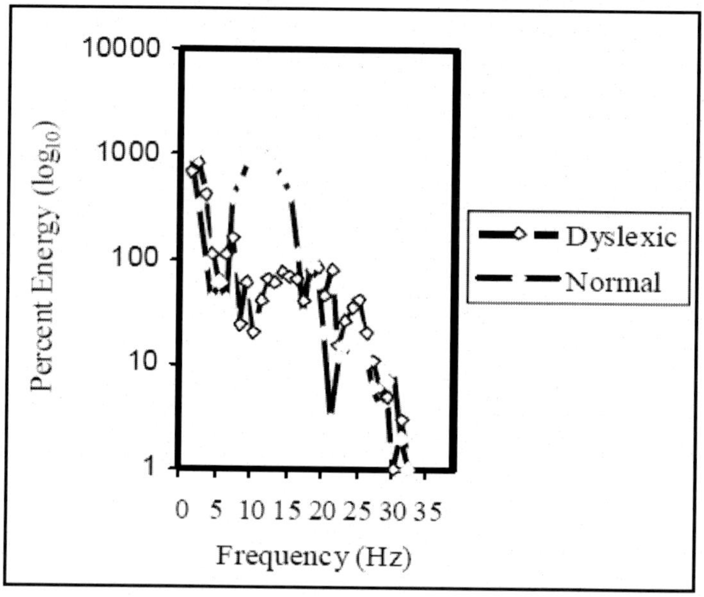


Figure 1. Mean values of EEG autospectral density by frequency order from $P_3$-$O_1$ electrode placements for normal and dyslexic subjects. (From Leisman (20).

In one study (19) left parieto-occipital EEG leads recorded a frequency spectrum in dyslexics that is consistently different from the spectrum obtained from normals. It is suggested that these effects represent significant differences in the functional organization of these areas. EEG coherence values indicate that normals have significantly greater sharing between hemispheres at symmetrical locations. Dyslexics demonstrate significantly greater sharing within hemisphere than do normals as evidenced in figure 1 and in Table 1. The data supports the notion that developmental dyslexia is a functional hemispheric disconnection syndrome. Other conditions in the spectrum of disorders that we are discussing yield similar results.

This spectrum of childhood disorders that we are discussing generally relates to an increase or decrease in activation of the brain and the balance of activation between brain regions. These conditions result from two primary system effects: 1) primary arousal deficit or imbalance, and 2) a specific activation deficit, imbalance, or asynchrony. The brain is driven by sensory input. We know that the brain receives more simultaneous sensory input than it can possibly consciously process (19, 20, 22-24). In general the more stimulation a brain cells receive the better their function allowing it to process more information faster, for longer periods of time (25-28). Therefore all sensory input is important although not all of it can be consciously processed and perceived. In fact, without subconscious baseline stimulation higher conscious processing of sensory stimuli would be difficult if not impossible.

Before higher brain centers can develop, the lesser supportive brain structures must develop. In the cortex, Luria (29) thought that lateralized cortical functions progress from primary cortical areas to secondary and tertiary areas as the child matures (29). Going back even further we see that development of cortical areas and the cortex itself are dependent on the anatomic and functional development of subcortical areas especially the cerebellum and the thalamus. Studies suggest that intact cerebellar functioning is required for normal cerebral functional and anatomical development (30, 31). The same has been seen for the thalamus - that intact thalamic function is necessary to cortical development and function (32). Developmental dysfunction of the same brain areas as seen in acquired disorders such as post-traumatic aphasia may be the basis of developmental learning disabilities and neurobehavioral disorders (33, 34).

**Table 1. Average frequency (in Hz), power (in dB), left-right asymmetry of power (in dB) between hemisphere and within hemisphere coherence values at $P_3$-$O_1$/$P_4$-$O_2$ locations for dyslexics and normals**

| | | Dyslexic | | | | | | Normal | | |
|---|---|---|---|---|---|---|---|---|---|---|
| S | Freq (Hz) | Power (dB) | L-R (dB) | Bilat. Coher. | W/in Coher. | Freq (Hz) | Power (dB) | L-R (dB) | Bilat. Coher. | W/in Coher. |
| 1 | 09.2 | 12 | -03 | -- | 1.1 | 09.2 | 28 | -- | -- | 0.8 |
| 2 | 10.4 | 21 | -04 | -- | 1.8 | 10.8 | 24 | -- | 2.4 | -- |
| 3 | 11.7 | 22 | 10 | -- | 2.4 | 12.7 | 18 | -- | 1.9 | -- |
| 4 | 09.8 | 18 | 04 | -- | 1.6 | 10.9 | 20 | -4 | 1.3 | -- |
| 5 | 10.8 | 17 | 03 | -- | 1.4 | 08.6 | 16 | -- | 1.9 | -- |
| 6 | 10.6 | 24 | -01 | -- | 0.8 | 08.9 | 08 | -- | 1.8 | -- |
| 7 | 10.6 | 28 | -05 | -- | 1.5 | 11.2 | 11 | -- | 2.4 | -- |
| 8 | 11.2 | 12 | -07 | -- | 2.1 | 11.7 | 13 | -2 | 1.5 | 1.8 |
| 9 | 12.0 | 19 | -04 | -- | 1.9 | 10.0 | 12 | -- | 1.3 | -- |
| 10 | 09.8 | 14 | -- | 0.7 | 0.6 | 10.7 | 15 | -1 | 1.3 | 0.9 |
| 11 | 10.8 | 25 | -02 | -- | 1.0 | 10.6 | 11 | -- | 1.2 | 1.4 |
| 12 | 11.7 | 22 | -- | 1.0 | -- | 12.0 | 09 | -- | 0.8 | 1.1 |
| 13 | 08.7 | 13 | -01 | -- | 0.9 | 11.7 | 07 | -- | 1.0 | -- |
| 14 | 09.0 | 27 | 08 | -- | 2.1 | 08.9 | 11 | -- | 1.9 | -- |
| 15 | 10.7 | 13 | -04 | -- | 2.4 | 09.5 | 10 | -- | 1.7 | 0.6 |
| 16 | 10.3 | 08 | -06 | -- | 1.8 | 08.8 | 11 | -2 | 2.1 | -- |
| 17 | 09.5 | 22 | -07 | -- | 2.0 | 08.6 | 14 | -- | 1.4 | -- |
| 18 | 12.2 | 20 | -07 | -- | 1.9 | 09.3 | 09 | -- | 1.8 | -- |
| 19 | 11.9 | 09 | -01 | -- | 0.9 | 12.4 | 12 | -- | 1.9 | -- |
| 20 | 08.4 | 15 | -04 | -- | 1.6 | 11.6 | 10 | -- | 0.9 | -- |

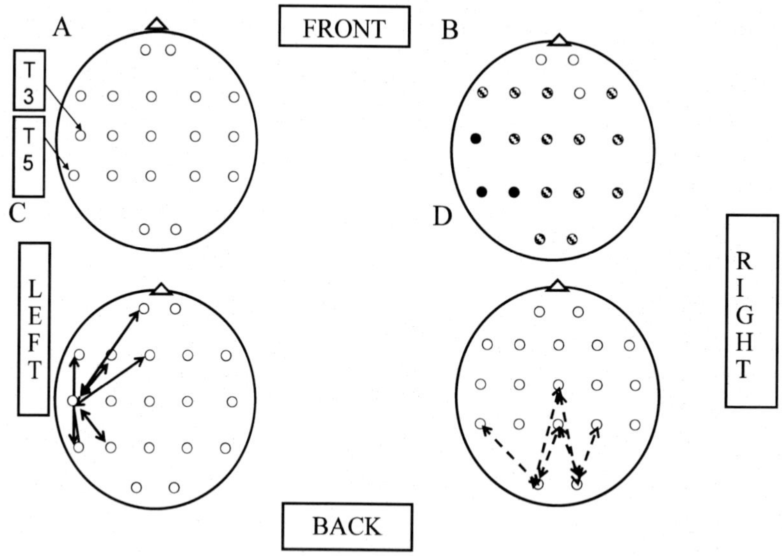


Figure 2. Schematic representation of the 19 electrodes represented by small circles (A-D). (A) T3 and T5 labels exemplify left temporal positions. (B) represents a significant change of amplitude among autistics relative to controls, represents activity at an electrode site not significantly different between autistics and controls, and represents amplitude significantly lower in autistics than in controls all at p<.01. (C) The solid lines that connect single electrode positions: demonstrate significant increases in coherence in autistics as compared to controls. (D) Represents significant decreases in coherence among autistics as compared to controls.

As Orton (35) had indicated, it is generally assumed that persons with learning disabilities have abnormal cerebral organization including atypical or weak patterns of hemisphere specialization (36-38). The developmental lag hypothesis proposed by Lenneberg (39) suggested that learning-disabled persons are slower to develop basic language skills and demonstrate weak hemispheric specialization for language tasks. In a reformulation of the progressive lateralization hypothesis (40), it may be that subcortical and antero-posterior progressions have a differential developmental course with learning disabled children and adults compared to control subjects or those with acquired syndromes.

Since learning disabled children exhibit deficient performance on a variety of tests thought to be a measure of perceptual laterality, evidence of weak laterality or failure to develop laterality has been found across various modalities (audio, visual, tactile) (41). It is thought these children have abnormal cerebral organization as suggested by Corballis (37) and Obrzut (38). The basic assumption is that dysfunction in the the central nervous system either prenatally or during early postnatal development, results in abnormal cerebral organization and associated dysfunctional specialization needed for lateralized processing of language function and non-language skills. It is thought that cortical and subcortical dysfunction which results from aberrant patterns of activation or arousal (34), inter- and intrahemispheric transmission deficits, inadequate resource allocation (42), or any combination of these may compromise hemispheric specialization in those with cognitive and behavioral deficits (41, 43-46).

Development of higher processing areas in the cerebellar cortex would develop after other more primary areas. For example, the lateral cerebellum would be dependent on proper development of the more midline areas in the inter-medial and medial zones first. Similarly, any region to which lateral cerebellum projected would be dependent on the effective development of the lateral cerebellum and it in turn would be dependent on the more medial cerebellar development. Therefore, if the medial aspects of the cerebellum do not develop adequately, then the lateral areas would still grow however, they may be smaller or atrophic, and dysfunction would be expected.

The cerebellum is thought to be part of a neuronal system that includes the thalamus, basal ganglia, and prefrontal cortex (46). Anatomic and functional development of the nervous system is dependent on sensory input, which is associated with growth of a given brain area and its associated connectivities with other brain regions. Brain area growth and the capacity to make functional connectivities is highly dependent on: continued regional stimulation and by global stimulation through connected and coordinated function. If specific regions are inadequately stimulated, then we may see failure of anatomic or functional development in that region with a preservation of basic lower level functionality. Higher functions that depend on greater areas of integrated stimulation may be lost or dysfunctional. If the sensory loss develops after a critical period, these areas may still be smaller due to atrophy or reverse plasticity, with either global or specific effects depending on the modality of dysfunction. In children with learning disabilities or affective disorders, there are specific areas of the nervous system that have been noted in imaging studies to be smaller than normal (32-34). Most often, these areas involve the prefrontal cortex, basal ganglia, thalamus, and cerebellum.

Some neurophysiological experts regard the central nervous system as partly a closed and part open system (31). An open system is one that accepts input from the environment, processes it, and returns it to the external environment. A closed system suggests that the basic organization of the central nervous system is geared toward the generation of intrinsic images and is primarily self-activating and capable of generating a cognitive representation of the outside environment even without incoming sensory stimuli. Although it is possible that a certain level of activation or stimulation will be intrinsic to single neuronal cells and the nervous system as a whole, this stimulation does not seem adequate to sustain a conscious, awake, individual. Behaviorally, arousal is a term used to describe an organism that is prepared to process incoming stimuli. From a physiologic standpoint, arousal also refers to the excitatory state or the propensity of neurons to discharge when appropriately activated (neuronal preparation).

A non-aroused organism is comatose (20). Therefore, an aroused alert individual that is prepared to process information is in a state dependent on sensory input with an attendant intrinsic excitability. Remove stimulation and the individual will eventually lose conscious awareness and become comatose or at least inattentive. The majority of brain activity associated with arousal comes from the ascending reticular activating system. The majority of this activity is relayed by the non-specific thalamic nuclei or intralaminar nuclei.

All sensory perception is based on the effectiveness of the arousal level of nonspecific, mostly subconscious, activity of the brain. There can be no specific sensory modality perception like vision or hearing without a baseline arousal level. The more stimulation or greater frequency of stimulation the more aroused an individual will be. Low frequency stimulation of midline thalamic non-specific nuclei produces inattention, drowsiness, and sleep accompanied by slow wave synchronous activity and so called spindle bursts. High frequency stimulation on the other hand has been shown to arouse a sleeping subject or alert a waking organism (47-49). Specific sensory perception and processing is dependent on specific thalamic relays, if one of the specific thalamic nuclei are damaged such as the lateral geniculate body, that specific sensory modality is lost (e.g., blindness) but it does not result in loss of other specific nuclei input like hearing. However, if lesions of the non-specific intralaminar nuclei exist, patients cannot perceive or respond to any input by the specific intact nuclei even though those pathways are intact. In essence, the person does not exist from a cognitive standpoint (31).

Luria (29) postulated that the brain was divided into three functional units: 1) the arousal unit, 2) the sensory receptive and integrative unit, and 3) the planning and organizational unit. He subdivided the last two into three hierarchic zones. The primary zone is responsible for sorting and recording incoming sensory information. The secondary zone organizes and codes information from the primary zone. The tertiary zone is where data are merged from multiple sources of input and collated as the basis for organizing complex behavioral responses (50). Luria's dynamic progression of lateralized function is similar to Hughlings Jackson's Cartesian coordinates with respect to progressive function from brainstem to cortical regions (51).

Satz and colleagues (40), have suggested that developmental invariance describes the lateral (x-axis) dimension of asymmetry, whereas current formulation of equipotentiality and the progressive lateralization hypothesis better describes vertical (subcortical-cortical) and horizontal (antero-posterior) progression during infancy and early childhood. Interestingly it has been noted that most research designed to address laterality issues in developmental disabilities (i.e., learning disabilities) has not dealt systematically with subcortical-cortical development or antero-posterior progression, all based on the concept of arousal unit.

The arousal unit is really the non-specific thalamic nuclei. We know that arousal is dependent on external and internal environmental sensory input. The largest proportion of subconscious sensory input passes between the thalamus, cerebellum, and dorsal column from slowly adapting receptors found in muscles with a preponderance of slow-twitch fibers - or slowly adapting muscle spindle receptors. The highest percentage of these is found in anti-gravity postural muscles especially muscles of the spine and neck (52). The receptors, which provide the major source of input to the brain, only receive sensory information. These receptors only work when muscles are stretched or contracted with gravity being the most frequent and constant sensory stimulus.

In summary, brain development and the adequacy of it continued functioning is dependent on sensory input. Specific sensory perceptual processes like vision and hearing are dependent on non-specific sensory input. This, in turn, creates a baseline arousal and synchronization of brain activity (consciousness). This is a form of constant arousal and is dependent on a constant flow of sensory input from receptors that are found in muscles of the spine and neck. These receptors receive the majority of their stimulation from gravity, creating a feedback loop that forms the basis of most if not all of brain function. Sensory input drives the brain, and motor activity drives the sensory system. Without sensory input the brain cannot perceive or process input. Without motor activity provided by constant action of postural muscles a large proportion of sensory stimuli are lost to further processing. This loop is the somatosensory system.

Higher processing is also dependent on the baseline sensory functions. For example, it has been shown that when performing a complex task, it is likely that transfer of motor commands to produce a final output is preceded to some degree, by transfer of information between association areas, which in turn may precede transfer between sensory regions (53).

## The relationship between motor function, sensation and consciousness

It is clear that the sensory-motor system then cannot be separated. A dysfunction of the sensory system results in a motor weakness or coordination deficit and a decrease in motor tone or coordination which in turn decreases the sensitivity of the muscle receptor and therefore the frequency of firing of the sensory pathways. The ability to sense body movement or position in space relative to gravity is known as proprioception, or the sense of subconscious touch. Proprioception is dependent on the amount of force or functional state of somatosensory receptors of joints, tendons, and especially muscle spindle receptors. These are pressure receptors similar to skin touch receptors for tactile sensation, the only major difference is in the frequency of stimulation and the resultant conscious or subconscious perception. Muscle tone may be defined as the resistance of stretch of muscles. Muscle tone is a product of the output of the brain or its level of activation and arousal. Output of the brain is directly related to input plus arousal level. Effective muscle tone is characteristic of an aroused individual. Proprioception and muscle tone are therefore related. The adequacy of proprioception results from the effective sensitivity of muscle spindle receptors. High sensitivity of muscle spindles is due to effective muscle tone, which in turn results from the adequacy of brain output.

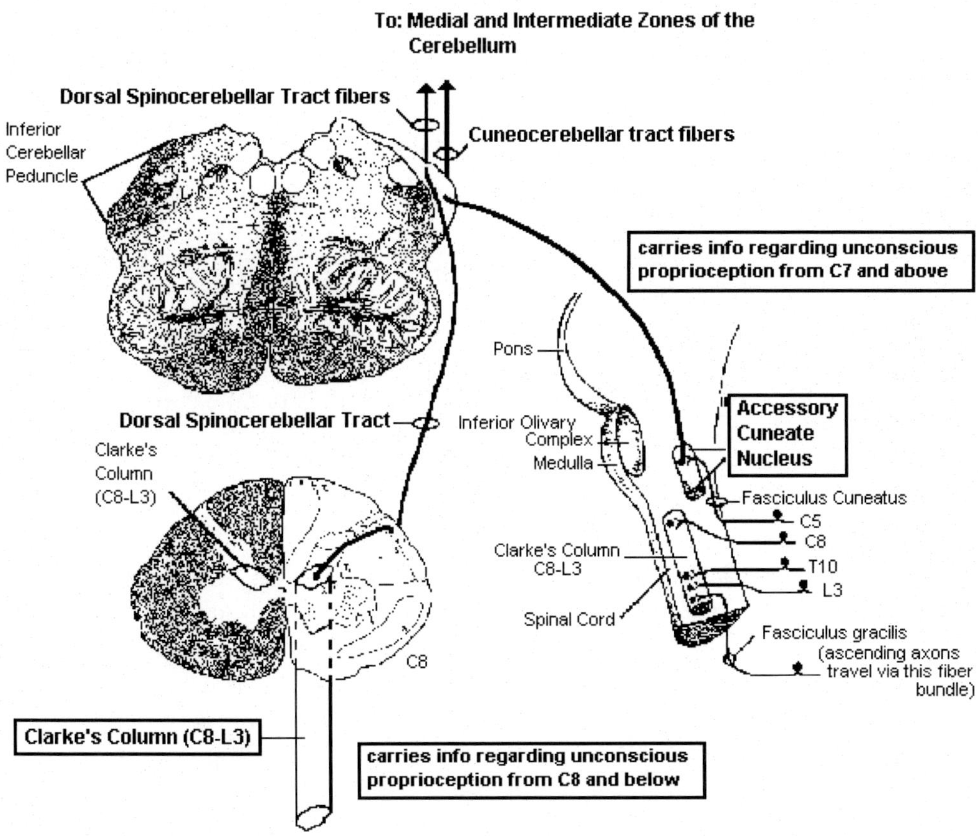


Figure 3. Proprioceptive pathways (cf. Leisman (57, 58)).

Of all the sensory input, proprioception constitutes the largest part. Many researchers have noted that in learning disabled children, there often exists poor proprioception and low muscle tone. Symptoms of poor proprioception and low muscle tone include poor balance, posture, clumsiness, and poor coordination (54, 55).

Jean Ayers (56) recognized over thirty years ago that these children demonstrated a variety of problems that she thought were related to what she called poor sensory integration. She noted then that these children possess different degrees of sensory deficits including hearing, visual, tactile, and proprioceptive. Associated with these symptoms included speech and language deficits, motor dysfunction, learning disabilities, and emotional problems. She thought that the vestibular system was the principle source of the dysfunction. Ayres arrived at this conclusion because she recognized that gravity plays a significant role in proprioception and further concluded that the major gravity receptors, which control balance, were primarily concentrated in the vestibular system. While her clinical observations were keen, we now recognize, however, that the majority of proprioceptive and gravity data arises from spinal and neck muscles, joints, and their sensory input to the cerebellum.

While vestibular receptors do not change their sensitivity, the cerebellum may alter it responsiveness to the vestibular apparatus based on the cerebellum's baseline arousal level, which results mostly from spinal and neck motor activity (60).

These midline motor structures of the spine are connected to the midline cerebellar structures in the medial zone and fastigial nuclei of the cerebellum and send sensory input directly back.

The cerebellum stimulates these midline muscles bilaterally. Signals then project to midline non-specific nuclei in the thalamus, which then project to the entire cortex (57, 58). This cerebellar feedback mechanism also connects through the vestibular nuclei and proceeds to primarily affect the proximal trunk muscles. They also ascend to effect the coordination of eye muscles. The intermediate and lateral cerebellum send more specific information about extremity and distal muscles, which goes to specific thalamic nuclei that are connected to the somatosensory cortex, prefrontal cortex, and association cortices on the contralateral side of the body. These specific areas of neocortex especially the frontal lobe then send fibers downwards to the ipsilateral brainstem reticular formation which then sets global muscle tone of all muscles on that side, both spinal and postural, as well as distal extremity muscles. It also sets the balance of muscle tone between anterior and posterior compartment muscles on the ipsilateral side of the body to help promote an upright bipedal posture.

Cerebellar lesions have been recognized since Gordon Holmes as resulting in problems with proprioception and motor tone. Some of these symptoms effect the bilateral coordination of muscles of the spine and eyes and occur primarily at the level of the cerebellum, and always occur bilaterally due to both contralateral and ipsilateral fibers (62). However, unilateral dyscoordination, unilateral decreases in muscle tone in both postural and extremity muscles and the balance of vestibular activity occur at the level of the cortex, dependent on contralateral cerebellar input plus arousal activity (57, 58). Levinson (63), in his study of almost 4,000 learning disabled subjects, showed that 94.1 percent presented with what he termed cerebellar-vestibular dysfunction. His data suggested that learning disabilities and dyslexia are C-V based and represent one disorder, that this C-V dysfunction continues with increasing age and that the symptomatic overlap within subjects and samples appear to reflect a common C-V basis rather than a group of separate neurophysiological disorders. He went on to state that a variety of so called "pure" disorders and terms such as dyslexia, dysgraphia, dyscalculia, dysphasia, dysnomia, dyspraxia, attention deficit disorder (ADD), perceptual-motor disorder, etc. merely reflect highly selected learning disabled symptoms and samples. Although he recognized cerebellar dysfunction, he related many of these aforementioned problems to a primary source in the inner ear of the vestibular system. He also did not consider asymmetric cerebral lateralization and its development as a significant factor. Therefore, a sensory deficit of proprioception and subsequent abnormality of muscle tone may reflect a global decrease in global cerebellar, thalamic, and cortical arousal levels.

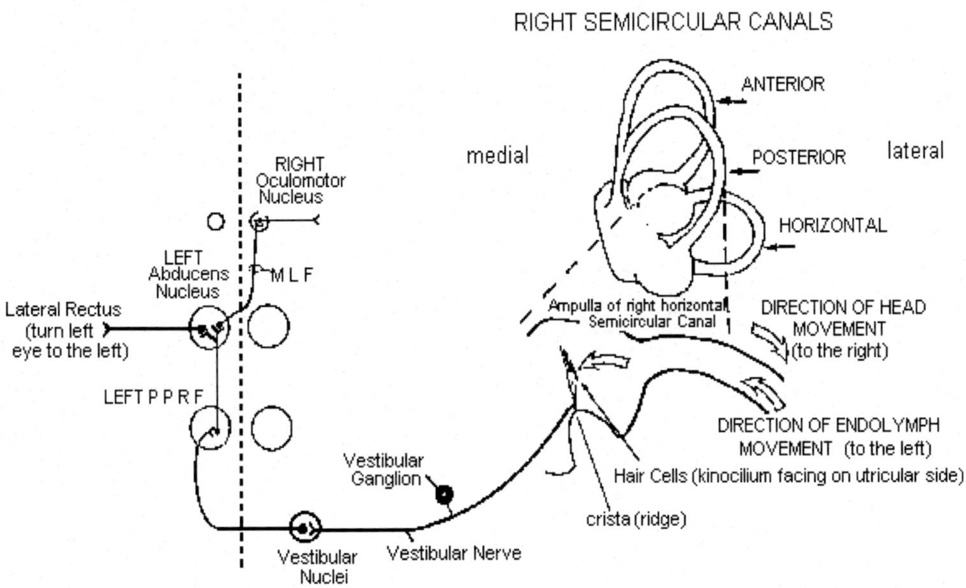


(A)

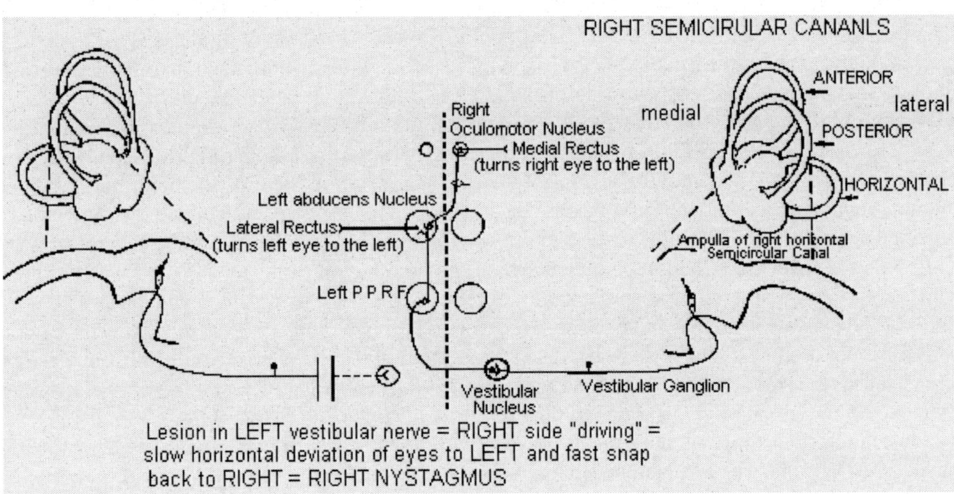


(B)

Figure 4. (Continued)

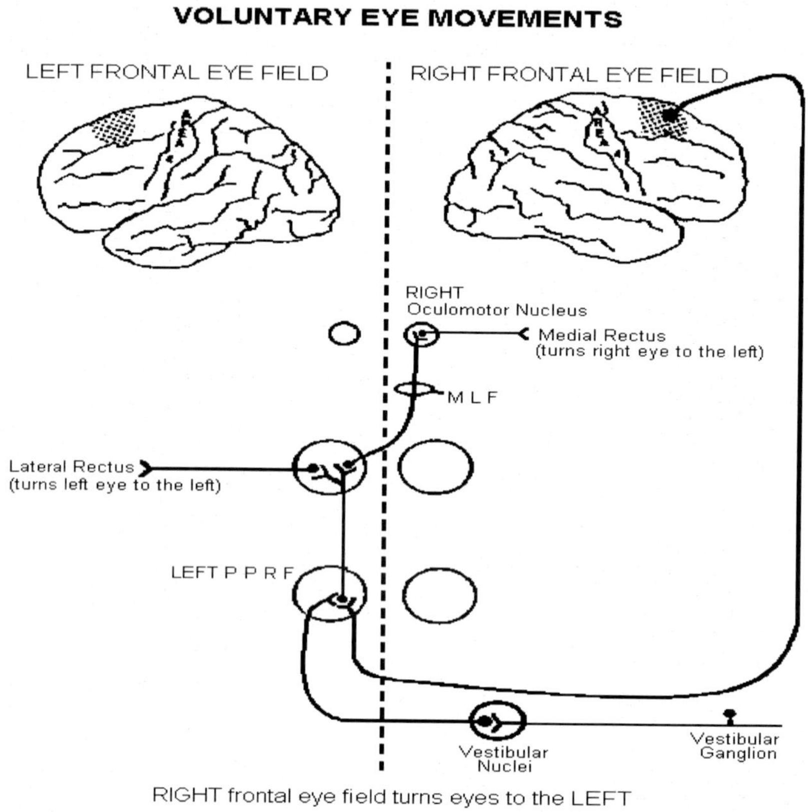


(C)

Figure 4. Compensatory eye movements induced by the vestibular apparatus, opposing head movements or changes in head position and act to keep the fovea of the retina on an object of interest. (A) Rotatory movement of the head to the right results in a increase in discharge of the right vestibular nerve, an increase in firing of the right vestibular nuclei, an increase in firing of neurons in the left paramedian pontine reticular formation (PPRF), an increase in firing of both small and large neurons in the left abducens nucleus and reflex turning of the left eye to the left (via left lateral rectus; Cranial nerve VI) and the right eye to the left (via ascending MLF input to the right medial rectus; Cranial nerve III). This is called the vesibulo-ocular reflex, critically important for stabilizing visual images in the presence of a continuously moving head. (B) Results of a lesion in the left vestibular nerve on eye movements. Such a lesion puts the right vestibular nerve in "control." This imbalance results in the eyes being pushed slowly to the left (right vestibular nerve turns on right vestibular nuclei, which turns on the left PPRF, which turns on the left abducens which turns both eyes to the left). When the eyes are pushed as far left as possible, they snap back very quickly to the right by mechanisms not fully understood. The eyes then slowly move to the left again, and this vicious cycle continues. This nodding back and forth is called nystagmus (to nod). A lesion of the left vestibular nerve will result in a right nystagmus. Thus, the right (intact) vestibular nerve is "driving" the left PPRF and left abducens to move the eyes slowly to the left, after which they reflexively snap back to the right. (C) Pathways involved in voluntary turning of both eyes horizontally to the left to see a new object of interest, called a left horizontal saccade. The left lateral and the right medial rectii contract synchronously. The two eyes then move together (conjugately) to the left, using a pathway beginning in the frontal eye fields of the cerebral cortex (area 8). This is a cortical area that lying rostral to the primary motor area (area 4). To voluntarily move eyes to the left, information from right frontal eye fields is conveyed to the left (contralateral) PPRF. The right frontal eye field directs the left PPRF to turn on both large and small neurons in the left abducens nucleus. The left eye then turns left (laterally) and the right eye turns left (medially). This is a voluntary left horizontal saccade (59).

Other specific sensory deficits may be result from the asymmetric arousal of these areas, which would present with specific localized perceptual dysfunction. Since proprioception is a subconscious sense, processed subconsciously through the cerebellum, thalamus and somatosensory cortex, when cortical proprioceptive input is decreased we are not consciously aware of the loss or dysfunction. However there are symptoms that we may experience when the proprioceptive input becomes too low or imbalanced. Dysequilibrium, or the feeling of unsteadiness of gait, is one primary symptom, poor balance, dizziness, or vertigo can be manifest if the cerebellum does not modulate vestibular input effectively.

In the past, most of the emphasis for balance dysfunction, such as vertigo, nystagmus, or motion sickness, had been placed on the vestibular apparatus of the inner ear. However, research suggests that as humans evolved from quadrupeds to bipeds the emphasis of control of balance, posture, and the coordination of head and eye movements was shifted from the inner ear to the spinal muscles and joints. Wyke (61) notes that during the course of the evolution of the erect from the quadrupedal posture, there has been a shift in the relative perceptual and reflexogenic significance of the mechanoreceptors in the labyrinth of the internal ear and those located in the cervical spinal joints in favor of the latter.

This evolutionary decrease in the functional significance of the vestibular system in man was first suggested by Rudolf Magnus (64) and is powerfully illustrated by the later clinical observations of Purdon Martin (65) which show, *inter alia*, that this system in man is of no significance at all in static postural circumstances or in the production of reflex righting reactions. In this connection, it may be relevant to note that the cervical articular mechanoreceptors became functionally active in the developing human fetus long before the vestibular mechanoreceptors (61). Wyke goes on to note that patients experience a feeling of postural instability and unsteadiness of gait in situations of poor lighting after these individuals have been provided with a cervical collar that affects their neck joints and muscles (61).

He also notes that based on neuropsychological study (61) showing that, "precision of voluntary control of arm movement in the absence of vision is markedly impaired by rotation of the head and neck to right and left of central position."

It has also been observed by de Jong and colleagues (66), and others (57, 58) that local anesthetic infiltration of cervical spinal and other joints in normal individuals results in a feeling of static body dysequilibrium (often with vertigo). Also noted is kinesthesia, upon which the accurate control of voluntary movements including walking depends even in the presence of a normally functioning vestibular system (61).

In regard to proprioceptive input and its relationship to various sources of input, Carpenter and colleagues (67) states "by far the most important proprioceptive information needed for the maintenance of equilibrium comes from neck joint receptors and muscles." Guyton (52) also notes "mechanisms governing equilibrium and orientation in three dimensional space proprioception are largely reflexive and subconscious in character and depend on input from several sources.

The most important of these are as follows: kinesthetic sense conveyed by spino-cerebellar system from receptors in muscles, tendons, and joints. Sense provided by the vestibular organ of the inner ear and visual input from the retina."

The reason input of spinal muscles and joints is so important is that they are made up of slowly adapting tonic receptors that continuously fire to the cerebellum and brain. The sheer volume of stimulation because of continual firing more than any other source of stimulus to the brain may be why the spinal muscles and joint have more neurons than the rest of the nervous system. The spinal muscles and joints process more information than any other region of the body, and is the only continuous source of stimulus to the cerebellum and brain, not the inner ear or the eyes, only the muscles that are forced to resist the forces of gravity.

To understand the effects of gravity on the nervous system we will review studies on the effects of micro-gravity on organisms and humans. In one study, the ultra-structure of somatosensory, visual, and olfactory cortex of the brain in rats exposed to space flight for 7 days ("Cosmos - 1667" biosatellite) and 14 days ("Cosmos - 1887 and - 2024" biosatellites) as well as rats of ground-based synchronous control and Vivarium control groups has been studied (68). The flight organisms showed similar changes in the ultra-structure of all the brain cortex regions under study. The observed differences were primarily due to the extent of observed changes, the relationship distribution density of changed structures, and specific features of their localization in the corresponding brain areas. These changes were most distinct in the structural components of the neuropile-presynaptic axon terminals, dendrites, synapses, as well as glial components. Studies revealed light and dark degeneration of axon terminals, destructive changes in the postsynaptic areas of dendrites, as well as enlargement of area occupied by glial components in the cortical neuropile.

These changes of the ultra-structure in the somatosensory cortex of the flight organisms were noted to be more pronounced than those in the visual cortex. In the olfactory cortex, of flight organisms the ultra-structural changes are less expressed than in the neocortical areas under study and are mainly localized at the sites of Axo-spinal contacts. Ultra-structural changes were observed to depend on the duration of space flight. Changes of the ultra-structure in the brain cortex of flight rats reflect the morphological-functional rearrangement of a system of inter-neuronal contacts that develop due to the loss (dark degeneration of axon terminals) or decrease (light degeneration) of the functional activity of some synapses. The gradually developing light degeneration of terminals is the result of deficient afferentation in weightlessness.

In another study, cytochemical and morphometrical analyses were performed of motor neurons in the lumbar enlargement of the spinal cord (LESC) and sensitive neurons in the lumbar inter-vertebral ganglia (LIVG) in rats after 19 - 32 day space flight on board Cosmos - 605, - 782 - 936 biosatellites. Results revealed a decreased content of RNA, protein, body and nuclei volume in motor neurons, and the content of RNA and protein in large living LIVO neurons. The investigators also noted that results support a conclusion of hypofunction of LIVO neurons in weightlessness. This conclusion, in turn, is thought to reflect a decline of afferent impulsation in weightlessness arising from proprioceptors of muscle joints and tendons of the hind limbs. In addition, results show that in rats after space flight on Cosmos - 2044 and 6 - 8 demonstrated a 12 percent decrease in the volume of the nucleolus in LESC motor neurons and a 33 percent decline in the number of peri-neuronal glial cells, as compared to ground based synchronous control rats. The investigators conclude that these results provides evidence for the hypofunction of motor neurons in weightlessness and suggests similar data previously obtained for rats in longer space flight (69).

These studies demonstrate that with loss of gravitational force the spinal cord, brain, and especially neocortex, show rapid structural changes and atrophy. This is as a direct result of the loss of the constant flow of proprioceptive input from muscles, tendons, and joints involved in maintaining posture. In humans in space flight or micro-gravity situations such as under water, vertigo, nystagmus and motion sickness are of the most concerning problems.

The primary source of these symptoms has been studied. Human data was collected on the peculiarities of sensory interaction under varying experimental conditions including micro-gravity.

Aizikov and colleagues (70) attempted to determine the most significant afferent input to the cerebral cortex. They stated, “The main role here appears to be the postural reflexes caused by an exposure of musculo-articular and vestibular systems to the gravitational field of earth and by forming during the life a subjective vertical. In this case of great importance is still antigravity musculature with its more powerful input of information as compared with that of the vestibular system. Thus owing to an integrative function of the brain cortex there exists gravitational vertical which by its nature is a peculiar balance of vestibular sensitivity, muscular sense and vision.” They continue by indicating that the greatest protective effect against experimental motion sickness is produced by a procedure, which uses activation of basal proprioceptive-tactile coordinates of the subjective vertical and consecutive tension of antigravity muscles, followed by tension of the antagonists. They point out that this is associated not only with a several hundred percent increase of tolerated duration of swinging (from 4 to 10 mm.) but also with a marked (5 points versus a baseline of 13) decrease of vegetative symptoms (motion sickness). They further note that with the aid of muscular tension, it is possible to eliminate illusions appearing during tilts and rotation as well as at the end of the procedure on a rotating chair.

The effect of electrical muscle stimulation is markedly smaller than that of muscular tension stimulation. Analysis of the protective anti-motion sickness effect of the muscular activity was tested with the administration of the drug scopolamine (71). It was revealed that the effectiveness of the muscular tension procedures was enhanced with a simultaneous administration of scopolamine and that the drug clearly potentiated the effect of muscular tension. The authors concluded that volitional efforts that accompany a purposeful motor act or muscular tension hinders or blocks completely spatial disorientation illusions and decreases significantly the severity of the vegetative vestibular response (VVR). The investigators thought that, “ascending proprio-tactile efferent impulses developing from muscle tension of the spine and lower extremities provide information on body position irrespective from vestibular sendings but they are adequate to overcome the negative effect of the latter.” Furthermore, the investigators go on to state that they think that an integration of these polysensory inputs is realized in coordinating structures as the cerebellum and cortex of the brain. They recommend that based on the results of this study muscular tension should be used for normalizing vestibular-motor interactions as the means of non-drug prevention of motion sickness.

What we have seen in these studies is that motion sickness, a severe symptom of loss of proprioceptive input, is a common finding in micro-gravity situations. That the loss of proprioceptive input is mostly the result of postural antigravity of the muscles of the spine and lower extremity and this presents with a a more powerful effect than loss of vestibular input and active contraction, and use of these muscles can completely compensate for the loss. We also see that this loss of proprioceptive input also results in nystagmus of the eyes and an inability to efficiently control eye movement. Loss of proprioceptive input can also result in significant abnormal autonomic reactions, which again can be alleviated by increasing proprioceptive input from those specific muscles. We have also seen that the loss of this input is thought to be mediated centrally through the cerebellum and cortex. This loss of input in rats has been shown to cause rapid light and dark degeneration of neurons in widespread areas of the brain - but especially the neocortex. Areas of neocortex involved include the somatosensory and visual areas especially.

Therefore, in children that present with signs and symptoms of proprioceptive loss, which includes, disorders of balance and gait, abnormal muscle tone - especially hypotonia, nystagmus, vertigo, dysequilibrium, nausea, motion-sickness symptoms, etc., these symptoms are due essentially to a primary dysfunction of cerebellar-thalamo-cortical input. The primary source of input to the cerebellum of proprioceptive input is from muscles, joints, and tendons of spine and lower extremity, and postural antigravity muscles. This input is more significant than vestibular input and can even compensate for vestibular loss. Therefore, anything that may decrease the ongoing proprioceptive input of postural antigravity muscles and/or vestibular input as seen in micro-gravity experiments can result in sensory loss, degeneration or reverse plastic changes in the cerebellum and neocortex. Such conditions have the possibility of affecting any or all other brain regions but especially neocortical functions.

## Sensory effects on functional connectivity, consciousness, and cognitive function

### *Tactile function*

Ayers (56) and others (54, 55) have noted that children with learning disabilities and behavior disorders often have altered sense of touch or tactile sensations. Most often, there exists a decrease in tactile sensitivity in these children, but others also appear to have a hypersensitivity to touch. Interestingly, tactile sensory input or conscious touch input travels much the same path as proprioceptive input. Therefore, the same dysfunctioning mechanisms that affect proprioception can also affect tactile perception. Both senses are mainly activate and are processed in the somatosensory cortex, however for touch and spatial orientation there does appear to be asymmetric lateralization favoring the right hemisphere. The somatosensory cortex is proximal to the post-central gyrus and areas adjacent to it (Brodmann areas 1, 2, and 3). These areas receive input from somatosensory pathways originating in the thalamus, which transfer tactile information of, pain, temperature, and proprioception. The primary somatosensory cortex (SI) is immediately caudal to the central sulcus, the secondary somatosensory cortex (SII), which obtains most of its afferent input from SI, is located ventral to SI. Somatosensory inputs projecting to the posterior parietal cortex arise from SI and SII. Somatosensory input projecting to the thalamus and proceeding to the primary somatosensory cortex transverses two main pathways: the antero-lateral system for pain and temperature sense, and the dorsal column-medial lemniscal pathway, which carries information about tactile proprioception and movement sensation. Any process that physically disrupts the flow of information such as a lesion at the receptor, nerve, spinal cord, brainstem, cerebellum, thalamus, or cortical level can cause abnormalities in the attendant perceptual processes. Abnormal perception, decreased arousal, or imbalance of arousal may result even with a physically intact pathway.

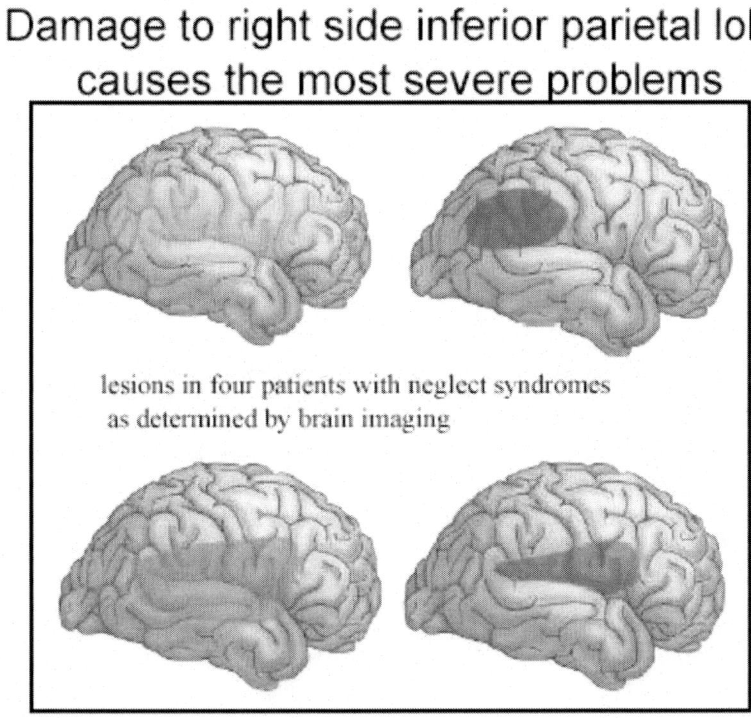


Figure 5. Cortical source of hemispatial neglect syndromes, most often seen after large areas of damage to right parietal lobe. It is a frequent consequence of stroke on the right side of the brain and thus neglect of everything on the left. It is also evidenced in other forms of brain dysfunction especially with a right hemisphere source. Patients ignore everything on the side opposite the lesion. It is not blindness. Patients recognize and label objects appropriately and thus it is a disturbance of spatial distribution of directed attention. Patients frequently bump into objects, tend a not to groom themselves, contralateral to the lesion. In the majority of patients, the lesion involves the supermarginal gyrus in the inferior parietal lobe at the temporo-parietal junction. Less frequently, damage or dysfunction to the dorsolateral premotor and medial frontal regions can also bring about hemineglect. Lesions confined to the primary motor, somatosensory, and visual cortices are not associated with neglect. The posterior parietal component provides an internal sensory mechanism, the limbic component regulates the spatial distribution, the frontal component coordinates the motor programs for scanning, reaching, and exploring, and the reticular component provides levels of arousal.

Arousal level or attention is the foundation of all perception and without proper arousal; any or all effective sensory perception can be impaired. These perceptual alterations and resultant inattention syndromes are known as neglect, and can occur with or without spatial awareness, tactile, visual and auditory sensations. In these cases, the physical pathways of the stimulus are intact but the cerebral cortex does not integrate or perceive the information, in essence rendering the stimulus non-existent to the individual. This can occur bilaterally, but more often, the result is a unilateral loss.

The asymmetric lateralization of the function, and the localization of the primary dysfunction will determine which sense will be most affected, this helps us to localize the primary problem. There are numerous studies of various asymmetries of tactile (haptic) perception, visual perception and of interference between two tasks performed at the same time (72). Tactile inattention is also known as pseudo hemi-anesthesia.

Vallar and colleagues (73) reported on a patient who had apparent contralateral hemi-anesthesia from a large right hemisphere cerebral infarction. Although the patient denied being stimulated on the left side, tactile stimulation did produce an electrochemical skin response. Three other patients were reported by the same author (73). All three had left hemi-anesthesia from right hemisphere lesions; however, all had normal evoked potentials recoded from the left side. This suggests that although the pathways were intact, the tactile sensations were not perceived due to lesions in the right hemisphere. Vallar and colleagues (73) used selective hemisphere anesthesia in 18 epileptic patients and found that contralateral tactile inattention was present in eight patients after right hemisphere injection of anesthesia but only in two subjects after left-sided injection.

Another form of tactile inattention is known as extinction to simultaneous stimulation. It has been reported that as patients with neglect or hemi-inattention symptoms improve, they may develop extinction to simultaneous stimuli. The difference is that individuals with inattention are not aware of tactile stimulation to the side opposite the impaired hemisphere. However, patients with extinction are aware of contralateral stimuli but are unable to perceive simultaneous bilateral stimulation, specifically failing to perceive the stimulus to the contralateral side. In most cases, studied contralateral extinction was more frequently associated with selective anesthesia of the right hemisphere than the left (74).

In spatial neglect, most commonly hemispatial neglect, patients with injury or dysfunction localized to one hemisphere may not be able to perform normally on spatial tasks. This is usually found in the contralateral hemi-space so that the stimuli to the left of the patient's body are neglected more often than those to the right side of the body (75). Neglect of the environment may also occur so that even when the individual lies on his or her side, the left half of the environment is neglected (76).

Spatial neglect is complex and can involve: 1) attentional disorders, 2) intentional or motor activation disorders, or 3) representational disorders (20). It has been hypothesized that hemispatial neglect may have four possible attention related causes: 1) contralateral spatial inattention, 2) ipsilateral attentional bias, 3) inability to disengage, and 4) reduced sequential attentional capacity or premature habituation. One theory (77) posits that that patients with left hemispatial neglect are unaware of stimuli presented to the left hemisphere because they may simply be less aware of stimuli on the left than on the right resulting in an ipsilateral bias with attention being drawn to that side and away from the neglected side. Another possibility for explaining neglect is that objects besides the critical stimulus in ipsilateral space draw the patient's attention with the bias becoming so strong that the individual may not be able to disengage their attention (78). It is also possible, as exemplified in one case, where bias or inattention may determine where stimuli are neglected, a limited sequential capacity or inappropriate habituation may also lead to hemispatial neglect (20, 79).

Hemispatial neglect is seen more frequently with right hemisphere lesions (80). Although several studies note that spatial neglect caused by right hemisphere lesions mostly affects the left side of space or body, it may also affect the right side of space (75). In humans, the inferior parietal lobe is more often associated with disorders of attention (21, 81). Temporo-parietal ablation in monkeys also results in contralesional attentional disorders, primarily extinction (82). Therefore, it is suggested by this research that tactile as well as spatial neglect can be a result of decreased or imbalanced arousal or attention. In the right hemisphere, a lesion or dysfunction can result in neglect that affects both sides of the body or space with the left being more frequently affected. The primary brain area reportedly responsible for the majority of cases is the inferior parietal lobe or temporo-parietal areas.

Functionally, decreased afferent input in the absence of a physical lesion could be another reason for neglect. In the parietal lobe, which is important in directing attention, it has been noted that the rate of cell firing appears to be associated with the importance of the stimulus to the monkey, so that important stimuli are associated with a higher firing rate than unimportant stimuli (82). It has been demonstrated that the activity of some parietal attentional neurons are spatially selective. However, the parietal lobe also receives input from other sensory modalities and the coding of spatial location is thought to be multimodal (83). The primary sensory cortices project only to the association cortex. These single modality primary sensory areas converge upon polymodal association areas in the monkey including the frontal cortex (periarcuate, prearcuate, and orbitofrontal) and both banks of the superior temporal sulcus (84). Multimodal association areas are important for sensory synthesis and cross-modal association. These multimodal convergence areas project to the inferior parietal lobe (85).

The cerebellum has also been noted to have a close connection to all association areas of the neocortex. The cerebellum has also been implicated in tactile learning and sensory tactile deficits besides its primary role in the processing of proprioceptive input. Leiner and colleagues (86) have stated that, "concomitant with the evolution of new association areas in the cerebral cortex, new neuronal connections evolved that descend (via enlarged structures in the brainstem) to new area 5 in the lateral cerebellum." It is further stated, "therefore, the neo-cerebellum can serve as a link between the posterior and frontal language areas of the cerebral neocortex in effect the cerebellum provides the cerebral cortex with an additional 'association area.'"

Blood flow studies during tactile learning of complicated geometrical objects show a high activation in the lateral cerebellum (87). The activation of the lateral cerebellum is thought to be due to cognitive processing during tactile learning, whereas the medial cerebellar activity relates more to the actual movement (88). The cerebellum has been specifically shown to be involved in sensory perception; this has been shown during chronometric tests (89) of timing functions. Cerebellar patients demonstrate deficits in perception of time intervals and judgment of velocity of a moving stimulus. It has been postulated that one role of the cerebellum is to modify motor performance to improve the efficiency of sensory processing by the rest of the nervous system by means of arousal.

Arousal is a physiologic state that prepares an organism for sensory processing by increasing sensitivity and signal-to-noise ratio (20). This is an extremely important concept because it forms the basis of all perception and perhaps even consciousness itself. The baseline arousal of all cortical areas makes all of these cells more active and therefore closer to threshold or more sensitive to incoming stimuli. The closer to threshold, the better the signal-to-noise ratio resulting global or specific effects on the brain. The results of such a process in turn could lower the effectiveness of global possessing of the brain or one specific function may be affected more than others. This can happen with an imbalance of arousal, where one side is too high in relationship to the other.

## Limbic influences on consciousness and cognition

The significance of the stimulus requires knowledge of the meaning of the stimulation and the motivational needs and goals of the individual (20). The limbic system provides the more primitive, motivation of immediate biologic needs, whereas the frontal lobe is involved with goal directed behavior. The difference between the limbic and frontal input to attentional or arousal systems, is that the frontal lobe may provide motivation and goals that are of a higher level beyond the basic biological needs of the child. It is thought that the frontal and limbic (cingulate gyrus) connections with the frontal lobe may provide the neuronal basis for the ability of motivational states to affect attentional systems and perception. Unilateral neglect in humans and monkeys can be induced by lesions in the dorsolateral frontal and prefrontal cortex (75) as well as with cingulate gyrus lesions (75). Affective behaviors have also been shown to be influenced by cerebellar dysfunction; especially midline cerebellar atrophy (90). The cerebellum is also known to be connected to the dorsolateral, frontal, and prefrontal cortex. Not only can the cerebellum affect global arousal, but it also has specific connections to association cortices for multi-modal sensory processing. It has strong specific connections to the somatosensory cortex in the parietal lobe, as well as the frontal lobe.

The overall neuronal preparedness and signal-to-noise ratio is dependent on arousal input. The cerebellum may be the largest contributor to the arousal system. The cerebellum also works to modify motor behavior to maximize all sensory input. Therefore, the hemispatial neglect can be seen with all sensory input, not just tactile and spatial, but also visual and auditory. Besides signal-to-noise ratio, neuronal synchrony is essential for sensory perception to exist (91-95).

Liederman (96) describes how synchronization dysfunction may result in a neglect syndrome for any sensory modality. She describes how cortico-cortical pathways can function to synchronize activity across remote cortical regions. This synchronization then is thought to have the effect of equilibratory activation between different regions. She is quoted, "thus disconnection symptoms such as those seen in split-brain patients can be accounted for mainly by two factors: the desynchronized and fragmented manner by which subcortical pathways permit inter-hemispheric integration and the diminished arousal state of the non-viewing hemisphere without the synchronizing influence of the cerebral commissures. The under activated hemisphere displays an internal neglect that is marked by an abnormality of processing of input after sensory reception it does not effectively process inputs to it (a) directly from the contralateral side of space, or (b) indirectly from the opposite hemisphere. These under-processed inputs are not consciously perceived though they are reacted to on an implicit level."

Synchronization of a hemisphere is thought to result from 40 Hz. oscillations that arise from the intralaminar thalamic nuclei. These subcortical oscillations in the thalamus have been traced back and are thought to originate from the cerebellum and dorsal column fibers that are thought to transmit information from slowly adapting receptors. These types of receptors are found most commonly in slow-twitch muscle fibers of postural spinal muscles. It is known that even in the intact brain the two hemispheres can maintain different arousal levels as well if not more than differences within adjacent areas of the same hemisphere. Large differences should not occur in a normally functioning intact brain. However, in situations where stimulus conditions cause the untrained or non-viewing hemisphere to be either busy or too minimally alert to adequately subserve inter-hemispheric integration (96) inter-hemispheric arousal differences may exist.

It has been demonstrated that right parietal lobe lesions cause a deficit of integration and not detection. It is thought that the neglect subjects do not have difficulty with directing their attention to a single-feature target. They do appear, however, to have difficulty with searching for conjunctions among distractions consisting of two elements, which together would constitute a conjunctive stimulus and patients present with deficiencies in their ability to integrate information after their attention has been focused on the features. They do not have the ability to use selective attention as the glue to bind these features (97).

Kinsbourne (98) thought that each hemisphere directs attention to the contralateral space and that a normal attentional system of one hemisphere inhibits the other hemisphere. Therefore, if one hemisphere is injured or less active, the other becomes attentionally hyperactive, and attention is biased to the side opposite the normal hemisphere. This may be one of the explanations for the increased sensitivity to touch that learning-disabled children exhibit. The right side of the brain is known to direct attention to both sides of the body, therefore if it were functionally attentionally hyperactive, the child may be hypersensitive to stimuli on both sides of the body and space.

Another reason for hypersensitivity of tactile stimulation maybe that proprioceptive and tactile input is inhibitory to pain input. Therefore, with decreased proprioceptive input, a child would be more sensitive to pain and therefore even touch would be painful. This would be compounded by the fact that loss of proprioceptive or arousal activity to the neocortex would cause a decrease in inhibition of limbic autonomic output, which in turn would result in increased sympathetic activity and increased adrenal catecholamine release. These substances sensitize alpha 2 receptors found in pain transmitting fibers, bringing the fibers closer to threshold globally. This may result in a child being hypersensitive to touch because of decreased stimulation or arousal.

Occupational therapists for years have used brushing techniques where they lightly brush the child's skin, the child eventually becomes "desensitized" to the stimulus, and the child will not be as defensive to touch. This may not be due to actual desensitization, but rather increased sensory input may result in an increased arousal and reciprocal inhibition of each hemisphere so that one is not hyperactive and one is not underactive. It may increase large afferent fiber input to produce inhibition of pain directly as well as inhibition of sympathetic output in the spinal cord, and brain.

In summary, sensory processing is a product of multiple factors. The baseline arousal level and signal-to-noise ratio or neuronal preparation, form the basis of all sensory perception. This can be globally deficient and/or specifically decreased in a limited area. It can be imbalanced from one side to the other with one side becoming hyperactive and the other hypoactive. Any decrease in arousal will affect at least one sensory perceptual process. The arousal level of a hemisphere is set by the subcortical structures especially the thalamus and cerebellum. They receive most of their input from muscle joint and tendon receptors in the postural and antigravity muscles. These receptors, which are continually transducing gravitational forces into the central nervous system, create the arousal level and the gamma oscillations that are the basis of all perception.

Hillyard (99) indicated, "What you are asking about is the nature of neuronal codes for sensory perceptual information. There is a general assumption that more activity-greater firing rates etc. -within a nerve cell population means that more information is being represented or processed by those cells. Conversely, a suppressed response reflects diminished processing. ... In simple low-level sensory signals, greater physical stimulus energy produces systematic increases in neuronal response amplitudes that are paralleled by elevations in the perceived stimulus magnitude. Also signal detection experiments in humans and monkeys have shown that moment-to-moment fluctuations in neuronal response amplitudes can predict precisely whether the person or organism detects a faint signal."

## Visual and auditory system influences on consciousness and cognition

Children with learning disabilities have also been noted to demonstrate various types of visual and auditory dysfunction. If we look at all sensory perception in light of Luria's theory (50) that the brain has three functional units: 1) the arousal unit, 2) the sensory receptive or integrative unit, and 3) the planning and organizational unit, and that the second and third are subdivided into three zones. The primary zone sorts and records incoming sensory stimuli, the secondary zone organizes and codes information from the primary zone, and lastly the tertiary zone is where data is merged from multiple sources of input and collated as the basis for organizing complex behavioral responses. These last two; especially the third or tertiary zones are what make humans unique. In regard to vision, the primary zone gives us the ability to see, to perceive light at its most basic level. The secondary zone allows us perform basic responses based on immediate biologic needs -the limbic response. Most organisms have evolved to this level. However, the human neocortex, which fits Luria's description of tertiary zone, gives us the ability to put a higher meaning to this stimulus, to go beyond basic primitive needs and motivations, and to utilize the stimulus to allow us to obtain higher more complex goals. This higher goal directed behavior is supported by the prefrontal cortex. This region allows us to put higher cognitive and emotional significance to a stimulus like light or sound. The parietal lobes allow us to integrate this information with other sensory stimuli before the meaning of it all is processed in the frontal cortex. This area of integration is the seemingly occurs in the temporal, parietal, and occipital cortices (approximately Brodmann's area 39). The primary zone would correspond to the primary visual cortex.

The final projection of the visual pathway is via the geniculo-cortical pathway. This group of axons exits the lateral geniculate nucleus of the thalamus and proceeds to the cerebral cortex terminating in the primary visual area of the occipital lobe (Brodmann's area 17). This area is regular and stippled in appearance hence its name the striate cortex. This area is also known as the primary visual area and it is thought to be the region of the cortex where the first level of visual processing takes place. If the signal-to-noise ratio is not high enough due to a decrease arousal in the occipital lobe, a child may appear to have a primary visual deficit, even though the eyes and the visual pathway may be intact.

A severe example of this is related by Malkowicz, Myers and Leisman (100) in which children who were apparently blind with no apparent reaction to the brightest light would have improved visual function coincident with improved movement ability. We had hypothesized that the pathways associated with vision in these children were always intact but for some reason this information was not summating to the level of perception in the brain.

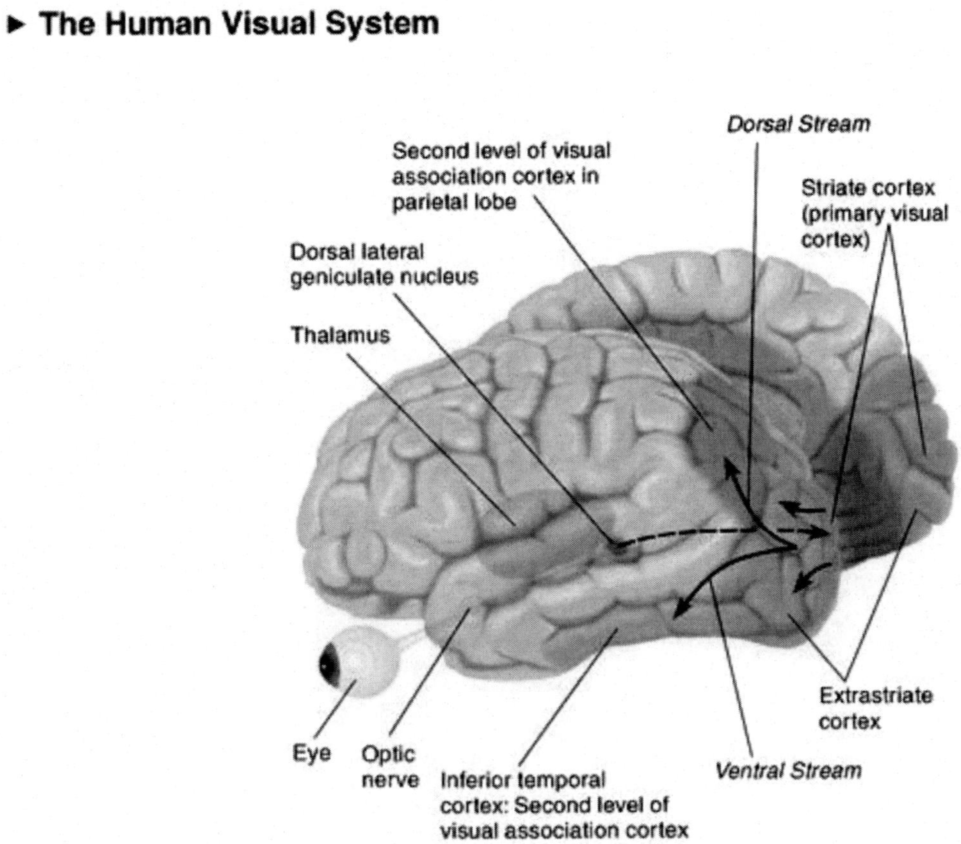


(A)

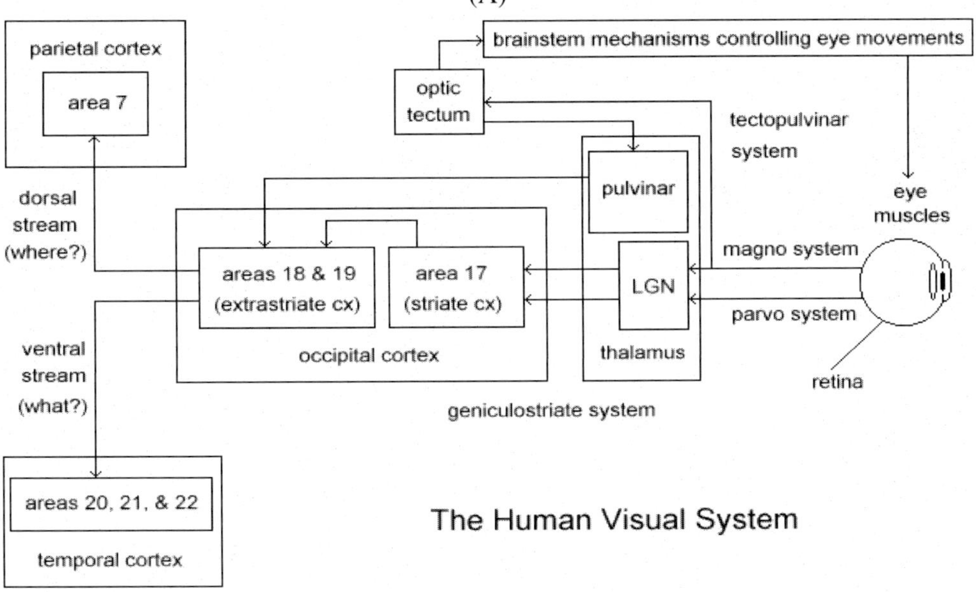


(B)

Figure 6. (Continued)

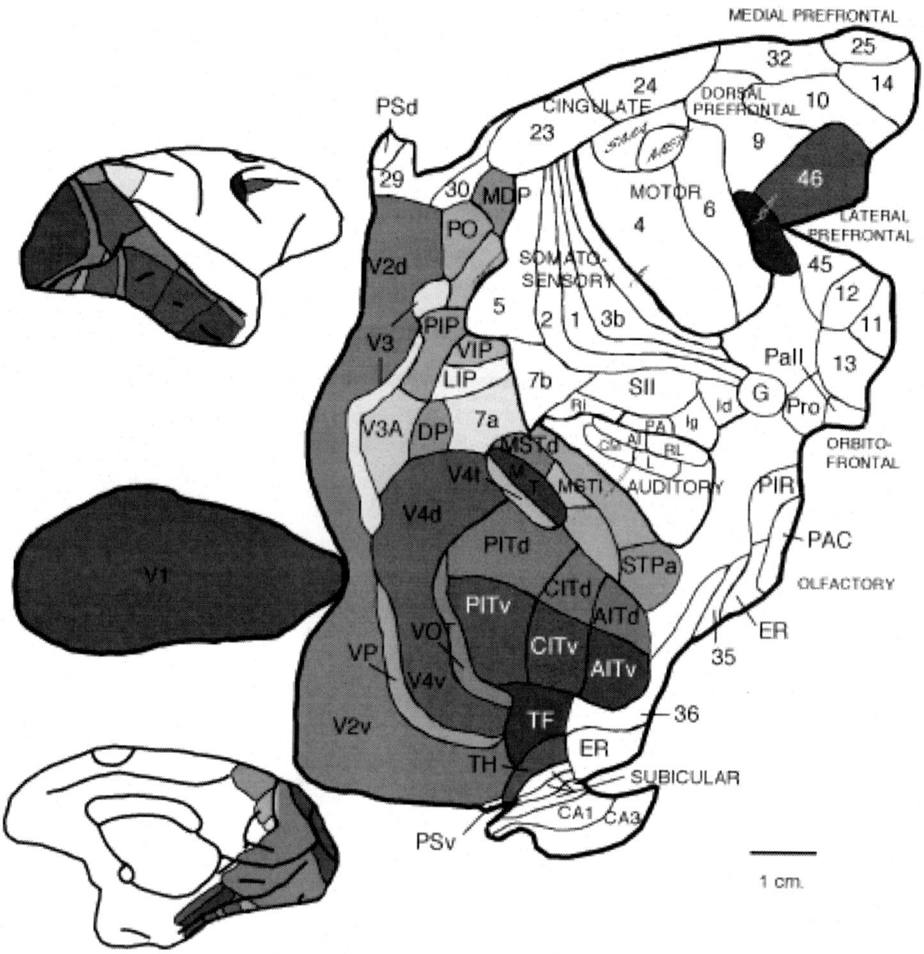


(C)

Figure 6. The human visual system. Goodale and Milner (1992) claim: “two cortical visual systems have evolved: a ventral stream for visual perception and a dorsal stream for the visual control of skilled actions.” (A) Damage to the Ventral Pathway: Their case of D.F. demonstrates a complete dissociation between visual form perception and visuomotor abilities. She can accurately reach for and grasp an object, which she cannot identify. D.F. suffered anoxia and subsequent damage to the ventrolateral regions of her cerebral cortex, with sparing of primary visual cortex and the dorsal pathway. Damage to the Dorsal Pathway: Optic ataxia, difficulty reaching for and grasping objects, often results from damage to superior portions of the parietal cortex. These patients can recognize and describe objects. Thus, there is a double dissociation between the ventral/dorsal pathways and the grasping/perceptual matching tasks. In the dorsal pathway, motion sensitive cells abound, particularly in the areas MT and MST. Cells in posterior parietal cortex show evidence of anticipating the retinal consequences of saccadic eye movements. Egocentric coding of these cells: Ventral pathway studies show that inferotemporal cortex cells are tuned to highly specific forms, for example one IT area is particularly responsive to face stimuli. These cells have extremely large receptive fields. These large cells are thought to underly object-centered representations. In studies of dorsal pathways in brain-damaged monkeys, deficits in visually guided reaching resulted from damage to the posterior parietal cortex. In studies of the ventral pathway, if the inferotemporal cortex is damaged or dysfunctioning bilaterally, the monkeys display severe difficulties in visual recognition and discrimination learning tasks. (B) The human visual system’s network of pathways. (C) Visual-fugal projections area.

While the aforementioned clinical observations were not examined under controlled circumstances, we can postulate that as these children increased their movement or crawling, they increased the tone of postural muscles and their feedback to the cerebellum and thalamus. This would increase the baseline arousal increase signal-to-noise ratio and neuronal sensitivity so that with greater degrees of motor activity the greater the degree of cerebellar feedback and the greater the effectiveness of sensory perception. The fact that the primary pathways were intact could also be considered a visual neglect syndrome that would be the same as tactile or spatial neglect, which would mean that the primary information may be effective but under-processed and therefore ignored or neglected. This however, would be more characteristically seen in a hemi-field of vision. Besides primary visual loss or visual neglect, there is an asymmetric distribution of visual processes. The specificity of symptoms of visual loss, such as object identification versus spatial localization, or global versus local effects, can help us to localize the problem to the right or left hemisphere and ventral or dorsal systems Ungerleider and Mishkin (101) proposed a model of cortical visual processing based on two parallel visual systems, one thought to be directed ventrally to the infero-temporal cortex, and one directed dorsally to the inferior parietal lobe. It has been shown in monkeys that lesions of inferior temporal cortex produce severe deficits in performance in a variety of visual discrimination learning but not in visuo-spatial tasks. However posterior parietal lesions cause severe impairments in visuo-spatial performance, such as in visually guided reaching and in judging which of two objects is closer to a visual landmark, however these lesions do not affect visual discrimination performance (101). Some cells in the parietal lobe are most active in the monkey when it fixes it gaze on an important object (fixation neurons) other cells fire when the organism is visually tracking a moving object that is important (tracking neurons) while others fire before a visual saccadic eye movement to a significant stimulus (saccadic neurons). Finally, there are neurons that fire when important stimuli present to peripheral vision (light-sensitive neurons) (82, 102).

The ventral visual pathway terminates in the inferior temporal lobe (area IT or TE). In TE area neurons, a small percentage of cells respond selectively to high order complex stimuli, such as faces or hands. Most of the neurons however respond specifically based on object features such as color, shape, and textures rather than specific objects. IT area cells are thought to make up a network of cells that appear to be involved with the representation of general object features. Lesions of the IT areas produce loss of perceptual constancies and loss of visual memories (103). It is thought that memories of visual inputs are limited to a habit learning system that involves the basal ganglia (103).

### *The dorsal visual pathway*

This system provides the basis for peripheral vision, motion perception, stereopsis, perception of three dimensionality based on perspective and shading, and most of the gestalt phenomena of linking operations (104). The dorsal pathway is thought to terminate in area PG of the inferior parietal lobe and intra-parietal sulcus. In monkeys it has been shown that a percentage of cells in the PG area fire when the organism fixates on interesting objects in a particular region in space (105). This is known as ambient vision (102). Some cells in area P6 have been shown to increase their firing rate when the organism expects a stimulus in a specific region of the visual field; this is called the enhancement effect (83). The posterior parietal cortex is involved in the control of spatial attention, lesions or dysfunction in this region impair the ability to orient attention to the contralateral side with presentation of invalid directional cues

(106). The two visual networks that have been described are parallel hierarchies of sequential neocortical cognitive representations, they are not exclusively neocortical however and they are dependent on the function of the limbic system. The ventral system has direct reciprocal connections to the amygdala and to the orbitofrontal cortex. The dorsal system connects to the cingulate gyrus, the hippocampus, and surrounding limbic areas. These connections are thought to provide the integration of emotional, motivational and interoceptive quality of visual perception (107).

Bilateral damage to both TE and the amygdaloid complex produce severe long lasting recognition loss (103). The affective components are added to visual stimuli by connections between neocortical aspects of the temporal lobe and amygdala. Without these connections, it is not possible to associate reward conditions with visual stimuli. The amygdala may also play a role in integrating perceptual and affective memories into a subjective experience (108).

There exist monosynaptic connections from the thalamus to the amygdala (108). The thalamo-amygdaloid system supports premature emotional reactions that are loosely coupled with the stimulus that do not require object recognition. Inputs to the amygdala from multi-modal association areas can be involved in evaluating object information integrated from different sensory modalities (108). The orbito-frontal cortex possesses direct reciprocal connections with the temporal pole and amygdala and is thought of to be the frontal extension of the ventral visual pathway. Severe impairments in visual object learning have been noted because of orbito-frontal lesions in monkeys (109). Learning and unlearning the emotional significance of sensory input may require close interaction with the amygdala and orbital region.

***Dorsal visual processing and limbic system and deficits in consciousness and cognition***

The convergence of limbic inputs from the cingulate-retrosplenial cortex with preprocessed sensory information may allow parietal neurons to recognize the motivational relevance in complex sensory events (85). Monkeys with unilateral cingulotomy display contralateral inattention in visual and somatosensory modalities (109). Right parietal or medial frontal infarcts including the cingulate cortex result in unilateral neglect for the left hemisphere (81) and significant inability with spatial memory in half the world (85). The cingulate cortex may mediate adaptively significant attention as opposed to more spatially oriented attention in the posterior parietal region. Bilateral cingulate infarcts in humans produce an akinetic state and attentional dysfunction. Bilateral para-hippocampal lesions result in decreased discrimination of complex geometric forms and faces.

The right hemisphere is more connected to the dorsal system. The right hemisphere's primary role in humans is visual-spatial behavior. Right posterior regions including the parietal lobe can disrupt visual-spatial behavior. Visual-spatial behavior that is typically disrupted includes visual judgment of line orientation (110), maze performance (111), and the ability to identify objects presented from an unusual visual perspective (112). Other functions of visual processing associated with right posterior damage includes constructional apraxia, dressing dyspraxia and prosopagnosia or disorders of face recognition (111), depth perception (113), spatial localization (111), identification of complex geometric shapes (114) and exploratory eye movements (21). The network of cortical and subcortical regions that control visual orienting in monkeys and humans are functionally part of dorsal visual system and include the posterior parietal region, the cingulate cortex, the dorsolateral frontal cortex, the pulvinar, and the inferior colliculus (85).

The right hemisphere stores global configurations of visual objects as opposed to local features or details of objects. Line orientations are oblique (21). The left hemisphere is associated with the ventral visual pathway. Lesions in the left occipital-temporal regions produce visual object agnosia (112). The left hemisphere is also superior for object identification shown from a usual viewpoint. The left hemisphere is better for line orientation when vertical, horizontal, or 45 degree diagonal orientations are used (21) generation of images of visual objects (115). Patients with left-hemisphere lesions are unable to assemble parts of visual image into a unified ensemble according to spatial and temporal relation such as above-below right-left (115), long term storage of categorical, prepositional, or semantic knowledge concerning an object (115), and analysis of local levels or detection of visual scene, sequential analysis of local information, or high spatial frequency.

***Auditory processing deficits in consciousness and cognition***

Many children with learning disabilities and behavioral disorders are also diagnosed with auditory processing problems. It is most commonly described as a central auditory processing disorder. In this case, many children have been diagnosed as having hypersensitivity to various auditory stimuli (116). Others have been thought to have decreased perception to sound. In most of these cases, it appears that the peripheral pathway is intact and that the problem lies in the central nervous system.

We now understand that spinal joints and muscles have the greatest concentration of receptors that respond to gravity and movement with the largest degree of activity arising from postural, antigravity muscles. We hypothesize that by increasing the movement of spinal joints and allowing those muscles to stretch and contract against the forces of gravity on a continuous basis, we would expect to increase the arousal level of the brain through the cerebellar, thalamic and spinal pathways. The result should be an increase in signal-to-noise ratio and the same level of sound that previously could not be perceived, now is better able to summate and be processed. This is one simple explanation.

The cerebellum and thalamus can influence the perception of sound in the same manner that they are thought to influence vision. The cerebellum and thalamus not only affect the arousal zone, but also the primary, secondary and tertiary zones, through connection to association cortices, prefrontal lobe, limbic system, and the effect on the ability to integrate and temporally bind auditory input with other sensory and emotional events to perceive and remember these events. Besides these global effects, we must consider the fact that as with visual and spatial functions, certain auditory functions are asymmetrically localized in the brain. These specific pathways can also be affected, and hemi-neglect symptoms may arise.

One method that is commonly used to test these asymmetric functions is the dichotic listening task. Dichotic listening is a measure of temporal lobe function (117), attention, and stimulus processing speed as well as a way to measure hemispheric language asymmetry (118). It is thought that auditory lateralization is probably not related to a single mechanism, but is thought to be related to several functions involving both perceptual and other cognitive factors (118). Hemispheric perceptors of sound are dependent on the level of activation and attention. Hugdahl has indicated that the level of right ear advantage (REA) in the DL task is significantly correlated with resting EEG asymmetry. Individuals with larger left-than-right EEG resting activation also had better recall from the right as compared to the left ear in DL

(118). DL is thought to be particularly effective at testing frontal-temporal functional integrity (118).

Dichotic listening has revealed a right ear advantage for consonant vowel (CV) syllables in about 80 percent of subjects and in 65 percent of left-handers. This REA has been found to be significant in children down to the age of five years. The REA for CV syllables is thought to correlate with the left hemisphere advantage for language skills. REA is thought to be related therefore to the integrity of the auditory system as well as to the structural organization of the two cerebral hemispheres. However, it is clear that dynamic cognitive and emotional factors can affect the level of the ear advantage. Also attention, transient changes in activation, and arousal have also been shown to influence the ear advantage. Emotional states especially the threat of negative events have been shown to affect the ear advantage; this is thought to be due to the right hemisphere advantage for negative emotions which change the balance between the hemispheres in activation level for processing of dichotic stimuli.

As with vision, an auditory bias to one side or the other may result in an auditory neglect. Kinsbourne (98) postulated that language activation of the left hemisphere might result in making the neglect associated with right hemisphere lesions more severe because it may increase the ipsilateral bias. On the other hand it is thought that language induced left hemisphere activation may make neglect from left hemisphere lesions less significant because it may decrease the ipsilateral bias. In contrast, emotional words elicit a right ear advantage (119). Stimuli such as pure tones and musical chords yield a LEA or right hemisphere advantage (71).

The REA/left hemisphere specialization for language processing has been postulated by Kimura (113) to be due to four factors: 1) the advantage of the contralateral over ipsilateral pathways in the auditory system, 2) the left hemisphere is preprogrammed to selectively attend to the right side of space, 3) ipsilateral perception is suppressed by contralateral input, and 4) input from the non-dominant hemisphere must travel across the corpus callosum to be processed by dominant hemisphere (120). This concept has significant relevance for examining cerebral organization in learning disabled populations. Issues of attention and arousal are the most intriguing factors known to interact with dichotic asymmetries in both normal and learning-disabled populations (41). Boliek and Obrzut (41) state that, "Evidence derived from neurobiological studies as well as data derived from our current investigations using behavioral paradigms, have led to the conclusion that for a large subset of learning-disabled children atypical cerebral organization and unusual patterns of laterality, attention and arousal may underlie deficits in auditory and visual, language and non language information processing abilities.

### *Motor system influences on consciousness and cognition*

A large percentage of children with learning disabilities demonstrate motor symptoms. These can range from poor tone, poor posture, slowness or unsteady gait, clumsiness, high tone, hyperactive motor behavior, weakness, poor coordination, imbalance of muscle tone, poor eye muscle control, tracking difficulty, poor handwriting, etc. These motor symptoms involve both voluntary and involuntary motor control. The sensory pathways of the nervous system that control motor activity involve the receptors in muscles, tendons and joints that transmit information about various aspects of movements to the cerebellum, thalamus, basal ganglia, somatosensory cortex and frontal lobe. The majority of efferent flow of information from the cerebral cortex is directed to the motor system, but the motor system can only respond appropriately based on sensory feedback, therefore it makes sense that the majority of subconscious input to the brain originates from the same motor system. Therefore, any interruption of the flow of this loop that sends sensory input from the motor system to the brain and then from the brain back to the motor system will have significant negative effects, not just on the sensory-motor system but to motor, sensory, emotional, cognitive, and autonomic functions as well. The majority of this sensory input and motor output is subconscious, and is processed in the cerebellum, thalamus, and basal ganglia. Many functions of the motor system are therefore reflexive, and are therefore a direct reflection of the adequacy of brain activity. For example, resting muscle tone is reflexive and subconscious and while we may be able to consciously modulate it, the baseline muscle tone is a reflection of base output in a structurally intact system.

High/normal tone is a reflection of a highly active, aroused brain that is prepared to process all the sensory input it can get. An individual with low/normal tone has a brain that has a low arousal, is not as active and not as prepared to process information. It would not be unusual to expect therefore that children with learning disabilities often have low muscle tone or motor dysfunction, especially when we consider that the majority of all incoming stimuli and antigravity motor information is processed in the cerebellum and this flow of input is essential to the baseline arousal of the cerebellum, thalamus, and cerebral cortex. If there is any disruption, dysfunction, or lack of development of this loop we would expect to see cerebellar motor symptoms usually demonstrated in most learning disabled children.

The basal ganglia, thalamus, and frontal lobe are intimately connected to one another processing mostly somatosensory and motor input. If there exists a dysfunction of this loop, we would expect to see typical basal ganglion motor symptoms of hypokinesia or hyperkinesia, as well as dysfunction of motor and non-motor functions of the frontal lobe. Although the global arousal and activity level is important, what is likewise important and more often at fault is an imbalance of brain and motor activity. It is essential that both sides of the brain and both sides of the motor system work together in a balanced coordinated way. This balanced function is a product of evolution, the survival of species, and related to the organism's ability to develop goal directed movement. To have goal directed controlled movement it is a prerequisite for an organism to be bisymmetric.

Bisymmetry appears to be an adaptation for motility and therefore applies especially to the locomotor system, including bones, joints and muscles, as well as those parts of the nervous system that controls their action (71). Therefore, balanced activity is of singular selective advantage for the motor system. To have a balanced bisymmetric organism and motor system, one must have a balanced and bisymmetric nervous system. Likewise, to have effective goal directed movement, the brain must integrate the sensory-motor loop with other brain functions that help motivate and direct movement as well as provide fuel and oxygen for that movement. The more goal directed the movement, the more integration is required, and the greater the requirement for stimulus processing to support the increasing size of the nervous system which is devoted primarily to sensory-motor functions. Any deviation from bisymmetry of the motor system results in an imbalance that may result in improper integration of brain function and over time creates an ever-increasing imbalance.

It has been shown that an increase in arousal or activation of one hemisphere (usually contributed by the stimulus) is typically accompanied by an inhibition of arousal in the opposite hemisphere, mediated at least partly by reciprocal inhibitory connections through the brainstem (96). Recent literature also states that when one hemisphere is maintained at a high level of arousal for an extended period, the result is an activation imbalance and the underutilized hemisphere becomes refractory (96). At the spinal cord level, especially in midline spinal muscles, increased activation, or tone, over one side will be associated with the inhibition of contralateral muscles, which will alter feedback through the cerebellum and thalamus to the cerebrum resulting in an imbalance of activation of these structures. In the periphery, the balance of muscle tone can be imbalanced not only from left to right but also in the anterior and posterior direction. In the motor system, the midline postural muscles of the spine and the ocular-motor muscles are primarily controlled reflexively by the medial zone of the cerebellum or spino-cerebellum. This process is mediated by the vestibular nuclei and the fastigial nuclei. These muscles have both decussating and non-decussating controlling efferent pathways so that there exists bilateral innervation or control. In normal situations therefore, these muscles should be equally balanced. However, activation of muscles on one side is usually coupled with inhibition of antagonist muscles on the other side. Decreased activation of the spino-cerebellum will normally result in decreased activation and coordination of the spinal and ocular-motor musculature.

Learning-disabled children quite often are seen to have poor postural tone, and ocular-deficiencies especially saccadic hyper- or hypo-metria (21). In infants, delays in the ability to roll over, head lift, and crawl may be a result of midline postural muscle tone deficiencies or hypotonia. In older children, the spinal muscles must be able to react as shunt stabilizers that are needed to create a stable base before spurt muscle activity of the extremities, therefore apparent weakness of extremity muscles may be due to failure of the spinal muscles to provide stability for extremity movement. Persistent tonic neck reflexes that have been noted in hyperactive and learning disabled children may be due to decreased activation of the cerebellum. Poor spinal muscle tone may lead to early fatigue of these muscles and may result in muscle pain, neck pain, and headaches in children. These children are also known to often sit in unusual postures, shift position, and may this be the cause of fidgety behavior. In an effort to compensate for their instability, they may hook their legs in their chairs.

In the extremities, muscles are innervated in an anterior and posterior distribution. This distribution of anterior compartment and posterior compartment control becomes reversed in the lower extremities during embryologic development so that in the upper extremities the anterior compartment muscles are neurologically the same as the posterior compartment muscles in the lower extremity. Voluntary motor activity is continually controlled contralaterally by the corticospinal and rubrospinal tracts. The reticulospinal tract regulates muscle tone ipsilaterally and this regulation involves all muscles ipsilaterally, which includes midline spinal or postural muscles as well as anterior and posterior compartment muscles. However, the reticulospinal tract also controls the normal balance of muscles so that anterior muscles of the upper extremity and posterior muscles of lower extremity are slightly less activated or more inhibited in relationship to their antagonist muscles. This ipsilateral increase of muscle tone as well as balance of activation of anterior and posterior compartment balance is thought to be a phylogenetic development in humans, which promotes an upright bipedal posture.

Reticulospinal output is under the direct control of descending neocortical activation especially frontal lobe output. Therefore, asymmetric activation of the neocortex may result in an imbalance of global motor tone as well as an imbalance of anterior and posterior compartment muscle activation and inhibition. In the spinal or postural muscles and ocular-motor muscles, this may result in an imbalance and in severe cases in spinal muscles this may result in a scoliosis or curvature of the spine. It may also result in a chronic head tilt to one side. In ocular-motor muscles, it may promote a stabismus or lazy eye that can be aggravated by a chronic head tilt. Subjective clinical reports often indicate that both strabismus and scoliosis are coincident, possibly a result of asymmetric hemispheric or neocortical activation or arousal. Both conditions are often associated with a history of learning disability (15). In the extremities, this may result in a fixed arm or leg on the side of decreased cortical activation or arousal. This results in antagonist muscle weakness as well as decreased arm or leg swing on the side of decreased cortical activation. This condition may also resemble or can be a form of hemi-motor neglect ipsilaterally.

Motor distribution and development appear to also be asymmetrically distributed in the cortex as observed by handedness. The left hemisphere appears to favor fine manual movements, and favors control of distal muscles whereas the right appears to be superior for control of proximal limb muscles and trunk musculature (122). The outflow of the intermediate regions of the cerebellum is directed to muscles involved with the distal portion of the limbs. The lateral region of the cerebellum is directed at areas of the cortex and basal ganglia that are involved with planning and animation of movement. There is thought to be an especially close relationship between the output nuclei of the lateral cerebellum, the dentate nuclei, and the premotor and supplementary cortices, which are directly implicated in the organization, planning, and modification of motor activities (123).

Basal ganglia dysfunction results in movement disorders of which we have described two types, hyperkinetic and hypokinetic. Hyperkinetic disorders present with increased motor activity and tone. Hyperactivity in children is often referred to as childhood hyperkinetic disorder. Hypokinetic dysfunction is often seen as slowness of movement or hypotonia. Frontal lobe motor dyspraxia dysfunction is seen in paratonia, and neurological examination of hyperactive children suggests that they experience more difficulties with coordination and more overflow movements than in control children (124). Studies that used various tests of motor coordination, such as balancing, gesturing, copying, writing, maze tracing, and pursuit tracking reported more difficulties on the part hyperactive children (124).

It has also been noted that a conceptual model linking performance and hyperactivity requires the consideration of factors related to energy supply. It has been suggested that preparatory processes optimize motor adjustment. However, preparatory processes could only be effectively maintained for short period requiring energy resources of alertness or activation. One hypothesis for this is that a low event rate, which causes a longer foreperiod, taxes activation and therefore hyperactive children cannot maintain the activation and the preparatory processes necessary. In contrast, it is postulated that a high event rate, which has a shorter foreperiod, puts less demand on activation and therefore the preparatory processes remain optimized (125). This may explain why in a high event rate condition, hyperactive children perform as well as controlled children (126). It has been suggested therefore that hyperactive children are primarily defective in energy resources, and a motor deficit is a secondary consequence (125).

These results may be interpreted in the context of cerebral asymmetry. The right hemisphere is favored for low temporal frequency movement therefore decreased activation or arousal of the right hemisphere would result in a low event rate deficit and fatigability, whereas the left hemisphere which favors high temporal frequency movements would perform at normal levels. Barkley (127) interpreted performance impairments in complex motor coordination tasks, such as copying designs, writing, maze tracing, and pursuit tracking, as indicative of a motor-control deficit, which, he suggested, was a link to a more central deficit in behavioral inhibition. Behavioral inhibition has been recognized as a core deficit associated with hyperactivity (127).

Much has been written about the role of the basal ganglia in motor and cognitive functions (*cf.* 1). Five frontal-subcortical pathways connect areas of the frontal lobe (supplementary motor area, frontal eye fields, and the dorsolateral prefrontal, orbito-frontal, and anterior cingulate cortices) with the striatum, globus pallidus and thalamus in functional systems, that mediate volitional motor activity, saccadic eye movements, executive functions, social behavior, and motivation (128). It has been suggested that normal basal ganglia function comes from a proper balance between direct and indirect striatal output pathways, and therefore abnormal imbalance or differential involvement of these pathways can result in hyperkinesia or hypokinesia of the type seen in basal ganglia disorders (129).

Regarding motor activity and hemispheric asymmetry, it has been shown that the right hemisphere has a somatotopic representation for sensory input for both right and left sides of the body, as well as an attention control function for both sides of space. The left hemisphere, however, is thought to have a similar pattern for the control of motor activity and intention. Whereas the right hemisphere controls motor activity and intention for only the contralateral side of the body, the left hemisphere appears to have control over the right (contralateral) and left (ipsilateral) side of the body for motor activity and intention. This was seen as early as 1905 when Liepmann (130) reviewed results of 89 patients tested for signs of apraxia with unilateral hemiplegia. He found that right brain-injured patients had normal right hand function while their left hand was paralyzed, approximately half of the left brain-damaged patients showed signs of severe apraxia or dyspraxia when trying to function with their left hands while their right hands were paralyzed. The conclusion was that an intact left hemisphere was not only necessary for normal function of right-sided movements, but it was also important for the normal function of intentional actions on the left side. It appeared that the left hemisphere played an executive role in voluntary motor function for the entire body both left and right side (130).

Interestingly dopamine, which is thought to regulate movement and is intimately involved with mood and motivation, is asymmetrically distributed favoring the left hemisphere. Decreased dopamine activity has been implicated in attention deficit hyperactive disorder as well as a number of basal ganglia disorders including both hyperkinetic and hypokinetic. Dopaminergic brain innervation arises from neurons located in the mesencephalon forming two subsystems. In the cortex, there is extensive dopamine innervation in the prefrontal, premotor, and motor areas and a relatively sparse innervation in posterior regions. It appears that in general there is a preferential innervation in motor versus sensory cortices and association areas versus primary sensory areas. Therefore, it is assumed that dopamine is involved in higher integrative cerebral functions and in the regulation of cortical output activity especially in motor control (131) with conclusions based on anatomic studies and confirmed by findings from lesion and pharmacological studies. These studies show that the integrity of dopaminergic pathways is crucial for the selection and operation of appropriate motor responses and for the coordination of motor with sensory input.

Volkow and colleagues (132) studied brain scans of 30 healthy males and females spanning many adult ages. The brain scans measure dopamine, which they think regulates human behavior including movement, working memory, and the experience of pleasure and reward. They found a direct relationship between depleted stores of dopamine and a decline on tests that measure motor and cognitive abilities. In another study Glick, Ross and Hough (133) examined neurotransmitter concentrations in the left and right sides of various brain regions collected in postmortem studies of 14 normal human subjects. Results showed that dopamine content is significantly higher in the left globus pallidus than in the right globus pallidus. Wittling (131) states, "Neurotransmitters such as dopamine, being more intimately involved in the control of motor behavior and higher integrative functions, obviously favor the left side of the human brain, whose leading role in the control of these functions is undisputed."

Recent studies have described the first direct evidence that dopamine triggers the major symptoms of schizophrenia, including psychosis. Nora Volkow (*cf.* (134)) was quoted as saying "schizophrenia is caused by a very significant disruption of the dopamine system." The area of the brain thought to be targeted by the disease is the striatum, which is rich in dopamine. In schizophrenic patients, findings in visual half-field tasks seem to provide evidence of a left hemisphere dysfunction. Abnormalities in dopaminergic neurotransmission have been implicated in a number of neurologic and psychiatric disorders including schizophrenia, attention deficit hyperactivity disorder (ADHD), Tourette's syndrome (TS), autism, alcoholism, drug addiction, and Parkinson's disease (1, 128). In each of the different conditions, it has been noted that a large percentage of individuals have motor difficulty.

Ayers (56) noted that learning disabled, autistic, and children with ADHD had motor problems as a prominent feature. She thought that this was primarily a result of poor sensory integration especially from the inner ear vestibular system; this is probably because the majority of motor symptoms could best be described as cerebellar symptoms. Ayers referred to this problem as developmental dyspraxia and she is quoted as saying, "Developmental dyspraxia is one of the most common manifestations of sensory integrative dysfunction in children with learning disorders or minimal brain dysfunction." Ayers discussed five aspects of movements and movement disorders that were disrupted in learning disabled children: 1) smooth control of movement such as picking up a pin, 2) postural reactions such as rolling over or balancing on one foot, 3) patterns of movement that are programmed into the central nervous system (e.g., crawling or walking, 4) specific motor skills, (e.g., writing the alphabet), and 5) motor planning. Ayers felt that developmental dyspraxia is a brain dysfunction that decreases the organization of tactile, vestibular, and proprioceptive sensations and interferes with motor planning. The cerebellum in connection with the frontal lobes primarily performs motor planning. The cerebellum is also the brain region that processes tactile, vestibular, and proprioceptive sensations. Children with autism, ADHD, and patients with schizophrenia have all been shown to have structural changes and atrophy of the cerebellum (135). Some of these patients have been shown to have smaller areas of the cerebellum, basal ganglia, and frontal lobes than those not affected.

A subset of autism is PDD, pervasive developmental disorder. Autism is characterized by an inability of relating to other people. The autistic child is often described as being in its own world. Speech or communications is often limited and, if they learn to speak, it has been noted that their speech lacks prosody, or intonation. In addition, autistic children may have emotional problems; sometimes they may show too much emotion and other times there appears to be no emotion at all. It is estimated that autism is a disorder of the brain and behavior that affects 5 out of 10,000 children (3). Autistic children appear healthy but may stare into space for hours, throw tantrums, show no interest in people, and perform perseverative or repetitive activities, like head banging, they may also have their attention drawn to small details and they may have difficulty inhibiting or stopping their actions.

Recently it has been reported that autistic children have subtle abnormalities in body movements or motor activity that can allow diagnosis as early as three months of age. Teitelbaum and colleagues (136) described their findings obtained by examining videotapes of babies that were later diagnosed with autism. The infants apparently showed specific motor deficiencies, which included difficulty rolling over, sitting up, crawling, and walking. It is thought that examining motor symptoms may also help diagnose other developmental disorders like, schizophrenia or attention deficit disorder. Teitebaum's work is important because it reflects a reality about autism that has been missed. We tend to think that it is a problem with the mind. Now that we are really beginning to see how the brain works we know that the mind is embodied. Body is part of the mind and there's no way to separate. Teitebaum, in the same article, commented that he got the idea of looking at autism as a movement disorder partly because of his work with brain damaged organisms. As they recover, he said, they go through predictable stages that reflect fundamental aspects of brain organization. Because human babies also pass through predictable stages of development, he theorized that deficits in the brain might show up in early movements. He notes that none of the autistic babies learned to roll over as normal children did. In addition, unlike normal infants who usually learn to sit up at 6 months, autistic infants fall over easily falling to one side "like a log" and failing to break their falls with their hands. Abnormalities are also seen in crawling and every autistic child shows some degree of asymmetry in walking.

In infants, it is known that the cortex is not completely developed, especially the frontal and prefrontal lobes, which are thought to assist in the control of motor planning. In infancy, the control of movement is centered at the subcortical level, especially in the cerebellum (1). The cerebellum receives information from the motor system, the spino-cerebellum, or vermis. The lateral cerebellum is thought to be involved with higher cognitive function and is especially connected to the prefrontal cortex. The lateral cerebellum, or cerebro-cerebellum, receives most of its input from the cerebrum. Therefore, examining the cerebellum may give us an idea as to which problem is the primary. If the vermis shows an abnormality, lack of development, or atrophy, it is more likely that the motor system is at fault and the developmental lag starts with failure of development of the vermis or its presynaptic connections. If the vermis alone is smaller, then we can think that the problem arose principally after the development of the lateral cerebellum, but initiated by a dysfunction of the motor system. If the lateral cerebellum is affected, then either it can be the result of an intrinsic problem, or an inadequacy of stimulation from the frontal lobe to the lateral cerebellum.

In regard to ADHD, imaging studies over the past decade have indicated which brain regions might malfunction in patients with the condition and that may account for the symptoms. This work suggests that involvement includes the prefrontal cortex, part of the cerebellum, and areas of the basal ganglia. In a study in 1996, Castellanos and his colleagues (12) found that the right prefrontal cortex, the caudate nucleus, and globus pallidus are significantly smaller in children with ADHD. Castellanos' group also found that the vermis region of the cerebellum is smaller in ADHD children. Patients with schizophrenia and autism have also shown structural changes of the cerebellum (137). It has been noted that several arguments support the cerebellum as a site of pathological or abnormal function in schizophrenia. Traditional neuroscience however, still considers the cerebellum exclusively associated with control of motor and ocular-motor functions. This is thought to arise from research on human cerebellar function on patients with cerebellar lesions where motor and ocular-motor signs are the most pronounced clinical finding (138). Previously motor and ocular-motor abnormalities known to be present in schizophrenia have been ascribed to basal ganglia, limbic and neocortical dysfunction (138). Blueler in 1911 (139) noted gait abnormalities in schizophrenia patients. He especially noted the irregular space and timing of their steps. Another unpublished study observed 16 schizophrenic patients at psychiatric University Hospital Zurich appear to show movement abnormalities. It was postulated that the clinical pattern of these patients may correlate to Blueler's observations and that these clinical findings may be blamed on a dysfunction of the anterior vermis of the cerebellum.

Various visual-motor abnormalities especially of saccadic and smooth pursuit eye movements have been noted in schizophrenia, and an increase of dysmetric, mostly hypometric, saccades are a consistent finding in schizophrenia (14). Saccadic dysmetria is thought to be characteristic of lesions in the dorsal cerebellar vermis; hypermetric saccades are thought to result when lesions involve larger areas of the dorsal vermis and fastigial nucleus. A postmortem study (141) showed that an abnormally small anterior cerebellar vermis was significantly more frequent in brains of schizophrenics as compared to normal controls. Furthermore, the cerebellar cortices showed Purkinje cell losses of different degrees and thinning of the granular and molecular layers of the cerebellar vermis.

In regard to non-motor control, the same dependence on sensory input probably exists. Neuroanatomic and electrophysiologic studies show that the cerebellum is part of a neural system that includes the thalamus, basal ganglia, and frontal lobes (46). Ascending projections from the cerebellum to the hippocampus-amygdaloid complex arise primarily from the fastigial nucleus, are bilaterally arranged, and are mono- and polysynaptic (*cf.* 1). It is thought that it is through the polysynaptic connections that the projections reach the limbic system via the ventral tegmental area (AlO) of the mesencephalon (*cf.* 1). The paleo-cerebellum-limbic projections, which are the pathways from the anterior vermis and fastigial nucleus to several areas of the limbic system, have been shown to modulate sensory input to the hippocampus (*cf.* 1) and also shorten or stop seizure discharge produced by electrical stimulation of the amygdala and hippocampus (1). It has been shown that this is a bilateral descending hippocampal-cerebellar projection system ending mostly in the vermian portions of the cerebellum (1). Purkinje cells project from the cerebellar cortex by GABA and inhibit neurons of the deep cerebellar nuclei of the cerebellum (1). According to studies on intra-nuclear collateral neurons of the deep nuclei, these neurons most likely use glutamate as a transmitter and mediate excitation of mesencephalic dopaminergic neurons (1), thereby increasing mesolimbic and mesocortical activity. In addition, noradrenergic and serotonergic projections as well as cholinergic pathways from the fastigial nucleus to the septal region may mediate non-motor functions of the cerebellum (138).

It has been shown that the dopamine $D_3$ receptor is expressed not only in limbic structures but also has been noted in Purkinje cells of the cerebellar lobules IX and X (archi-cerebellum) in rat brain. It is therefore thought that the same neuronal substrates may be involved in motor control as well as in cognition and emotion.

In studies using PET scans of 25 hyperactive adults compared to a control group Zametkin and Ernst (142) found that there was less overall activity in the brains of hyperactive adults, especially in the premotor cortex and superior prefrontal cortex. The frontal lobes regulate goal directed behaviors, a hierarchy of reflexive movements, cross-temporal contingencies, approach and avoidance behaviors, response inhibition, and perseverations (79). Furthermore, the prefrontal cortices regulate goal-accomplishing movements (50). Along with the basal ganglia and cerebellum, these structures regulate primary motor output (79).

The goal directed movements regulated by the prefrontal cortex are complex and have multiple sequences. Luria suggested that following frontal lobe damage, subordinate reflexes are no longer integrated seamlessly into goal directed movements (50). Frontal damage or dysfunction produces two characteristic defects. First patients with frontal damage may have difficulty initiating movements without guidance of explicit stimuli. Clinically these patients are passive and apathetic, reminiscent of children with autism or depression. Second, these patients may have difficulties inhibiting responses to stimuli. Clinically they are distractible and react randomly to environmental stimuli. This is more typical with children with ADHD. Many patients with frontal damage show features of both kinds of deficits (77). They do not know when to move or when not to move (79). The difference is that the primary symptom probably lies in an asymmetric dysfunction of the prefrontal region. Autistic children for example are thought to have left brain deficits, which normally produce approach behavior, therefore with decreased activation avoidance behaviors are exhibited. This would be seen as a lack of ability to appropriately perform intentioned movement, disability in initiating movement or of approach movement. Children with right brain deficits show decrease in avoidance behavior, which is typical of right frontal lobe involvement. This decrease in effective avoidance movement translates to increased approach movements, typical of a hyperactive child.

The right brain also governs attention, and with deficits in response inhibition, the child's ability to focus attention will likewise be deficient with an oftentimes seen consequence of perseverative or repetitive movements, all typical of right brain deficits. Right-brain involved children will demonstrate increased levels of approach movements and repetition that they find difficult to stop, whereas with the intention- governing, left-brain, those children with primary activation impairment in this hemisphere we observe lack of initiative, motivation, or effective intentional movements. Depression, shyness, and lack of initiative or motivation are typical of left-brain decrease in activation or arousal. Increase activation or arousal on one side or the other produces the exact opposite reaction in each hemisphere.

What seems to be demonstrated is an imbalance in the complimentarity of the right and left hemispheres as well between the frontal and parietal lobes of the same hemisphere and attendant subcortical structures. For instance, increase firing of the basal ganglia and thalamus activating one hemisphere will produce hyperkinetic movements and increased activation of that hemisphere. Decreased basal ganglia and thalamic firing may produce hypokinetic movement and decreased firing of frontal areas on that side. Depending on whether the decrease or increase is right or left frontal will determine whether the child exhibits increase avoidance or approach movements. Again, the frontal lobe controls goal directed movement and behavior.

An individual's approach to environmental stimuli is an important aspect of goal-directed behaviors. Dense interconnections between prefrontal cortices and somatosensory, visual, and auditory cortices provide the neural substrate for integration of and sensations (143). Based on monkey studies, it has been postulated that inhibitory interactions between parietal and frontal cortices mediate the approach to and avoidance of stimuli (*cf.* 1). Therefore, it is thought that individuals can choose to approach or avoid environmental stimulation by modulating parietal and frontal lobe activity (79). An important study of patients with frontal lobe disease by Beversdorf & Heilman (144) compared motor dysfunction to cognitive dysfunction using standard tests of frontal lobe cognitive function. This study compared the motor and non-motor functions of the frontal lobe to see if there was a correlation between the two. In the past the motor and non-motor function of the frontal lobe were considered separate and therefore did not relate directly to one another. This study suggests that there is a direct and equal relationship between motor and non-motor deficits of the frontal lobe. Therefore, the degree of cognitive or behavioral dysfunction correlates directly to an individual's motor dysfunction. Therefore, it is postulated that in patients with diffuse prefrontal dysfunction, the inability to inhibit simple movements to simple external stimuli may correlate with the inability to inhibit complex social behaviors in response to complex internal stimuli. If this correlation is accurate, then a motor dysfunction could result in cognitive and emotional dysfunction and vice versa. This also has powerful therapeutic implications because it should follow that improved sensory-motor function should result in improved cognitive and behavioral function of the frontal lobe.

## DISCUSSION

There exists a specific group of children who exhibit noticeable deficiencies performing tasks that require *semantic-linguistic* or *visuo*-spatial skills or both. Characteristics of children with developmental learning disabilities have been well documented over the last few decades and have often been compared to adult patients with known brain lesions (41). It has also been noted that in general these learning disabilities do not respond to classroom education remediation. It has further been hypothesized that these disabilities may be related to a neurodevelopment process primarily affecting the left hemisphere (41).

Laterality hypotheses have been promoted mostly based on studies of infants, children, and adults with known lesion sites. Developmental dysfunction of the same brain areas as seen in acquired disorders, may be the basis of learning disabilities (33, 34). It is generally accepted that individuals with learning disabilities demonstrate abnormal cerebral organization, which includes abnormal or weak patterns of hemispheric specialization (37, 38, 121). It has been shown that learning disabled children exhibit decreased performance on a number of tests thought to measure perceptual laterality, and it has been shown that weak laterality has been found across several modalities including auditory, visual, and tactile as well as two combined modalities such as verbal-manual tasks. It has been proposed that these children exhibit abnormal cerebral organization (34, 37).

The basic assumption is that abnormal structural development of the central nervous system, developed prenatally or during early postnatal development, causes abnormal cerebral organization and associated functional specialization that is necessary for lateralized processing of language and non-language information. It is thought that cortical and subcortical dysfunction develops from abnormal patterns of activation or arousal (34), inter- and intra-hemispheric transmission deficits, or inadequate resource allocation. Decreased or abnormal patterns of activation or arousal will result in a delay or dysfunction of cerebral structure and function that will result in a number of functional problems that contribute to learning disability. It is important to understand the nature of functional disconnection not only to better understand autism spectrum disorder, but to also be able to comprehend how disconnectivities between brain regions informs our understanding of conscious experience.

It is not known which portions of the brain are responsible for cognition and consciousness; what little is known points to substantial interconnections among the brainstem, subcortical structures and the neocortex. Thus, the 'higher brain' may well exist only as a metaphorical concept, not in reality. We have also seen that the role of cortex is (1) interface between the world/body and the conscious self; (2) integration of sensory input & motor output. Functional disconnectivities then represent the behavioral traits observed and reconnectivities may be engineered. The cortical integrating mechanism implicates the temporal-parietal junction (TPJ).

We know that the core region of vestibular cortex is situated at the TPJ including the posterior insula the implication is that the TPJ and cortical areas along the intraparietal sulcus combines information from tactile, proprioceptive, and visual input in coordinated reference frames. The TPJ allows for the perception of the entire body and its parts, biological motion, mental body self-imagery proving the TPJ's role in multisensory perception. This view that the TPJ is responsible of a large degree of functional connectivity has been confirmed by numerous studies represented in figure 5.

Providing a basis for organized connectivities being responsible for adequacy of function and that disorders of those networks can be responsible for defects in conscious experience exemplified, in our case, by autism, we can provide a *gedanken* experiment on the so called *Sprague Effect* (145). The complete removal of posterior visual areas of a hemisphere in the cat (parietal areas too) renders the animal profoundly and permanently unresponsive to visual stimuli in the half of space contralateral to the cortical tissue removal. The cat is blind in the same way as would a human with radical damage to the geniculostriatal system. If one were then inflict additional damage on such a severely impaired animal at midbrain level, then the ability of the cat to orient and localize stimuli in the formerly blind field would be restored. This would be accomplished by removing the contralateral *superior colliculus* or by severing fibres in the central portion of the *collicular commissure*. Adding damage in the brainstem to the cortical damage "cures" a behavioural effect of massive cortical damage. The *Sprague Effect* is a consequence of secondary effects generated at the brainstem level by unilateral cortical removal. The damage deprives the ipsilateral superior colliculus of its normal cortical input. Damage unbalances collicular function via indirect projection pathways, those chiefly from the *substantia nigra* to the *colliculus*, which crosses the midline in a narrow central portion of the collicular commissure. The "restorative" interventions partially correct this imbalance, allowing the collicular mechanism to resume at least part of its normal functional contribution to behaviour, with partial restoration of vision as a result.

The disorganization of brain function can be viewed in the context of functional disconnectivity which, when viewed in a more global form leads us to a better understanding of the nature of human consciousness in the context of interregional communicative ability within the brain and nervous system.

## REFERENCES


[1] Melillo R, Leisman G. Neurobehavioral disorders of childhood: an evolutionary approach. New York: Springer, 2009.

[2] Leisman G, Melillo R. Cortical asymmetry and learning efficiency: a direction for the rehabilitation process. In: Randall SV, ed. Learning disabilities: new research. Hauppauge, NY: Nova Science, 2006:1-24.

[3] Melillo R, Leisman G. Autistic spectrum disorders as functional disconnection syndrome. Rev Neurosci 2009;20:2:111-32.

[4] Aylward EH, Minshew NJ, Goldstein G, Honeycutt NA, Augustine AM, Yates KO, et al. MRI volumes of amygdala and hippocampus in non-mentally retarded autistic adolescents and adults. Neurology 1999;53(9): 2145-50.

[5] Blatt, GJ, Fitzgerald CM, Guptill JT, Booker AB, Kemper TL, Bauman ML. Density and distribution of hippocampal neurotransmitter receptors in autism: an autoradiographic study. J Autism Dev Disord 2001;31(6):537-43.

[6] Hardan AY, Minshew NJ Keshavan MS. Corpus callosum in autism. Neurology 2000;55(7):1033-6.

[7] Hardan AY, Minshew NJ, Harenski K, Keshavan MS. Posterior fossa magnetic resonance imaging in autism. J Am Acad Child Adol Psychiat 2001;40(6): 666-72.

[8] Hardan AY, Minshew NJ, Mallikarjuhn M, Keshavan MS. Brain volume in autism. J Child Neurol 2001;16(6):421-4.

[9] Saitoh O, Courchesne E. Magnetic resonance imaging study of the brain in autism. Psychiat Clin Neurosci 1998;52(Suppl):S219-22.

[10] Aoyama F, Iida J, Inoue M, Iwasaka H, Sakiyama S, Hata, K, et al. Brain imaging in childhood and adolescence-onset schizophrenia associated with obsessive-compulsive symptoms. Acta Psychiat Scand 2000;102(1): 32-7.

[11] Rosenberg DR, Dick EL, O'Hearn KM, Sweeney JA. Response-inhibition deficits in obsessive-compulsive disorder: an indicator of dysfunction in frontostriatal circuits. J Psychiatr Neurosci 1997;(22):29-38.

[12] Castellanos FX, Giedd JN, Berquin PC, Walter JM, Sharp W, Tran T, et al. Quantative brain magnetic resonance imaging in girls with attention-deficit/hyperactivity disorder. Arch Gen Psychiatr 2001;58(3):289-95.

[13] Singer HS, Reiss AL, Brown JE, Aylward EH, Shih B, Chee E, et al. Volumetric MRI changes in basal ganglia of children with Tourette's syndrome. Neurology 1993;43(5):950-6.

[14] Leisman G, Ashkenazi M. Aetiological factors in dyslexia: IV. Cerebral hemispheres are functionally equivalent. Int J Neurosci 1980;11:15-164.

[15] Galaburda AM, Sherman GF, Rosen GD, Aboitiz F, Geschwind N. Developmental dyslexia: Four consecutive patients with cortical anomalies. Ann Neurol 1985;18:222-33.

[16] Kaufmann WE, Galaburda AM. Cerebrocortical microdysgenesis in neurologically normal subjects: a histopathologic study. Neurology 1989;39(2 Pt 1):238-44.

[17] Duane DD. Neurobiological correlates of learning disorders. J Am Acad Child Adolesc Psychiatry 1989;28(3):314-8.

[18] Geschwind N, Levitsky W. Human brain: left-right asymmetries in temporal speech regions. Science 1968;161:181-7.

[19] Leisman G. Coherence of hemispheric function in developmental dyslexia. Brain Cognit 2002;48:425-31.

[20] Heilman KM, Watson RT. Intentional motor disorders. In: Levin HS, Eisenberg HM, Benton AL, eds. Frontal lobe function and dysfunction. New York: Oxford University Press, 1991:199-213.

[21] Leisman. G. The role of visual processes in attention and its disorders. In: Leisman G, ed. Basic visual processes and learning disability. Springfield, IL, Charles C Thomas, 1976:7-123.

[22] Broadbent DE. The role of auditory localization in attention and memory span. J Exp Psychol 1954;47:191-6.

[23] Broadbent DE. Perception and communication. New York: Plenum, 1958.

[24] Broadbent DE. Information processing in the nervous system. Science 1965; 150(695):457-62.

[25] Venables PH. The Emanuel Miller memorial lecture 1987. Childhood markers for adult disorders. J Child Psychol Psychiatry 1989;30(3):347-64.
[26] Pascual R, Figueroa H. Effects of preweaning sensorimotor stimulation on behavioral and neuronal development in motor and visual cortex of the rat. Biol Neonate, 1996;69(6):399-404.
[27] Szeligo F, Leblond CP. Response of the three main types of glial cells of cortex and corpus callosum in rats handled during suckling or exposed to enriched, control and impoverished environments following weaning. J Comp Neurol 1977;172(2):247-63.
[28] Van Praag H, Kempermann G, Gage FH. Neural consequences of environmental enrichment. Nat Rev Neurosci 2000;1(3):191-8.
[29] Luria AR. Higher cortical functions in man. New York: Basic Books, 1966.
[30] Rae C, Karmiloff-Smith A, Lee MA, Dixon RM, Grant J, Blamire AM, et al. Brain biochemistry in Williams syndrome: evidence for a role of the cerebellum in cognition? Neurology 1998;51(1):33-40.
[31] Llinas RR. Neurobiology. Thorny issues in neurons. Nature 1995;373(6510):107-8.
[32] Castro-Alamancos MA. Role of thalamocortical sensory suppression during arousal: focusing sensory inputs in neocortex. J Neurosci 2002;22(22):9651-5.
[33] Dawson G. Brief report: neuropsychology of autism: a report on the state of the science. J Autism Dev Disord 1996;26(2):179-84.
[34] Obrzut JE. Hemispheric activation and arousal asymmetry in learning disabled children. In: Obrzut JE, Hynd GW, eds. Neuropsychological foundations of learning disabilities: A handbook of issues, methods, and practice. San Diego, CA: Academic Press, 1991:179-98.
[35] Orton ST. Reading, writing and speech problems in children. New York: Norton, 1937.
[36] Bryden MP. Dichotic studies of the lateralization of affect in normal subjects. In: Hugdahl K, ed. Handbook of dichotic listening: Theory, methods, and research. Chichester: Wiley, 1988.
[37] Corballis MC. Human laterality. New York: Academic Press, 1983.
[38] Obrzut JE. Defident lateralization in learning-disabled children: Developmental lag or abnormal cerebral organization? In: Molfese DL, Segalowitz SJ, eds. Brain lateralization in children: Developmental implications. New York: Guilford, 1988:567-89.
[39] Lennenberg EH. Biological foundations of language, New York: Wiley, 1967.
[40] Satz P. Developmental dyslexia: An etiological reformulation. In: Pavlidis G, ed. Perspectives on dyslexia. Vol. I. Neurology, neuropsychology and genetics. New York: Wiley, 1990:3-26.
[41] Boliek CA, Obrzut JE. Perceptual laterality. In: Davidson RJ, Hugdahl K, eds. Brain asymmetry. Cambridge, MA: MIT Press, 1995.
[42] Keshner EA, Peterson BW. Motor control strategies underlying head stabilization and voluntary head movements in humans and cats. Prog Brain Res 1988;76:329-39.
[43] von Plessen K, Lundervold A, Duta N, Heiervang E, Klauschen F, Smievoll AI, et al. Less developed corpus callosum in dyslexic subjects--a structural MRI study. Neuropsychologia 2002;40(7):1035-44.
[44] Frank Y, Pavlakis SG. Brain imaging in neurobehavioral disorders. Pediatr Neurol 2001;25(4):278-87.
[45] Cohen L, Dehaene S, Chochon F, Lehéricy S, Naccache L. Language and calculation within the parietal lobe: a combined cognitive, anatomical and fMRI study. Neuropsychologia 2000;38(10):1426-40.
[46] Evarts EV, Thatch WT Jr. Central control of movement. VI. Strategies and tactics in research on central control of movement. Neurosci Res Program Bull 1971;9(1):113-8.
[47] Chiron C, Pinton F, Masure MC, Duvelleroy-Hommet C, Leon F, Billard C. Hemispheric specialization using SPECT and stimulation tasks in children with dysphasia and dystrophia. Dev Med Child Neurol 1999;41(8):512-20.
[48] Arnulf I, Bejjani BP, Garma L, Bonnet AM, Houeto JL, Damier P, et al. Improvement of sleep architecture in PD with subthalamic nucleus stimulation. Neurology 2000;55(11):1732-4.
[49] Halboni P, Kaminski R, Gobbele R, Zuchner S, Waberski TD, Herrmann CS, et al. Sleep stage dependant changes of the high-frequency part of the somatosensory evoked potentials at the thalamus and cortex. Clin Neurophysiol 2000;111(12):2277-84.
[50] Luria AR. The working brain. New York: Basic Books, 1973.

[51] Kinsbourne M, Hiscock M. The normal and deviant development of functional lateralization of the brain. In: Mussen P, Haith M, Campos J, eds. Handbook of child psychology, 4th ed. New York: Wiley, 1983.

[52] Guyton AC. Textbook of medical physiology. Philadelphia, PA: Saunders, 1986.

[53] Banich MT. Interhemispheric processing: Theoretical considerations and empirical approaches. In: Davidson RJ, Hugdahl K, eds. Brain asymmetry. Cambridge, MA: MIT Press, 1995.

[54] Zemon V, Conte MM, Camisa J. Stimulus orientation and contrast constancy. Int J Neurosci 1993;69(1-4):143-8.

[55] Kohen-Raz R. Application of tetra-ataziametric posturography in clinical and developmental diagnosis. Percept Mot Skills 1991:73(2):635-56.

[56] Ayers AJ. Sensory integration and learning disabilities. Los Angeles, CA: Western Psychological Services, 1972.

[57] Leisman G. Cybernetic model of psychophysiologic pathways: II Consciousness of effort and kinesthesia: J Manip Physiol Therapeut 1989;12(3):174-91.

[58] Leisman G. Cybernetic model of psychophysiologic pathways: III Impairment of consciousness of effort and kinesthesia. J Manip Physiol Therapeut 1989;12(4):257-65.

[59] Harting JK. The global brainstem, 1997. URL: http://www.medsch.wisc. edu/anatomy/ bs97/text/bs/contents.htm

[60] Matsushita M, Xiong G. Uncrossed and crossed projections from the upper cervical spinal cord to the cerebellar nuclei in the rat, studied by anterograde axonal tracing. J Comp Neurol 2001;432(1):101-18.

[61] Wyke B. Cervical-articular contributions to posture and gait: their relation to senile disequilibrium: Age Ageing 1979; 8:251-8.

[62] Ramnani N, Toni I, Passingham RE, Haggard P. The cerebellum and parietal cortex play a specific role in coordination: a PET study. Neuroimage 2001;14(4):899-911.

[63] Levinson HN. The cerebellar-vestibular basis of learning disabilities in children, adolescents and adults: hypothesis and study. Percept Mot Skills 1988;67(3):983-1006.

[64] Magnus R. Korperstellung. Berlin: Springer 1924. (German)

[65] Martin JP. The basal ganglia and posture. London: Pitman Medical, 1967.

[66] de Jong P, de Jong M, Cohen B, Jongkees L. Ataxia and nystagmus induced by injection of local anesthetics in the neck. Ann Neurol 1977;1:240-6.

[67] Carpenter MG, Allum JH, Honegger F. Vestibular influences on human postural control in combinations of pitch and roll planes reveal differences in spatiotemporal processing. Exp Brain Res 2001;140(1):95-111.

[68] Dyachkova LN. Ultrastructural Characteristics of Plastic Changes in the Brain Cortex of Rats Exposed to space flight. Physiologist 1991;34(Suppl 1):185-6.

[69] Polyakov IB, Drobyshev IV, Krasnov IB. Morphological changes in the spinal cord and intervertebral ganglia of rats exposed to differential gravity levels. Physiologist 1991;34(Suppl):S187-8.

[70] Aizikov GS, Kreidich YV, Grigoryn RA. Sensory interaction and methods of non-medicinal prophylaxis of space motion sickness. Physiologist 1991;34(Suppl):S220-3.

[71] Gordon CR, Gonen A, Nachum Z, Doweck I, Spitzer O, Shupak A. The effects of dimenhydrinate, cinnarizine and transdermal scopolamine on performance. J Psychopharmacol 2001;15(3):167-72.

[72] Hiscock M, Kinsbourne M. Phylogeny and ontogeny of cerebral lateralization. In: Davidson RJ, Hugdahl K, eds. Brain asymmetry. Cambridge, MA: MIT Press, 1995:535-78.

[73] Vallar G, Bottini G, Sterzi R, Passerini D, Rusconi ML. Hemianesthesia, sensory neglect and defective access to conscious experience. Neurology 1991;41:650-2.

[74] Meador K, Loring DW, Lee G., Brooks BS, Thompson WO, Heilman KM. Right cerebral spedalization for tactile attention as evidenced by intracarotid sodium amytal. Neurology 1998;38:1763-66.

[75] Heilman KM, Valenstein E. Mechanisms underlying hemispatial neglect. Ann Neurol 1979;5:166-70.

[76] Ladavas E. Is the hemispatial deficit produced by right parietal damage associated with retinal or gravitational coordinates? Brain 1987;110:167-80.

[77] Heilman KM, Watson RT. Intentional motor disorders. In: Levin HS, Eisenberg HM, Benton AL, eds. Frontal lobe function and dysfunction. New York: Oxford, 1991:199-213.

[78] Posner MI. A framework for relating cognitive to neural systems. Electro encephalography Clin Neurophysiol 1986;38(Suppl):155-66.

[79] Chatterjee, A. Feeling frontal dysfunction: facilitory paratonia and the regulation of motor behavior. Neurology 1998;51(4):937-9.

[80] Costa LD, Vaughan G Jr, Horwitz M, Ritter W. Patterns of behavioral deficit associated with visual spatial neglect. Cortex 1969;5(3):242-63.

[81] Heilman KM, Watson RT, Valenstein E, Damasio AR. Localization of lesions in neglect. In: Kertesz A, ed. Localization in neuropsychology. New York: Academic Press, 1983:445-70.

[82] Lynch JC. The functional organization of posterior parietal association cortex. Behav Brain Sci 1980;3:485-534.

[83] Robinson DL, Goldberg ME, Stanton GB. Parietal association cortex in the primate: sensory mechanisms and behavioral modulations. J Neurophysiol 1978;50:1415-32.

[84] Pandya DM, Kuypers HGJM. Corticocortical connections in the rhesus monkey. Brain Res 1969;13:13-36.

[85] Mesulam MM. Attention, confusional states and neglect. In: Mesulam MM, ed. Principles of behavioral neurology. Philadelphia, PA: FA Davis, 1985: 125-68.

[86] Leiner HC, Leiner AL, Dow RS. The human cerebro-cerebellar system: its computing, cognitive, and language skills. Behav Brain Res 1991;44:113-28.

[87] Roland. PE, Eriksson L, Widen. L, Stone-Elander S. Changes in regional cerebral oxidative metabolism induced by tactile learning and recognition in man. Eur J Neurosci 1989;1:3-18.

[88] Fox PT, Raichle ME, Thach WT. Functional mapping of the cerebellum with positron emission tomography. Proc Nat Acad Sci USA 1985;82:7462-6.

[89] Posner MI, Petersen SE, Fox PT, Raichle ME Localization of cognitive operations in the human brain, Science 1988;240:1627-31.

[90] Gutzmann H, Kuhl KP. Emotion control and cerebellar atrophy in senile dementia. Arch Gerontol Geriat 1987;6:61-71.

[91] Koch P, Leisman G. A continuum model of activity waves in layered neuronal networks: A neuropsychology of brain stem seizures. Intern J Neurosci 1990;54(1/2):41-62.

[92] Koch P, Leisman G. Wave theory of large-scale organization of cortical activity. Intern J Neurosci 1996;86:179-96.

[93] Koch P, Leisman G. A layered neural continuum architecture in attentional and seizure disorders. Intern J Neurosci 2000;107(3-4):199-232.

[94] Koch P, Leisman G. Effect of local synaptic strengthening on global activity-wave growth in the hippocampus. Intern J Neurosci 2001;108(1-2): 127-46.

[95] Leisman G, Koch P. Continuum model of mnemonic and amnesic phenomena. J Intern Neuropsychol Soc 2000;(6):589-603.

[96] Flannery KA, Liederman J. Is there really a syndrome involving the co-occurrence of neurodevelopmental disorder talent, non-right handedness and immune disorder among children? Cortex 1995;31:503-15.

[97] Prather P, Jarmulowicz L, Brownell H, Gardner H. Selective attention and the right hemisphere: a failure in integration, not detection. Presented at the International Neuropsychology Society Meeting, San Diego, CA, 1992.

[98] Kinsbourne M. The cerebral basis of lateral asymmetries in attention. Acta Psychol 1970;33:193-201.

[99] Hillyard SA. Event-related potentials and human information processing. In: Edelman G, Smith BH, eds. Encyclopedia of neuroscience, 2nd ed. Amsterdam: Elsevier, 1999:679–82.

[100] Malkowicz D, Myers G, Leisman, G. Rehabilitation of cortical visual impairment in children. Intern J Neurosci 2006;16(9):1015-33.

[101] Ungerleider LG, Mishkin M. Two cortical visual systems. In: Ingle DJ, Goodale MA, Mansfield RJW, eds. Analysis of visual behavior. Cambridge MA: MIT Press 1982:549-86.

[102] Motter BC, Mountcastle VB. The functional properties of the light-sensitive neurons of the posterior parietal cortex studied in waking monkeys: sparing and opponent vector organization. J Neurosci 1981;1:3-26.
[103] Mishkin M, Malamut B, Bachevalier J. Memories and habits: Two neural systems. In: Lynch G, McGaugh JL, Weinberger NM, eds. Neurobiology of learning and memory, New York: Guilford, 1984:65-77.
[104] Livingstone MS, Hubel DH. Psychophysical evidence for separate channels for the perception of form, color, movement and depth. J Neurosci 1987;7: 3416-68.
[105] Mountcastle VB. Brain mechanisms in directed attention. J R Soc Med 1978;71(1):14-28.
[106] Posner MI, Inhoff AW, Friedrich FJ, Cohen A. Isolating attentional systems: A cognitive-anatomical analysis. Psychobiology 1987;15.107-21.
[107] Liotti M, Tucker DM. Emotions in asymmetric corticolimbic networks. In: Davidson RJ, Hugdahl K, eds. Brain asymmetry. Cambridge, MA: MIT Press,1995:389-423.
[108] Ledoux JE. Emotion. In: Plum F, ed. Handbook of physiology. The nervous system. Vol 5. Higher cortical functions. Bethesda, MD: American Physiological Society, 1987:419-59.
[109] Leisman G, Koch P. Networks of conscious experience: Computational neuroscience in an understanding of life, death, and consciousness. Rev Neurosci 2009;20(3):151-76.
[110] Benton AL, Varney NR, Hamsher Kd. Lateral differences in tactile directional perception. Neuropsychologia 1978;35(6):354-67.
[111] De Renzi E, Faglioni P, Villa P. Topographical amnesia. J Neurol Neurosurg Psychiat 1977;40:498-505.
[112] Warrington EK. Neuropsychological studies of object recognition. Philos Trans R Soc London 1982;298:15-27.
[113] Kimura D. Functional asymmetry of the brain in dichotic listening. Cortex 1967;3:163-78.
[114] Umilta C, Bagnara S, Simion F. Laterality effects for simple and complex geometrical figures, and nonsense patterns. Neuropsychologia 1978;16:43-9.
[115] Kosslyn SM. Seeing and imaging in the cerebral hemispheres: A computational approach. Psychol Rev 1987;94:148-75.
[116] Geffen GM, Sjoberg G, Mason C, Smyth D, Butterworth P. Manual of the Queensland University Auditory Word Memory Test (QUAWMT), Brisbaine, Australia: Queensland University, 1992.
[117] Spreen O, Strauss E. A compendium of neuropsychological tests. New York: Oxford University Press, 1991.
[118] Hugdahl K. Dichotic listening: Probing temporal lobe functional integrity. In: Davidson RJ, Hugdahl K, eds. Brain asymmetry. Cambridge, MA: MIT Press, 1995.
[119] Ely PW, Graves RE, Potter SM. Dichotic listening indices of right hemisphere semantic processing. Neuropsychologia, 1989;27:1007-15.
[120] Bradshaw JL, Nettleton NC. Monaural asymmetries. In: Hugdahl K, ed. Handbook of dichotic listening. New York: John Wiley, 1988:45-69.
[121] Bryden MP. Does laterality make any difference? Thoughts on the relation between cerebral asymmetry and reading. In: Molfese DL, Segalowitz SJ, eds. Brain lateralization in children: Developmental implications. New York: Guilford, 1988:509-25.
[122] Peters M. Handedness and its relation to other indices of cerebral lateralization. In: Davidson RJ, Hugdahl K, eds. Brain asymmetry. Cambridge, MA: MIT Press, 1995.
[123] Halsband U, Ito N, Tanji J, Freund HJ. The role of premotor cortex and the supplementary motor area in the temporal control of movement in man. Brain, 1993;116:243-266.
[124] Shaywitz SE, Shaywitz BA. Diagnosis and management of attention deficit disorder: A pediatric perspective. Pediatr Clin North Am 1984;31:429-57.
[125] Leung PWL, Konnolly KJ. Do hyperactive children have motor organization and/or execution deficits? Dev Med Child Neurol 1998;40:600-7.
[126] Van der Meere J, Vreeling HJ, Sergeant J. A motor presetting study in hyperactive, learning disabled and control children. J Child Psychol Psychiat 1992;33,1347-54.
[127] Barkley RA. Behavioral inhibition, sustained attention and executive functions: constructing a unifying theory of ADHD. Psychol Bull 1997;121:65-9.

[128] Cummings JL. Anatomic and behavioral aspects of frontal-subcortical circuits. Ann NY Acad Sci 1995;769:1-13.

[129] Alexander GE, Crutcher MD, Delong MR. Basal ganglia–thalamocortical circuits. Parallel substrates for motor, oculomotor, (prefrontal) and (limbic) functions. In: Uylungs HBN, Van Eben CG, DeBruin JPC, Corner MA, Feenstr, MGP, eds. The prefrontal cortex, its structure, function, and pathology. Amsterdam: Elsevier, 1990:266-71.

[130] Liepmann H. Das krankheitshild der apraxie (motorischen/asymbolie). *Monatsschr Psychiatr Neurol* 1900;8:15-44. *(German)*

[131] Wittling W. Brain asymmetry in the control of autonomic-physiologic activity. In: Davidson RJ Hugdahl K, eds. Brain asymmetry. Cambridge, MA: MIT Press, 1995:305-57.

[132] Volkow ND, Logan J, Fowler JS, Wang GJ, Gur RC, Wong C, et al. Association between age-related decline in brain dopamine activity and impairment in frontal and cingulate metabolism. Am J Psychiatry 2000;157(1):75-80.

[133] Glick SD, Ross DA, Hough LB. Lateral asymmetry of neurotransmitters in human brain. Brain Res 1982;234:53-63.

[134] Vastag B. Pay Aatention: Ritalin acts much like cocaine. JAMA 2001;286:905-6.

[135] Fatemi SH, Halt AR, Realmuto G, Earle J, Kist DA, Thuras P, et al. Purkinje cell size is reduced in cerebellum of patient with autism. Cell Mol Neurobiol 2002;22(2):171-5.

[136] Teitelbaum P, Teitelbaum O, Nye J, Fryman J, Maurer RG. Movement analysis in infancy may be useful for early diagnosis of autism. Proc Natl Acad Sci USA 1998;95(23):13982-7.

[137] Ojeda N, Ortuño F, Arbizu J, López P, Martí-Climent JM, Peñuelas I, et al. Functional neuroanatomy of sustained attention in schizophrenia: contribution of parietal cortices. Hum Brain Mapp 2002;17(2):116-30.

[138] Martin P, Albers M. Cerebellum and schizophrenia: a selective review. Schizophr Bull 1995;21(2):241-50.

[139] Bleuler E. Dementia praecox or the group of schizophrenias. New York: International Universities, 1911.

[140] Leviel V, Chesselet M, Glowinski J, Cheramy A. Involvement of the thalamus in the asymmetric effects of unilateral sensory stimuli on the two nigrostriatal dopaminergic pathways of the cat. Brain Res 1981;223:257-72.

[141] Weinberger DR, Berman KF, Ladarola N, Driesen N, Zec RF. Free frontal cortical blood flow and cognitive function in huntington's disease. J Neurol Neurosurg Psychiatry 1988;51:94-104.

[142] Zametkin AJ, Ernst M. Problems in the management of attention-deficit-hyperactivity disorder. N Engl J Med 1999;340(1):40-6.

[143] Barbas H, Pandya DN. Architecture and intrinsic connections of the prefrontal cortex in the rhesus monkey. J Comp Neurol 1989;286(3):353-75.

[144] Beversdorf DQ, Heilman KM. Facilitatory paratonia and frontal lobe functioning. Neurology 1998;51:968-71.

[145] Sprague JM. Interaction of cortex and superior colliculus in mediation of visually guided behavior in the cat. Science 1967;153:1544-7.

In: Considering Consciousness Clinically
Editors: Gerry Leisman and Joav Merrick
ISBN: 978-1-63484-260-0


*Chapter 15*

# EPILEPSY AND CONSCIOUSNESS

***Stefano Cavanna[1,*] and Andrea E Cavanna[2,3]***
[1]Department of Radiology, University of Turin Medical School,
Turin, Italy
[2]Department of Neuropsychiatry, BSMHFT and University of Birmingham, Birmingham,
United Kingdom
[3]Department of Neuropsychiatry, Institute of Neurology, UCL,
London, United Kingdom

## ABSTRACT

Pathophysiological alterations of the conscious states are not uncommon across neurological conditions. In epilepsy, the assessment of consciousness has a central role for the phenomenological description of the ictal states and the diagnostic classification of the seizures. This paper reviews the clinical picture of the seizure types which are characteristically accompanied by altered conscious states, i.e., generalized seizures and complex partial seizures. Useful insight into the neural correlates of consciousness can be gained from the neurophysiological and neuroimaging studies investigating the brain mechanisms of seizure-induced alterations of consciousness.

## INTRODUCTION

Researchers with philosophical, psychological and medical background have long been engaged in the quest for univocal definition for the elusive and multifaceted concept of consciousness. From a clinical and practical perspective, consciousness has traditionally been considered equivalent to the waking state and the ability to perceive, communicate and interact with the environment or other individuals. When referring to epilepsy, the term

[*] Correspondence: Andrea E Cavanna MD, PhD, Department of Neuropsychiatry, BSMHFT and University of Birmingham, The Barberry National Centre for Mental Health, 25 Vincent Drive, Birmingham B152FG, United Kingdom. E-mail: a.cavanna@ion.ucl.ac.uk

'consciousness' indicates the patients' responsiveness during the ictal state. However, such a definition fails to account for other possible causes of impaired responsiveness (e.g., forced attention, ictal aphasia and other transient disturbances of sensory processes and memory) (1). Moreover this definition does not take into account the variations in the subjective contents of ictal consciousness (2). Recent research has highlighted the difference between two dimensions of consciousness: the level of general awareness (quantitative feature) and the subjective content of experience (qualitative feature), which is important for clinical practice and is supported by converging evidence from neurological and neurophysiological studies (3, 4).

## Consciousness: Level and contents

The neural substrates underpinning consciousness can be divided into those necessary for the creation of the content of conscious experiences and those required for the maintenance of the level of conscious states (5). The content of consciousness includes a variety of subjective experiences such as sensations, emotions, intentions, memories and feelings and is the sum of the interactions between endogenous and exogenous factors, like internal attention and the experiences derived from the environment, with associated viscero-motor reactions. Temporal cortex lesions have been associated with alterations in subjective conscious experiences, especially affect and emotions, and further neurophysiological experiments illustrated the key role of the medial temporal lobe structures for the conscious recall of past events and memories. The level of consciousness (wakefulness/arousal) is controlled by ascending ponto-meso-diencephalic reticular pathways and widespread thalamo-cortical projections. Lesions involving these areas produce alterations in level of consciousness that range from impaired awareness to coma and persistent vegetative state (6, 7).

Further evidence has been provided by functional neuroimaging studies: positron emission tomography studies of healthy subjects during slow wave sleep, drug-induced anaesthesia and hypnotic states consistently demonstrated a pattern of selective thalamic hypometabolism. Consequently, the upper brainstem-diencephalic activating system has been established as a neuroanatomical foundation of conscious awareness. In epilepsy, the spread of ictal discharge to sub-cortical structures generates abnormal or disrupted activity in the thalamo-cortical networks and correlates with complete loss of consciousness.

Clinical neurologists traditionally refer to the level of consciousness when reporting the phenomenological description of epileptic seizures associated with 'loss' or 'impairment' of consciousness. Given that the content of consciousness is subjective and personal, it is frequently underestimated in clinical practice. This situation could be attributed partly to the problems surrounding definitions and partly to miscommunication between patients and their physicians. Integration of both the objective level and the subjective contents of conscious states has been recognized as fundamental for obtaining a clear and complete understanding of the clinical alterations of consciousness in the different types of epileptic seizures. Consequently, recent studies have proposed an integrated dimensional model of consciousness, thereby allowing for a comprehensive assessment of the ictal conscious state (8).

According to this bi-dimensional model, different grades of alteration of consciousness can be identified. The most dramatic alteration is its temporary extinction in the generalized seizure, characterized by complete unresponsiveness and absence of ictal subjective experience. Complex partial seizures produce a more variable picture; seizures originating from the temporal lobe, for example, generate intense subjective experiences as a result of perceptive and affective features affecting the contents of ictal consciousness. Contrary to this, in simple partial seizures the level of general awareness is typically preserved, with the contents of consciousness selectively affected by a blend of visual, auditory, somatosensory and mnemonic experiences (9).

## Generalized seizures

Generalized tonic–clonic seizures (GTCS, or 'grand mal' epilepsy) are characterized by unresponsiveness and convulsions, and occur as a result of the widespread activation of both cerebral hemispheres. The tonic phase of GTCS starts with upward eye deviation and axial muscle contraction, in association with a typical electroencephalographic (EEG) pattern (10-20 seconds of diffuse high frequency activity). The following clonic phase shows a rhythmic limb contraction with poly-spike-and-wave discharges at EEG, generated as a result of the activity of large groups of neurons (8). These seizures can either start in a generalized form (generalized *ab initio*) or be subsequent to a propagation of the epileptic discharge from a focal area of the cortex (secondarily generalized). Both types are invariably associated with complete loss of content and level of consciousness.

The most common causes of epileptic-induced loss of consciousness are GTCS in association with typical childhood absences ('petit mal' epilepsy). Absence seizures are characterized by a sudden interruption of voluntary behavior, including slowing or interruption of speech, and cessation of activities such as chewing or walking. The clinical picture includes unresponsiveness and short-lasting staring, usually for 5-10 seconds. Occasionally eyelid fluttering or mild myoclonic spasms may transpire and simple behaviors such as repetitive tapping or counting could be unimpaired during the seizures, whereas more-complex tasks discontinue (10). Like GTCS, absence seizures typically determine a complete loss of both the level of general awareness and consciousness contents. Recovery is usually sudden, whereby previous activity is resumed and there is no significant post-ictal deficit (11).

The dramatic impairment of consciousness that occurs during GTCS usually lasts for a few minutes. Convulsive episodes are typically followed by profound lethargy and confusion that persist for a variable period, lasting from minutes to hours (12, 13).

Animal studies of GTCS based on blood-flow, metabolic and electrophysiological mapping produced different results about the brain structures involved. Some of the studies indicated homogenous involvement of the whole brain (14) whereas other experimental studies demonstrated more regional changes (3, 8). Recently single photon emission computed tomography (SPECT) ictal–interictal imaging studies of cerebral blood flow in secondary GTCS have demonstrated focal involvement of the brain, often in regions of seizure onset (9). Further studies of spontaneous secondary GTCS in patients with epilepsy (9) and GTCS induced by electro-convulsive therapy in patients with treatment-refractory depression (15) revealed that cerebral blood flow increases during the seizure in specific focal brain regions, mainly in the thalamus and upper brainstem as well as lateral frontal and parietal cortex. On the other hand, a reduced cerebral blood flow has been demonstrated in the anterior and posterior cingulate gyrus and in the lateral frontal and parietal cortex during post-ictal phase. Interestingly the intervening regions of the primary sensory and motor cortices are usually spared, which may support the idea that the motor manifestations of GTCS may be mediated by brainstem circuitry. In the rare situations in which GTCS is confined to the bilateral sensorimotor cortex, consciousness is usually unimpaired as is within secondary GTCS following propagation from a temporal focus (8, 16).

Over the last few years, investigations in patients with GTCS, using a combination of EEG recording along with functional MRI (fMRI), have reached excellent standards of spatial and temporal resolution (17, 18). Preliminary EEG-fMRI investigations have suggested that generalized spike-wave seizures could selectively involve particular networks and spare others. These studies have demonstrated a decrease in cortical signal in the anterior and posterior midline regions, and lateral frontal and parietal association areas associated to bilateral thalamic activation (19). As a result of these findings, many authors have criticized the idea that loss of consciousness in absence seizures could be caused by involvement of the entire brain in the seizure discharge (20). The emerging picture is that loss of consciousness in absence seizures results from a disruption of normal information processing in specific brain regions due to focal involvement of the bilateral fronto-parietal association cortex and related sub-cortical structures (3, 8).

## Complex partial seizures

In partial epileptic seizures (focal seizures), abnormal discharges may remain localized to the specific area where it takes origin or can secondarily spread to other parts of the brain. Usually clinical manifestations correlate to the area of the cortex in which the seizure originates, the extent of its propagation and the duration of the attack. According to consciousness assessment, partial epileptic seizures can be classified into two categories: simple partial seizures, in which consciousness is preserved, and complex partial seizures, which are characterized by a loss of consciousness. Complex partial seizures can present with a variable degree of consciousness impairment. In the majority of cases they originate from the temporal lobe, frequently associated to pathological changes such as mesial temporal sclerosis.

Complex partial seizures of temporal lobe origin typically commence with premonitory symptoms (lip-smacking automatisms, rising abdominal sensation or fear) referred to as 'epileptic aura' (21). These seizures can last from 10-15 seconds to 1-3 minutes. During this period of time, the patient progressively loses contact with the environment, showing unresponsiveness and fixed stare. EEG recordings are characterized by 5-7 Hz rhythmical epileptiform activity from the temporal lobe, with some bilateral slowing. When the seizure ends it is still possible to present with a degree of impairment of consciousness for several minutes, known as postictal period.

John Hughlings-Jackson first observed that epileptic activity arising from the temporal lobe can create subjective experiential phenomena in the patient's mind (22). These experiences range between mnemonic, affective and composite perceptual phenomena, like hallucinations and illusions involving most commonly sight and hearing. The affective components of experiential phenomena, also called 'epileptic qualia' (1), include both unpleasant (fear, guilt, sadness) and pleasant (euphoria, joy, excitement) subjective feelings, along with symptoms of depersonalization (altered sense of self) and derealization (altered experience of the external world). Specific alterations of the contents of consciousness can occur also as an isolated phenomenon in simple partial seizures with experiential symptoms. Although experiential phenomena were originally described following stimulation of the temporal neocortex, subsequent studies have suggested that they can be elicited during medial temporal lobe stimulation, discharges and seizures. Specifically, activation of the limbic components of the medial temporal lobe, including the amygdala, have been proposed to be responsible for the affective component of experiential phenomena (1, 3). These ictal manifestations have been an informative source of evidence on regional brain function and raise relevant theoretical questions, in particular that of whether they represent a direct manifestation of ictal activity or are rather the result of disinhibition of connected neural systems by the ictal activity.

SPECT and EEG studies have demonstrated that in complex partial seizures bilateral involvement of the association cortices is important for loss of consciousness (23-25). A 'network inhibition hypothesis' has been formulated to explain how consciousness could be impaired within complex partial (4, 23). This hypothesis suggests that focal seizures that arising in the medial temporal lobe could spread to subcortical structures (ponto-mesencephalic reticular formation and medial diencephalon), disrupting their activating function on the cerebral cortex. This results in widespread inhibition of non-seizing regions of the frontal and parietal association cortex. Fronto-parietal network inhibition is ultimately responsible for the loss of consciousness in the late ictal and immediate postictal phase of some complex partial seizures. The results of an increasingly large number of studies provide support to this sophisticated model of selective network inhibition. In addition, functional imaging studies using ictal SPECT have highlighted the pivotal role of medial temporal and midline sub-cortical connections in limbic complex partial seizures with experiential contents (25). Further investigations with SPECT techniques have identified consistent changes outside the temporal lobe, namely increases in cerebral blood flow in the upper brain stem and medial thalamus and hypoperfusion in the anterior and posterior midline regions and fronto-parietal association cortex (26).

An ictal-interictal investigation in patients with surgically confirmed mesial temporal sclerosis tested this model through analysis of cerebral blood flow changes while performing continuous video-EEG monitoring (27). It was found that seizures associated with loss of consciousness (complex partial seizures) induced increases in cerebral blood flow in the temporal lobe and in midbrain sub-cortical structures, including mediodorsal thalamus and upper brainstem, accompanied by decreases in the frontal and parietal association cortex bilaterally (lateral prefrontal, anterior cingulate, orbital frontal, and lateral parietal cortex). In contrast, partial seizures which remained confined to the temporal lobes were found to be associated with preservation of consciousness (3, 8).

Ictal EEG recordings obtained from patients during temporal lobe seizures with impaired responsiveness showed marked slowing in bilateral frontal and parietal association cortices, which was particularly prominent in the late ictal phase and extending into the early postictal period (28). Taken together, the results of these studies provide solid support to the hypothesis that loss of consciousness in temporal lobe seizures could arise from a widespread inhibition of the fronto-parietal cortex, consequent to an abnormal activity in the midline cortical structures (diencephalic activating systems and upper brainstem).

Furthermore, cases of patients with specific epileptogenic lesions of the mesial temporal lobe have consistently shown that the contents and the level of consciousness may vary separately (29). For example, limbic status epilepticus can be characterized by high levels of arousal associated with diminished contents of consciousness (30).

## CONCLUSION

The concept of consciousness is central to epileptology, despite the methodological difficulties concerning its application to multifaceted ictal phenomenology. Both aspects of consciousness (level and content) could be affected to different degrees during almost any type of epileptic seizures. Furthermore, the differences in ictal semiology between patients with epilepsy can offer unique chances for understanding the relationship between impaired conscious state and altered brain function. Different neural mechanisms have been shown to underlie the level and the content of consciousness. Alteration of the general level of awareness seems to relate to either primary (generalized seizures) or secondary (focal seizures) involvement of subcortical structures. This in turn leads to transient disruption of fronto-parietal and midline interhemispheric associative networks. On the other hand, the qualitative features of consciousness (subjective contents) are mainly regulated by the activity of limbic components of the temporal lobe.

Information on cerebral localization of seizures, acquired with neurophysiological investigations and functional neuroimaging studies, will prove useful in the formulation of refined diagnostic and therapeutic protocols for epileptic seizures. The importance of dissecting epilepsy-induced impairments of consciousness along the level-versus-content dichotomy should not be underestimated. The investigation of the specific neurobiological changes in the networks involved in impairment of consciousness in epilepsy could lead to the development of targeted treatment strategies, such as new medications and deep brain stimulators aimed at preserving consciousness in patients with medically refractory epilepsy.

Further investigations in both humans and animal models will be necessary to improve our understanding of the brain mechanisms underlying impairment of consciousness in different neurological conditions. Particular attention should be paid to the investigation of the differences and similarities of brain involvement between conditions primarily affecting the general level of awareness (coma, vegetative states, generalized seizures) and conditions associated with more complex changes in the subjective contents of experience (complex partial seizures).

## ACKNOWLEDGMENTS

This work is dedicated to the loving memory of Dr M Ordicchio.

## REFERENCES


[1] Monaco F, Mula M, Cavanna AE. Consciousness, epilepsy and emotional qualia. Epilepsy Behav 2005;7:150-60.

[2] Cavanna AE. Seizures and consciousness. In: Schachter SC, Holmes GL, Kasteleijn-Nolst Trenite DGA, eds. Behavioral aspects of epilepsy: Principles and practice. New York, Demos, 2008:99-104.

[3] Cavanna AE, Monaco F. Brain mechanisms of altered conscious states during epileptic seizures. Nature Rev Neurol 2009;5:267-76.

[4] Cavanna AE, Bagshaw AP, McCorry D. The neural correlates of consciousness during epileptic seizures. Discov Med 2009;8:31-6.

[5] Blumenfeld H. Epilepsy and consciousness. In: Laureys S, Tononi G, eds. The neurology of consciousness. Amsterdam: Elsevier, 2009:247-60.

[6] Critchley HD. Neural mechanisms of autonomic, affective, and cognitive integration. J Comp Neurol 2005;493:154-66.

[7] Alkire MT, Hudetz AG, Tononi G. Consciousness and anesthesia. Science 2008;322:876–80.

[8] Northoff G. What the brain's intrinsic activity can tell us about consciousness? A tri-dimensional view. Neurosci Biobehav Rev 2013;37(4):726-38

[9] Blumenfeld H, Varghese GI, Purcaro MJ, Motelow JE, Enev M, McNally KA, et al. Cortical and subcortical networks in human secondarily generalized tonic-clonic seizures. Brain 2009;132:999-1012.

[10] Gummadavelli A, Kundishora AJ, Willie JT, Andrews JP, Gerrard JL, Spencer DD, et al. Neurostimulation to improve level of consciousness in patients with epilepsy. Neurosurg Focus 2015;38(6):E10. doi: 10.3171/2015.3.FOCUS1535.

[11] Laureys S, ed. The boundaries of consciousness: neurobiology and neuropathology. Amsterdam: Elsevier, 2005.

[12] Zappulla RA. Epilepsy and consciousness. Semin Neurol 2007;17:113–9.

[13] Tononi G, Koch C. The neural correlates of consciousness: an update. Ann NY Acad Sci 2008;1124:239–61.

[14] Engel J Jr, Kuhl DE, Phelps ME. Patterns of human local cerebral glucose metabolism during epileptic seizures. Science 1982;218:64-6.

[15] Enev M, McNally KA, Varghese G, Zubal IG, Ostroff RB, Blumenfeld H. Imaging onset and propagation of ECT-induced seizures. Epilepsia 2007; 48:238–44.

[16] Nogueira RG, Sheth KN, Duffy FH, Helmers SL, Bromfield EB. Bilateral tonic–clonic seizures with temporal onset and preservation of consciousness. Neurology 2008;70:2188–90.

[17] Hamandi K, Salek-Haddadi A, Laufs H, Liston A, Friston K, Fish DR, et al. EEG-fMRI of idiopathic and secondarily generalized epilepsies. Neuroimage 2006;31:1700-10.

[18] Laufs H, Lengler U, Hamandi K, Kleinschmidt A, Krakow K. Generalized spike-and-wave discharges and resting state brain activity by using eeG/fMri in a patient with absence seizures. Epilepsia 2006;47:444–8.

[19] Van Luijtelaar G and Sitnikova E. Global and focal aspects of absence epilepsy: the contribution of genetic models. Neurosci Biobehav Rev 2006;30:983–1003.

[20] Blumenfeld H, Taylor J. Why do seizures cause loss of consciousness? Neuroscientist 2003;9:301-10.

[21] Alvarez-Silva S, Alvarez-Silva I, Alvarez-Rodriguez J, Perez-Echeverria MJ, Campayo-Martinez A, Rodriguez-Fernandez FL. Epileptic consciousness: concept and meaning of aura. Epilepsy Behav 2006;8:527-33.

[22] Vignal JP, Maillard L, McGonigal A, Chauvel P. The dreamy state: hallucinations of autobiographic memory evoked by temporal lobe stimulations and seizures. Brain 2007;130:88–99.

[23] Norden AD, Blumenfeld H. The role of subcortical structures in human epilepsy. Epilepsy Behav 2002;3:219-31.

[24] Lux S, Kurthen M, Helmstaedter C, Hartje W, Reuber M, Elger CE. The localizing value of ictal consciousness and its constituent functions: a video-EEG study in patients with focal epilepsy. Brain 2002;125:2691–8.

[25] Lee KH, Meador KJ, Park YD, King DW, Murro AM, Pillai JJ, et al. Pathophysiology of altered consciousness during seizures: subtraction SPECT study. Neurology 2002;59:841-6.

[26] McNally KA, Paige AL, Varghese G, Zhang H, Novotny EJ Jr, Spencer SS, et al. Localizing value of ictal-interictal SPECT analyzed by SPM (ISAS). Epilepsia 2005;46:1450-64.

[27] Blumenfeld H, McNally KA, Vanderhill SD, Paige AL, Chung R, Davis K, et al. Positive and negative network correlations in temporal lobe epilepsy. Cereb Cortex 2004;14:892-902.

[28] Blumenfeld H, Rivera M, McNally KA, Davis K, Spencer DD, Spencer SS. Ictal neocortical slowing in temporal lobe epilepsy. Neurology 2004;63:1015-21.

[29] Shin WC, Hong SB, Tae WS, Kim SE. Ictal hyperperfusion patterns according to the progression of temporal lobe seizures. Neurology 2002;58:373-80.

[30] Engel J. A proposed diagnostic scheme for people with epileptic seizures and with epilepsy: report of the ILAE Task Force on Classification and Terminology. Epilepsia 2001;42:796-803.

In: Considering Consciousness Clinically
Editors: Gerry Leisman and Joav Merrick

ISBN: 978-1-63484-260-0


*Chapter 16*

# SHAKEN BABY SYNDROME AND CONSCIOUSNESS

***Dovilė Grinkevičiūtė*, Lina Jankauskaitė, Rimantas Kėvalas and Vaidotas Gurskis***
Department of Pediatrics, Lithuanian University of Health Sciences, Kaunas, Lithuania

## ABSTRACT

In this chapter we aim to study and identify the cases of child abuse and signs of their presentation as well as to determine the relationship between consciousness and shaken baby syndrome in children under 36 months of age. A total of 385 patients met the "high-risk" criteria for child abuse and were divided into two groups: 51 (13.2%) abused and 334 (86.8%) non-abused children. The abused children were significantly younger than non-abused (mean age 6 vs. 14 months); 74.5% (n=38) were younger than 1 year. In 21 (80%) cases, shaken baby syndrome was identified. Seizures, somnolence or collapse, decreased level of consciousness, vomiting, episodes of respiratory arrest or cyanosis, and an indefinite head lump were the main complaints among children with shaken baby syndrome. Retinal hemorrhages were documented in 18 (35.3%) cases of the abused group and only 2 (0.8%) cases of the non-abused group. Physicians examining a child aged less than 3 years with unexplainable respiratory arrest, seizures, decreased level of consciousness should be aware of child abuse.

## INTRODUCTION

Physical abuse in children is a challenging condition for a clinician to be diagnosed. It is a condition that recognized on time can be life-saving. The identification of suspected abuse is essential not only to treat the present condition, but also to protect the child from a

* Correspondence: Dovilė Grinkevičiūtė, Department of Pediatrics, Lithuanian University of Health Sciences, Eivenių 2, Kaunas 50009, Lithuania. E-mail: dovilgrin@hotmail.com

subsequent, perhaps more serious, trauma. Despite the variety of different legislation regarding child abuse, children maltreatment remains underdiagnosed and underreported in the countries worldwide (1).

There are 4 classes of child maltreatment: physical abuse, sexual abuse, psychological abuse, and neglect. Physical abuse is characterized by physical injury (e.g., bruises, fractures, tissue disruption), which result from hitting, punching, beating, kicking, biting, burning, shaking, or otherwise harming a child (2). When evaluating a child who is suspected of being physically abused, it is important to remember that findings appearing to be abusive may result from other causes (3). Besides, very young children can present with milder, nonspecific clinical signs when having experienced maltreatment (4). Discrepancies between the history and clinical findings on a physical examination, denial, and socio-familial risk factors should suggest the likelihood of presumable non-accidental injury.

Shaken baby syndrome (SBS) is referred to as a constellation of inflicted injuries in young children characterized by repeated acceleration-deceleration injury with or without blunt head impact (5). It is also known as "shaken infant syndrome," "infant whiplash syndrome," "shaken/impact syndrome," or more simply, "inflicted/non-accidental/intentional or abusive head injury" (6, 7). Injuries associated with SBS include retinal hemorrhages, intracranial bleeding, skull fractures, and skeletal fractures (8). Head injury is the major cause of death in infancy among the fatalities attributed to child abuse, and it is the leading element of long-term physical and psychological disability (9). Based on different sources, mortality rates range from 13% to 30% (5, 7, 9). Permanent neurological sequelae are observed in up to 50% of survivors of maltreatment cases (7, 10). The brains of infants and young children are more prone to a head injury as the result of angular deceleration than are the brains of adults. The features contributing to the susceptibility mentioned above are as follow: an infant head is relatively large, heavy, and unstable; the neck musculature is weak; the infant skull is relatively flat permitting the brain to move more readily within the skull; the skull is thin and pliable; infants and young children have relatively soft brain with high water content (8).

In our study we aimed to identify the cases of child abuse and signs of their presentation as well as to determine the relationship between consciousness and SBS in children aged less than 36 months.

## OUR STUDY

The retrospective case history analysis was conducted in the Pediatric Units of the Hospital of Lithuanian University of Health Sciences (former Hospital of Kaunas University of Medicine), Lithuania.

All pediatric patients admitted and treated in the Pediatric Intensive Care Unit, the Pediatric Neurosurgery Unit, and the Pediatric Surgery Unit during the 5-year period and meeting one of the "high-risk" criteria for child abuse – age of less than 12 months with the presence of any trauma or age of less than 3 years with the presence of head trauma or any bone fractures – were enrolled in the study. Physical abuse was identified when injuries were unexplained, unexplainable, and implausible or injuries were incompatible with the history given by parents or caregivers. In the retrospective analysis, patients' characteristics, trauma circumstances, main complaints/reasons for seeking medical advice, symptoms at presentation, injuries associated with SBS, and outcome were assessed. The patients were divided into two groups: abused and not abused.

Data were analyzed with the SPSS 13 programme for Windows. For comparison of nonparametric criteria, the chi-square criterion ($\chi^2$) was used. The means of quantitative variables were compared using the Student's t test. Data are expressed as mean ± standard error mean (SEM). Statistical significance was set at $P < 0.05$.

# OUR FINDINGS

A total of 385 patients (162 female and 223 male) met the "high-risk" criteria for child abuse; 13.5% (n=51) of the patients were identified to be abused. The mean age of the patients in the abused group was 6 ± 1.4 months, and 38 (74.5%) patients were aged less than 1 year. The patients in this group were significantly younger when compared with their counterparts in the non-abused group (mean age, 14 ± 0.5 months) ($P < 0.05$). Both the groups were matched for gender ($P > 0.05$). Only 11 (30.5%) children in the abused group had a history of trauma ($P < 0.001$). In 21 (80%) cases of maltreatment, SBS was identified.

## Trauma circumstances

The majority of children in the non-abused group sustained domestic trauma. In the group of abused children, trauma occurred most commonly under unclear circumstances. The distribution of abused and non-abused children by trauma circumstances is shown in Table 1.

**Table 1.** Distribution of abused and non-abused children by trauma circumstances

| | Non-abused n (%) | Abused n (%) |
|---|---|---|
| Car accident | 35 (9.1)* | 0 |
| Domestic trauma | 292 (75.8)* | 5 (1.3) |
| Violence from the parents | 0 | 6 (1.6) |
| Violence from other people | 0 | 4 (1.0) |
| Violence in education place | 1 (0.3) | 0 |
| Unclear circumstances | 5 (1.3) * | 34 (8.8) |
| No data | 1 (0.3) | 2 (0.5) |
| Total | 334 (86.8) | 51 (13.2) |

*$P < 0.05$ comparing non-abused and abused children.

## Main Complaints and Symptoms on Presentation

Neurological symptoms were the main reason for seeking medical advice in the abused group (Figure 1).

Decreased level of consciousness, respiratory arrest, and seizures observed on presentation were more frequent in the inflicted trauma than the accidental injury group ($P < 0.001$) (Figure 2).

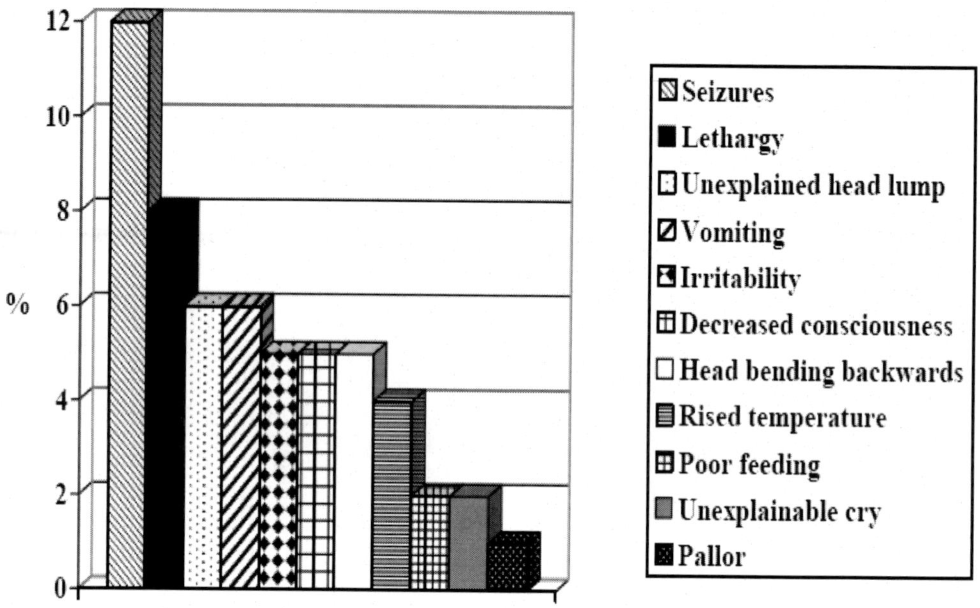


Figure 1. Main reasons for seeking medical advice in the abused group.

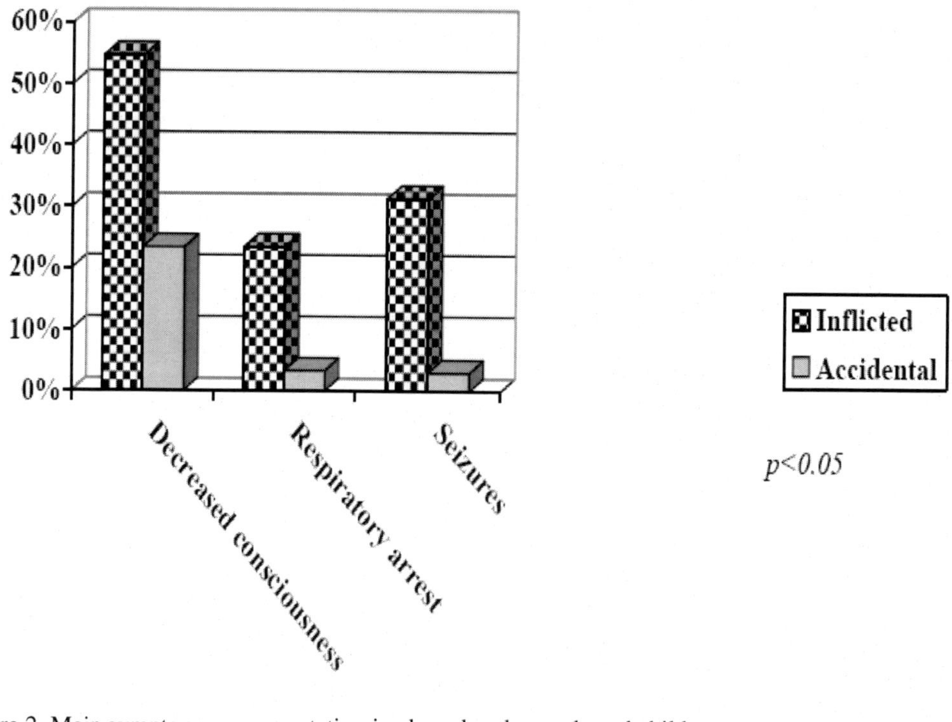


Figure 2. Main symptoms on presentation in abused and non-abused children.

## Injuries Associated with SBS

Injuries associated with SBS were investigated in the study as well. Retinal hemorrhages were documented in 18 (35.3%) cases of the abused group and only 2 (0.6%) cases of the non-abused group. No retinal hemorrhages were found in 26 (51.0%) and 229 (68.6%) abused and non-abused children, respectively; however, 7 (13.7%) cases of inflicted trauma and 103 (30.8%) cases of accidental trauma did not undergo any testing ($P < 0.001$).

Computed tomography (CT) of the head showed intracranial bleeding in 17 (33%) and 7 (2%) cases of the inflicted and accidental trauma groups, respectively. Five (1.5%) non-abused and 2 (3.9%) abused patients were found to have evidence of other diffuse brain lesions on CT. CT scans were not performed in 19 (38%) children of the abused group and 255 (76%) children of the non-abused group ($P < 0.001$).

Skull fractures were confirmed with 2 directional x-ray films of the skull and/or head CT scans; skeletal fractures, with x-ray films. There were 17 (33.3%) cases of skull fractures, 1 (2.0%) case of rib fractures, and 6 (11.8%) cases of multiple fractures in the abused group. The patients in this group had no long bone fractures. Meanwhile in the non-abused group, skull, long bone, rib, and multiple fractures were found in 109 (32.6%), 59 (17.7%), 3 (0.9%), and 11 (3.3%) children, respectively. No fractures were documented in 27 (52.9%) abused and 152 (45.5%) non-abused patients ($P < 0.05$).

The injuries of internal organs were observed in 4 (7.8%) cases of inflicted and 8 (2.4%) cases of accidental trauma groups ($P < 0.05$). The same percentage of abused and non-abused children was found to have facial injuries: 49.0% (n=25) and 45.8% (n=153), respectively ($P > 0.05$).

## Outcome

The mean duration of hospitalization was significantly greater in the abused than the non-abused group (12 ± 1.4 days versus 6 ± 0.4 days, $P < 0.05$).

Artificial ventilation was required in 16 (31.3%) and 17 (5.4%) cases of inflicted and accidental trauma, respectively. The duration of artificial ventilation did not differ significantly comparing the groups: it was 71.4 ± 19.5 hours and 77.9 ± 10.5 hours in the abused and non-abused groups, respectively accordingly ($P > 0.05$).

The patients in the abused group had significantly increased mortality when compared with the non-abused group (13.5% versus 0.9%, $P < 0.05$).

# Discussion

Our study showed that the children identified as abused were very young. Most of the studies indicate that confirmed cases of abuse are mainly found among children aged less than 3 years (7, 11-13). Children at the age of <12 months are most likely to experience non-accidental injuries (6, 7, 14). They are vulnerable both due to their unique anatomical and physiological characteristics, and socio-familial status. The data on true incidence of inflicted injuries or SBS are scarce not only in Lithuania, but also all over the world. The reported numbers of non-accidental trauma cases are only the tip of the iceberg (15). The underreporting of the incidence of SBS could be largely attributed to the fact that a large proportion of the cases occur indoors. Some abused children are not even brought to medical or health care professionals. The establishment of a correct diagnosis is another problem. It is a condition always necessary to think about in the appropriate circumstances, but it is also severe in psychological aspect when being misdiagnosed.

Numerous guidelines and scales have been developed for the evaluation of suspected inflicted trauma (16, 17). Many buts remain. There is still a great number of false positive and underdiagnosed cases and this needs deeper consideration. Another side of the discussion is trauma circumstances and presenting symptoms. Our study showed that most of the children in the abused group sustained trauma under unclear circumstances, while domestic trauma was mentioned as a major cause of injury in the non-abused group.

Several retrospective analyses demonstrated that no history of trauma in 64%–97% of abusive head trauma cases was offered (10, 18). Discrepancies between the history and findings, opinion changing, denial with evident signs of an injury, or presence of socioeconomic risk factors should be the warning signs when differentiating inflicted trauma cases from accidental ones. The symptoms on presentation should suggest the possible cause for seeking medical advice, but most of them can be seen along with other pathologies. In our study, the most common complaints for referring to a medical professional were neurological alterations: seizures, lethargy, irritability, vomiting, or decreased level of consciousness. Most of the abused children will be presented to medical professionals only when caregivers consider symptoms as urgent.

It has been reported that 91% of abused children developed symptoms directly after the injury (6). Our study showed decreased consciousness, seizures, and respiratory arrest to be the main symptoms observed on primary examination. With reference to different literature, the initial findings during a physical examination can vary from assessed as normal to a life-threatening event, which requires resuscitation (13, 15, 18, 19). Excluding or confirming the diagnosis of inflicted injury is always debatable. Other causes should be considered simultaneously. Bleeding disorders and vasculitides can manifest with different bruises and neurological symptoms. Osteogenesis imperfecta and neoplasms manifesting with multiple or spontaneous bone fractures are the entities that may be confused with child abuse. SBS can mimic viral and bacterial neuroinfection. Moreover, some cultural practices at first glance can appear as child abuse (3).

Taking an accurate history of the disease and a thorough primary examination are the essential steps suggesting existing child abuse. Unfortunately a comprehensive history is rarely provided on presentation. The triad of clinical features – retinal hemorrhage, intracranial hemorrhage, and skeletal fractures – has been suggested to be indicative of inflicted trauma (6, 8). According to different data, a unilateral retinal hemorrhage is considered as the most pathognomonic sign; however, the presence of bilateral or multiple hemorrhages is more significant in suspecting SBS (20, 21). The findings of retinal hemorrhages on an ophthalmologic examination always arouse suspicion of inflicted trauma, but do not confirm the diagnosis; therefore, so the absence of retinal hemorrhages cannot be taken as a basis to reject the diagnosis of SBS. In some retrospective series, 60%–85% of retinal hemorrhages were shown to be associated with an abusive head injury (6, 22); therefore, the role of an ophthalmologist having experience with pediatric patients is unquestioned.

Another study carried out in Canada reported that the findings of retinal hemorrhages were associated with more severe head trauma (15). The results of our study showed that retinal hemorrhages were 30-fold more common in abused than non-abused children; however, half of abused children had no retinal hemorrhages at all. According to our study, intracranial bleeding was found more frequently in abused children so it is in line with the results of the studies carried out worldwide. The character of intracranial lesions in general remains open to question since arrival to the health care institution is mostly delayed. Most of the studies suggest neuroimaging to be first line investigation when inflicted trauma is suspected (1, 19, 22), but the benefit of radiation versus CT should be also estimated.

MRI is suggested as a complimentary investigation, when abnormalities in CT scans are found (6, 19); however, in our study, neither abused nor non-abused children underwent MRI. The percentage of children with skull fractures was the same in both the groups. Skull fracture is not a pathognomonic feature of child abuse by itself as it is common both in accidental and inflicted trauma. Discrepancies between the disease history and pathological clinical findings may be suggestive of child abuse (20). Regarding other injuries, two retrospective studies reported that children diagnosed with an inflicted head injury frequently had rib, long bone, and cervical spine injuries, typically considered to be associated with abuse. Abdominal injuries were observed in 4% of the examined children. Other findings such as bruising, scratches, and beating marks are observed as well (6, 15). Our study showed that injuries of the face and internal organs were equally common in both patients' groups, but long bone fractures were documented only in the unintentional trauma group, while rib fractures were more common in the non-accidental trauma group. More surprisingly half of the patients in both groups had no fractures at all.

Various data sources suggest that the skeletal survey should be performed to every child aged less than 2 years, when a child is suspected to be a victim of abuse (6, 12, 19). Abusive head trauma is the main cause of death in children under 2 years of age. In our study, the mortality rate among children with non-accidental head trauma was 13-fold greater and these children stayed in the hospital 2 times longer when compared with children who sustained an unintentional head injury. We did not follow up our children for physical or neurological disability after SBS, but according to different studies, more than 50% of survivors have a persistent physical and/or neurological deficit (6, 13, 15, 19).

Although there are many guidelines and protocols indicating and suggesting the possible investigation plan when child abuse is suspected, the worldwide estimates show that this condition remains underdiagnosed and determines persistent child disablement or death. However, child abuse is preventable and diagnosed timely can be life-saving. Family education to prevent non-accidental injuries, medical staff training to recognize child abuse, medical professionals' cooperation composing an all-in-one team when inflicted trauma is suspected, and well-functioning legislation are the key components of protection from child abusive traumatism. We recommend that every child younger than 3 years with suspected child abuse should be carefully examined when unexplainable respiratory arrest, seizures, or decreased level of consciousness are present even though there are no any external findings.

## REFERENCES


[1] Endom EE. Physical abuse in children: diagnostic evaluation and management. Uptodate.com. URL: http://www.uptodate.com/contents/physical-abuse-in-children-diagnostic-evaluation-and-management

[2] Ricci LR, Botash AS, McKenney DM. Pediatrics, child abuse. Emedicine.com. URL: http://emedicine.medscape.com/article/800657-overview

[3] Boos SC, Endom EE. Differential diagnosis of suspected child abuse. Uptodate.com. URL: http://www.uptodate.com/contents/differential-diagnosis-of-suspected-child-abuse?source=see_link.

[4] Hymel KP, Hall CA. Diagnosing pediatric head trauma: guidance for pediatricians on distinguishing between accidental and inflicted injuries. Pediatr Annals 2005;34(5):358-70.

[5] Forbes B. Child abuse: Eye findings in children with abusive head trauma (AHT). Uptodate.com. URL: http://www.uptodate.com/contents/child-abuse-eye-findings-in-children-with-abusive-head-trauma-aht

[6] Christian C, Endom EE. Evaluation and diagnosis of abusive head injury in infants and children. Uptodate.com. URL: http://www.uptodate.com/contents/child-abuse-evaluation-and-diagnosis-of-abusive-head-trauma-in-infants-and-children

[7] Dias MS, Smith K, deGuehery Kathy, Mazur P, Li V, Shaffer ML. Preventing abusive head trauma among infants and young children: A hospital-based, parent education program. Pediatrics 2005;115;470-7.

[8] Christian C, Greenbaum VJ. Epidemiology, mechanisms, and types of abusive head injury in infants and children. Uptodate.com. URL: http://www.uptodate.com/contents/child-abuse-epidemiology-mechanisms-and-types-of-abusive-head-trauma-in-infants-and-children.

[9] Rubin DM, Christian CW, Bilaniuk TL, Zazyczny KA, Durbin DR. Occult head injury in high-risk abused children. Pediatrics 2003;111:1382-6.

[10] Bechtel K, Stoessel K, Leventhal JM, Oble E, Teague B, Lavietes S, et al. Characteristics that distinguish accidental from abusive injury in hospitalized young children with head trauma. Pediatrics 2004;114(1):165-8.

[11] Tung GA, Kumar M, Richardson RC, Jenny C, Brown WD. Comparison of accidental and nonaccidental traumatic head injury in children on noncontrast computed tomography. Pediatrics 2006;118(2):626-33.

[12] Mandelstam SA, Cook D, Fitzerald M, Ditchfield MR. Complementary use of radiological skeletal survey and bone scintigraphy in detection of bony injuries in suspected child abuse. Arch Dis Child 2003;88:387-90.

[13] Haviland J, Russel RIR. Outcome after severe non-accidental head injury. Arch Dis Child 1997;77:504-7.

[14] Chhabra A, Smergel E, Geller E. Child abuse. Emedicine.com. URL: http://emedicine.medscape.com/article/407144-overview

[15] King JW, MacKay M, Sirnik A, Canadian Shaken baby group. Shaken baby syndrome in Canada: clinical characteristics and outcome of hospital cases. CMAJ 2003;168(2):155-9.

[16] Lindberg DM, Lindsell ChJ, Shapiro RA. Variability in expert, assessments of child physical abuse likelihood. Pediatrics 2008;121:945-53

[17] Jenny C, Hymel KP, Ritzen A, Reinert SE, Hay ThC. Analysis of missed cases of abusive head trauma. JAMA 1999;281(7):621-6.

[18] Hettler J, Greenes DS. Can the initial history predict whether a child with a head injury has been abused? Pediatrics 2003;111:602-7.

[19] American Academy of Pediatrics. Shaken baby syndrome: rotational cranial injuries-technical report. Pediatrics 2001;108(1):206-10.

[20] Levin AV, Christian CW and committee in child abuse and neglect, section on ophthalmology. Clinical report-the eye examination in the evaluation of child abuse. Pediatrics 2010;126:376-80.

[21] Kellogg ND, Committee on child abuse and neglect. Evaluation of suspected child physical abuse. Pediatrics 2007;119:1232-41.

[22] Minns RA. Subdural haemorrhages, haematomas, and effusions in infancy. Arch Dis Child 2005;90:883-4.

In: Considering Consciousness Clinically
Editors: Gerry Leisman and Joav Merrick

ISBN: 978-1-63484-260-0


*Chapter 17*

# BRAIN AND CEREBRAL CORTEX DURING SEIZURES

***Valeriy N Zaporozhan*[1], *Leonid S Godlevsky*[1,*], *Georgiy N Vostrov*[2], *Evgeniy V Kobolev*[1], *Valeriy V Desyatsky*[1], *Irina A Kolker*[1], *Gilles van Luijtelaar*[3] *and Antonius RML Coenen*[3]**

[1]Odessa National Medical University, Department of Biophysics, Computer Sciences and Medical Devices, Odessa, Ukraine
[2]Odessa National Polytechnical University, Odessa, Ukraine
[3]Donders Center for Cognition, Radboud University, Nijmegen, The Netherlands

## ABSTRACT

The relationships between frontal, temporal, and occipital zones of cortex of both hemispheres and paleocerebellar cortex in Wistar and WAG/Rij rats were investigated with an application of multiple linear regression analyses. Taking into consideration the dependence of epileptiform manifestations on sleep-wakefulness cycle, passive wakefulness state was used for data collection.

The process of transition from absence to clonic seizure activity, which was provoked through the administration of sodium benzilpenicillin salt in WAG/Rij rats, was characterized as follows: 1) a preservation of high levels of interaction between brain structures in alpha band; 2) a pronounced decrease of interaction in delta and high-frequency rhythm bands; 3) moderate reduction of interaction between brain structures in the theta range. The increase of the number of connections of cerebellar cortex was marked in the course of transition from absence to clonic seizure activity, which might be in favor for the involvement of the cerebellum in the control of excitability of the brain.

---

[*] Correspondence: Professor Leonid S Godlevsky, National Medical University, 2 Valihovsky Lane, 65082, Odessa, Ukraine. E-mail: godlevsky@odmu.od.ua; godlevsky@ tekom.odessa.ua; g.vanluijtelaar@donders.ru.nl.

## INTRODUCTION

It might be assumed that functional links between brain structures are timely maintained in specific frequency bandwidths of the EEG signal. Such links, for example, might be identified in the course of epileptic activity development. Hence, the facilitative roles of the alpha rhythm as well as antiepileptic effects of high-frequency rhythms are well known (1-5). Therefore it is thought that the investigation of dynamic ratios between amplitudes of signals (in certain bandwidths) can be used to identify relations or mutual influences/ links between structures-sources of corresponding signals. Just with this aim multiple linear regression (MLR) method was used, which is able to identify these links and to qualify them as "positive" or "negative" (6-8). Presentation of the results of MLR application to ECoG signals was performed with so called polycycling multigraphs, which permit to present algebraic equations geometrically (7, 8). The usage of MRL in such way (the investigation of signals originating from numerous cortical zones) was expected to include the neurophysiologic principle of spatial summation, and therefore MRL was initially suspected to be highly susceptible for the detection of subtle mutual influences between areas under investigation. This expectation was in correspondence with the well known fact of reduction of threshold by a dosage of an epileptogen, when it is applied to large cortical zones; this effect can be explained on the basis of spatial summation (9). Hence, gathering information from different zones of brain, affected by an epileptogen, provides us with details, which are obviously missed when restricted zones are under inspection. Thus, early effects of the epileptogens can be detected.

The identification of the cerebellar paleocortex for the investigation was justified by facts of its well documented involvement in the control of epileptogenesis with the net result depending upon the level of epileptogenesis (3, 10, 11). Namely, the low power of epileptogenic excitation is quite susceptible to backward suppressive influences derived from cerebellar structures. More intensive epileptogenesis is prone to be intensified by cerebellar influences as far as local inhibitory circuitries are broken down by powerful epileptogenic effects (10). In any case cerebellar neurons are disregarded as ones which serve as sources of primarily induced epileptogenesis (12). Hence, the cerebellar cortex was chosen for the investigation as far as its role in the pathogenesis of epileptic syndromes might be regarded as suppressive at least in models with low or moderate levels of epileptogenicity (3, 10, 11). Opposite to paleocerebellar cortex, hemispheric cortical structures were regarded as those which served as targets for epileptogenic effects of penicillin. Hence, MRL data was analyzed in terms of the role of cerebellar structures in different models of generalized epileptogenesis.

WAG/Rij rats were used as a genetic model of absence epilepsy, and characteristic spike-wave discharges were regarded as an electroencephalographic equivalent of absence epilepsy (1, 5, 13). A second experimental situation investigated in WAG/Rij rats was the induction of seizures through the deterioration of GABA inhibition with benzilpenicillin (14, 15). Two stages in penicillin–induced epileptogenesis have been modeled. The first was characterized by absence-like manifestations (SWD bursts) and was supported by hyperexcitable states of cortical neurons, including inhibitory ones, while preserved GABA hyperactivated receptors resulted in typical generalized slow wave generation (2, 4). Further increase of epileptogenic stimuli was followed by the breakdown GABA control and exhaustion of local inhibitory mechanisms with generalized clonic seizures precipitated as a result.

Hence, with regard to the role played by GABA, the time-course of penicillin effects might be characterized as opposite: hyperexcitation and absence-like state are substituted with their collapse and seizures precipitation. Therefore MRL was expected to give "opposite" results with regard ECoG-expressed signs of two stages of penicillin induced epileptogenesis.

## OUR STUDY

Subjects were 6-months old WAG/Rij (n = 3) and Wistar (n = 4) rats. All animals were kept at a constant room temperature of 22°C with 12 an hr artificial dark/light cycle and free access to a standard diet and tap water.

Procedures involving animals and their care were conducted according to University guidelines that comply with international laws and policies (European Community Council Directive 86/609, OJ L 358, I, December 12, 1987; National Institute of Health *Guide for Care and Use of Laboratory Animals*, US National Research Council, 1996). Electrodes were implanted into frontal (AP = 1,5; L = 1,8), temporal (AP = -5,0; L = 6,0) and occipital (AP = -6,0; L = 2,5) zones of cortex of both hemispheres under Nembutal anesthesia (40,0 mg/kg, i.p.) in accordance to coordinate of stereotaxic atlas (16). Besides, bipolar electrodes (interelectrode distance-2,0 mm) were implanted into caudal part of paleocerebellar cortex under visual control.

Animals were allowed to recover from surgery for at least 7 days. The ECoG was recorded with a time constant of 0,3 sec, and the following bipolar recordings were made: 1-fronto-temporal; 2-temporo-occipital, and 3-fronto-occipital leads (Figure 1, A). Corresponding leads in right hemisphere were numerated as № 4-, 5-and 6. Seventh lead (№7) was used for bipolar registration of paleocerebellar activity.

Generalized seizure activity was induced with the sodium salt of benzilpenicillin solution, it was administered in a dosage of 300.000 IU/100 g of body weight (14). The ECoG of Wistar rats which underwent similar experimental conditions (sham operation) served as a control group.

ECoG registration in freely moving rats was performed with a sampling of 256/sec. The next frequency bandwidths were investigated: beta 1: 21,0-32,0 Hz.; beta 2: 14,2-18,3 Hz.; alpha: 8,0-12,8 Hz.; theta: 4,0-7,5 Hz. and delta: 0,5-3,9 Hz. The average amplitude of ECoG was used, which was calculated for an epoch of 10-second. Altogether 30 data points were obtained from 300 seconds of registration in each rat. The corresponding data points were averaged for all animals within the same groups and used for further analysis. The entire period (300 seconds) corresponded to the passive wakefulness state of the experimental animals. Mathematical models were created by computer analysis employing MLR and regression analyses.

The formation of a mathematical model was performed employing multiple linear regression and correlation. With the aim of creating mathematical models of each of the amplitude indices under investigation, we obtained the Y-plotted characteristic marked later on in equations (1.1.-1.7.) with YA1k, YA2k, YA3k, YA4k, YA5k, YA6k and YA7k-figures that were in good correspondence to above mentioned number order of bipolar leads. Y-data was calculated on the basis of other variable-amplitudes in the other six leads (X-plotted ones, marked as ax1, bx2, cx3, dx4, ex5, fx6 and gx7). The resultant data permit us to identify the direction and type of proper influence, and to depict it with the corresponding arrow on the multigraph.

As a result of such a process, equations pertinent to multiple liner regression and which were used regularly (on the basis of false-rotation) in our analysis received a typical form:

$$YA1k = Bo + bx2 + cx3 + dx4 + ex5 + fx6 + gx7 \quad (1.1);$$

$$YA2k = Bo + ax1 + cx3 + dx4 + ex5 + fx6 + gx7 \quad (1.2);$$

$$YA3k = Bo + ax1 + bx2 + dx4 + ex5 + fx6 + gx7 \quad (1.3);$$

$$YA4k = Bo + ax1 + bx2 + cx3 + ex5 + fx6 + gx7 \quad (1.4);$$

$$YA5k = Bo + ax1 + bx2 + cx3 + dx4 + fx6 + gx7 \quad (1.5);$$

$$YA6k = Bo + ax1 + bx2 + cx3 + dx4 + ex5 + gx7 \quad (1.6);$$

$$YA7k = Bo + ax1 + bx2 + cx3 + dx4 + ex5 + fx6 \quad (1.7);$$

Where, Bo is a constant factor. Coefficients “a,” “b,” “c,” “d,” “e,” “f,” “g” reflect the level of the influence upon the index which is under analysis of the rest of the members of equation (x1; x2; x3; x4, x5, x6, x7).

The regression coefficients indicate the amount of influence of a certain electrode on each of the other electrodes. The significance of coefficients of regression was determined by the standard deviations of coefficients of regression, the efficacy of regression as a whole (positive and negative links) was estimated by calculating the square coefficient of multiple correlation. In this way, positive and negative links were identified between leads (structures), as well as their direction. The level of statistical significance was accepted at 0,05 (when one-way directed influence was determined) and 0,1 (when two-way directed influences were determined). Geometrical presentation of the equations of MLR was performed in the form of polycyclic multigraphs containing directed positive and negative influences marked with arrows when they were significant. The error calculation was connected with the evaluating of the “power” of corresponding relations.

The multigraph analysis consisted of the following steps:

A. Creation of polycyclic multigraphs on the basis of relationship of average amplitudes of signals registered in every lead, with consequent determination of:
   a. Number of mutually positive (a) and negative (b) intrahemispheric links;
   b. Number and character of links between hemispheric structures and the cerebellar paleocortex.
B. The creation of polycyclic multigraphs in specific frequency bands with consequent analogous analysis as was made at “A.”

## OUR FINDINGS

Background ECoG activity of Wistar rats (control) was characterized as desynchronized beta activity with short and irregular slow-waves. Such activity corresponded to the period of passive wakefulness of animals (Figure 1A).

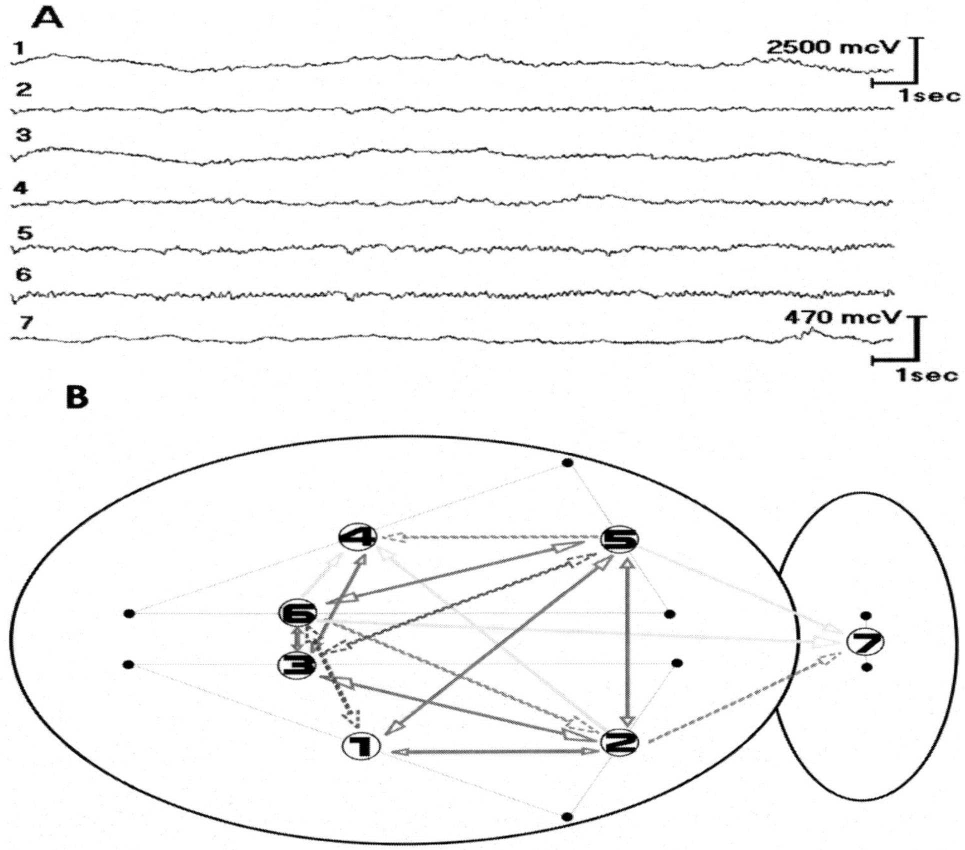


Figure 1. Characteristics of the spontaneous ECoG activity in Wistar rats (passive wakefulness). Marks: on "A" fragment and later on the same fragments of Figures 3, 5 and 7 the next leads are depicted: (1) fronto-temporal; (2) temporo-occipital, and (3) fronto-occipital ones in the left hemisphere (schematically are depicted above fragment "A"); with 4-, 5-and 6-the same leads in right hemisphere are marked; 7-bipolar lead of paleocerebellar cortex. Calibration: 2500 mcV, and for paleocerebellum (lead N7)-470 mcV. Time mark-1 second. A polycycling multigraph is presented at "B" fragment, which reflects relationships between brain structures in Wistar rats. Marks: figures in circles correspond to leads, which were marked on fragment "A." Solid lines (green color)-positive links, and interrupted lines (red color)-negative ones. The direction of influence is marked with an arrow (one way influence-with light green and orange, while two-ways influences-with dark green and red). Figures in circles are located between electrodes (small black points arranged in form of triangles), which serves for corresponded bipolar registration.

The multigraphs of the background ECoG activity in Wistar rats were characterized by the presence of mutual positive links between cortical zones of both left and right hemispheres (total number-2 and 1 correspondently), and 4 positive interhemispheric mutual links were present as well.

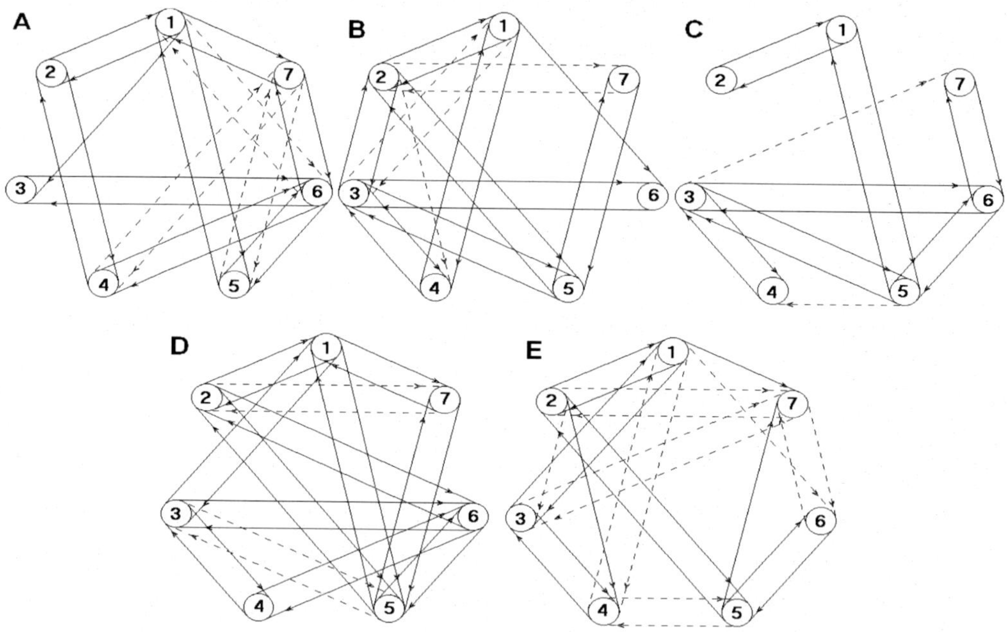


Figure 2. Polycycling multigraphs, which reflect relationships (links) between brain structures in Wistar rats, which were created in different bandwidths of EcoG. A-, B-, C-, D-and E-beta-2, beta-1, alpha-, theta-and delta-bands correspondently. Numbers in circles correspond to leads, solid lines-positive links, and interrupted lines-negative ones. The direction of influence is marked with an arrow.

Additionally, two mutual negative interhemispheric links were also identified. Meanwhile, paleocerebellar cortex did not engage links to hemispheres, but it received two positive and one negative link from hemispheral structures (see Figure 1B).

It was of interest to analyze the level of similarity of multigraphs, which were created for certain bandwidths, and to compare them with the initial multigraph, which was created on the basis of the background ECoG signal. Hence, the total number of mutually positive links between structures in theta-band was quite identical with the initial multigraph as far as 6 out of 7 mutual positive links were reproduced (see Figure 2). In the delta band 4 mutually positive links were reproduced in the range of delta activity, while 5 similar links were reproduced in the rest of the investigated bandwidths.

It should be stressed that a minimal number of negative links was identified in alpha frequency range, and in all cases they were one-side directed. Meanwhile in delta band 5 mutually negative links along with two one-side directed negative links were identified.

Mutual positive links between fronto-temporal and temporo-occipital zones of the left hemisphere were present in all frequency bands; this fact favors a stable functional interaction between these zones (see Figure 2).

It can be concluded that in Wistar rats during passive wakefulness functional relationships between brain cortical structures and paleocerebellar cortex are present mainly in the theta-band, as far as the largest number of positive links was identified in this bandwidth. At the same time, relations between structures, which were identified in alpha band, are characterized by a minimal number of mutual negative links, while negative links were most pronounced in delta band.

## ECoG in WAG/Rij rats

The background ECoG activity in WAG/Rij rats was characterized by generation of spike-wave discharges (SWD) with frequency of 7-10/sec and amplitude of discharges form 100 to 450 mcV (Figure 3A). The average duration of the SWD was 5 sec (with undulations from 1 to 30 sec). The frequency of SWD bursts generation was 15-20 per hour. A tremor of vibrissae along with the accelerated breathing was noted in rats during SWD. Reactions on gentle tactile stimuli were absent as well. Otherwise the behavior of rats during SWD was qualified as immobile, before and after SWD animals were mainly passive, the EEG showed mainly passive drowsiness. For the analysis all naturally occurring periods with SWD were used (Figure 3A). Hence, all measurements and EEG collection for further analysis was made during passive wakefulness state of rats.

Polycyclic multigraphs point to the existence of two mutually positive links between structures of the left hemisphere as well as a single mutually positive link in the right hemisphere (see Figure 3B). It should be stressed that such findings resemble those observed in Wistar rats. At the same time a total of 5 interhemispheric positive links was identified in WAG/Rij rats, which was greater than in Wistar rats, which displayed 4 similar links. Besides, there was only a single negative link while in Wistar rats 2 such links were found. The presence of mutual links of both positive and negative nature between paleocerebellum and cortical structures was noted in WAG/Rij rats, while in Wistar rats the cerebellum did not have an impact upon cortical structures.

Creation of polycycic multigraphs in different frequency-specific bands of WAG/Rij rats revealed the presence of two mutually positive links both in beta-1 and beta-2 bands, which were also present in the multigraph, which was created on the basis of background EcoG signal (Figure 4). Besides, one mutual negative link was identified in beta-1 band, which was present between cerebellum and occipital zone of the left hemisphere, and which was also present in the initial multigraph. In the alpha band four mutual positive links were noted, which were also present in the initial multigraph. Most numerous links common with the initial multigraph were found in delta and theta bands (6 out from 7) (see Figure 4). It is also worth to note that one mutual negative link was reproduced in the delta band, while two of them, which were common with the initial multigraph, were reproduced in the theta band (see Figure 4). In all, the data suggest that functional relationships between brain structures in WAG/Rij rats during periods of SWD are present in theta and delta bands. The smallest level of involvement is observed in beta-1, and especially beta-2 bandwidths.

Significant difference between Wistar and WAG/Rij rats under conditions of their passive wakefulness state was confined to the marked reduction of mutual negative links in the delta band (5 in Wistar against 2 in WAG/Rij rats) as well as an opposite ratio for mutual positive links (5 against 2 correspondently). These facts are in favor of the greater extent of synchronization of processes in WAG/Rij rats in both hemispheres during passive wakefulness in the delta band in comparison with Wistar rats. Interestingly, in high-frequency bands (beta-1 and beta-2) the total number of mutually positive links in Wistar rats exceeded the one's in WAG/Rij rats (7 and 5 correspondently), and this fact might be in favor for the lessening of the mechanisms of interhemispheric interaction in high-frequency bandwidth in animals with inherited absence epilepsy.

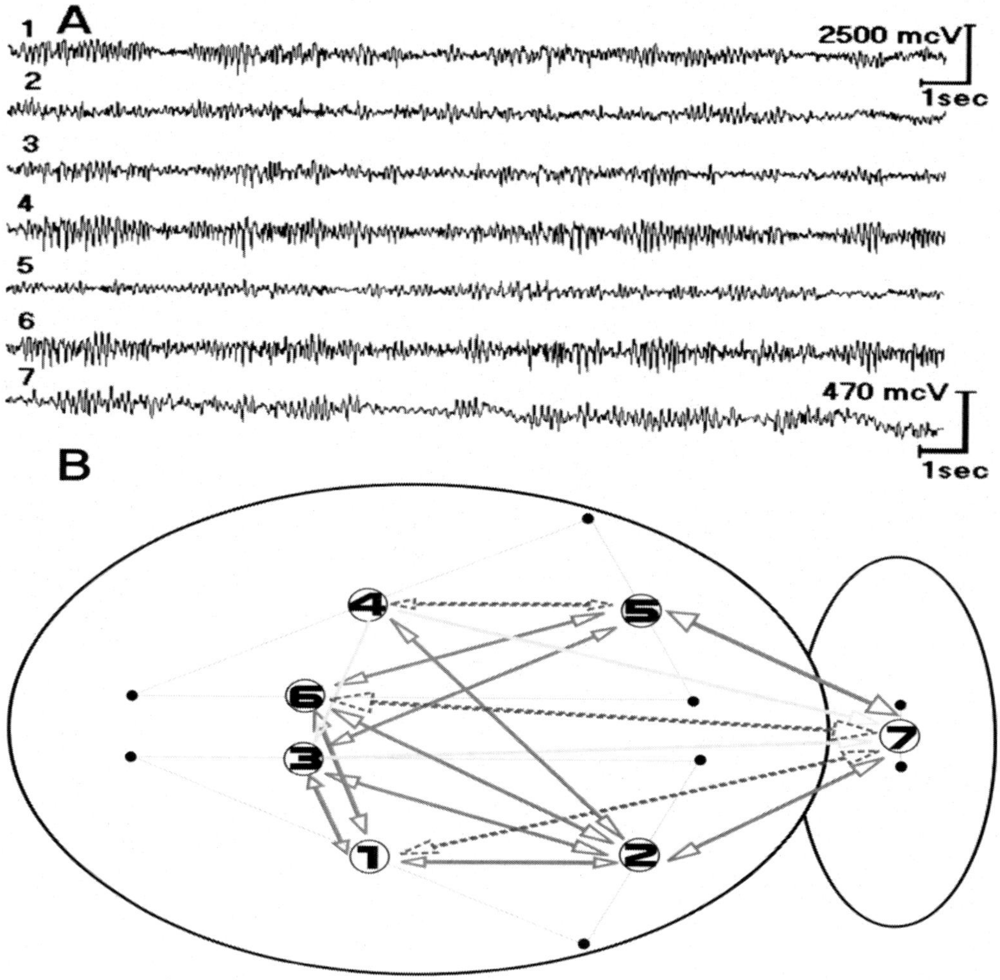


Figure 3. The characteristics of EcoG in WAG/rij rats (passive wakefullness). Marks: on A"-the development of SW burst, which correspond to period of freezing of animals with the tremor of vibrisses and head tilting. Fragment "B"-the same as on Figure 1.

## The influence of penicillin on the ECoG of WAG/Rij rats

The action of penicillin was followed by the net increase of the frequency of SWD bursts up to 3-6 per min in 270-400 sec from the moment of administration. The amplitude of certain discharges was from 300 to 700 mcV, while the duration of bursts was from 2 to 7 sec (see Figure 5,A). The frequency of SWD was from 7 to 10/sec. The amplitude of potentials registered in paleocerebellar cortex was from 120 to 300 mcV, and their frequency-7-8 discharges per sec (see Figure 5A, zone 7). Main characteristics of SWD bursts (frequency and duration) continued to be the same as before penicillin treatment.

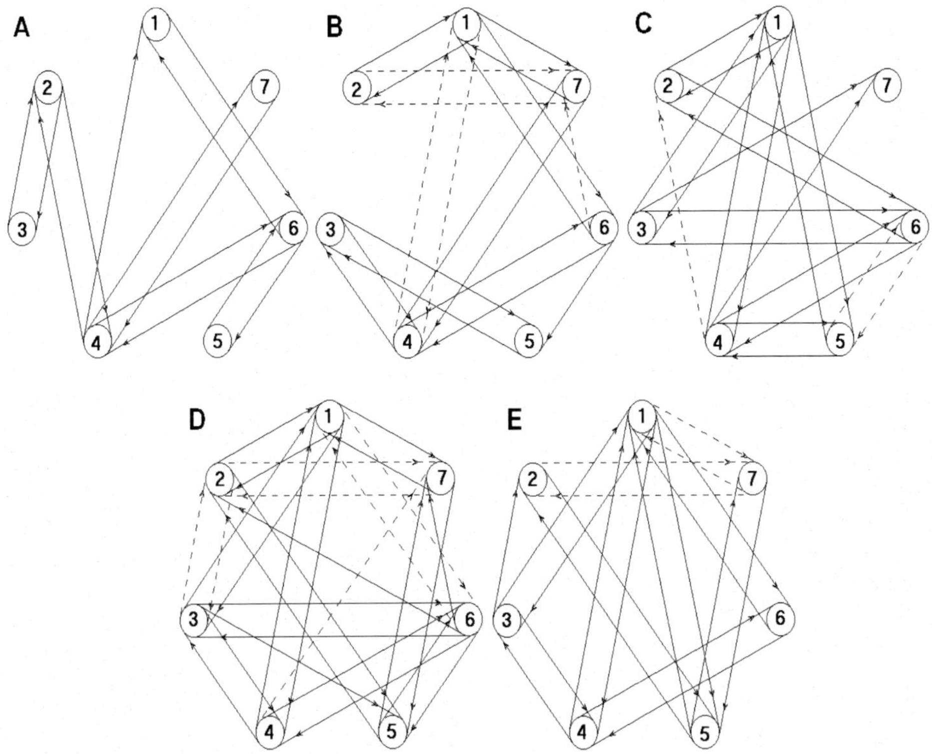


Figure 4. Polycycling multigraphs, which reflect relationships between brain structures in WAG/rij rats in different bandwidths of ECoG. Notes: the same as on Figure 2.

Polycycling multigraphs based on fragments of EcoG, as described above, revealed that all zones of cortex of the left hemisphere were united with mutual positive links. Such picture was not observed in the right hemisphere, where mutual negative type of links was prevalent (see Figure 5B). Negative relationships between paleocerebellar cortex on the one side and both fronto-temporal zone of the left hemisphere and fronto-occipital zone of the right hemisphere on the contrlateral side, were established. It is of interest to note that the interhemispheric positive mode of interaction was presented in the form of four mutual links, while negative interhemispheric links were absent (see Figure 5 B).

Multigraphs created at this stage of the development of epileptic activity revealed the disappearance of mutual links between cerebellar paleocortex and cortical zones of hemispheres, which were defined in beta-2 band (see Figure 6). The maximal number of mutual positive links, which were identical to those identified in the initial multigraph before penicillin administration, was reproduced again in alpha band (9 out of 10). Besides, in this band 2 out of 3 mutual negative links were preserved.

A substantial number of mutually positive links was also reproduced in the theta band, compared to the initial character of links (before penicillin administration) – 7 out of 10. The least reproducibility of mutual positive links (2 out of 10) was registered in the delta band. The general reduction of links was also characteristic for the delta band. 5 and 4 mutual positive links, which had been observed before penicillin administration, were kept in beta-1 and beta-2 bands respectively.

The creation of the next stage of the dynamics of electrographic manifestations was characterized by the appearance of spike discharges in the ECoG of WAG/Rij rats, while the number of classical SWD was substantially reduced. Such characteristics were registered firstly in 2 out of 3 rats in right hemisphere 450 and 820 sec after the administration of the epileptogen (Figure 7A). A marked reduction in the number of mutually positive interhemispheric links was observed at this stage of epileptogenesis (Figure 7B). Thus, if during the stage with SWD there were 4 interhemispheric links, at the stage of spikes appearance and suppression of SWD, there was only one interhemispheric link. There were three mutual positive links between paleocerebellar and hemispheral cortical zones.

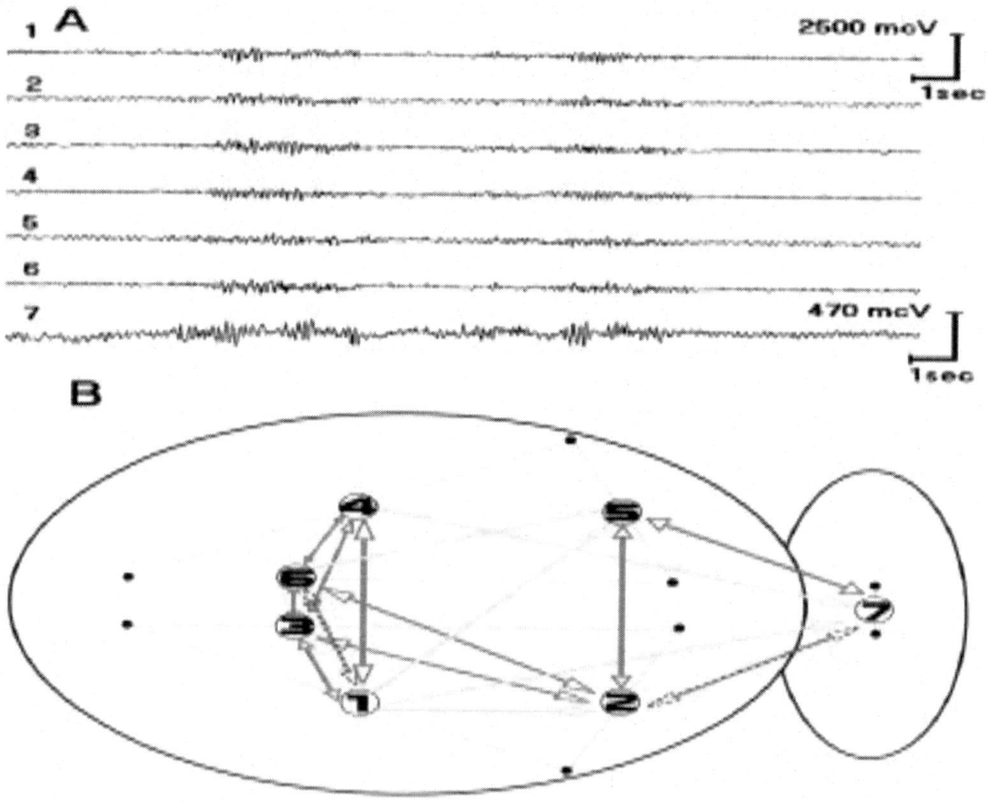


Figure 5. The activation of bursts of SWD in brain structures of WAG/rij rats under the influence of benzilpenicillin sodium salt, which was observed in 7 min from the moment of epileptogen i.p. administration (300.000 IU/ 100 g of body weight). Notes: on "A" and "B" are the same as on correspondent fragments on Figure 1.

Most pronounced reproducing of mutually positive links was observed in alpha band, when compared with the corresponding multigraph created before penicillin administration (5 out from 7) (Figure 8). Three mutual positive links were maintained in the theta band, while only two were common (in beta-2 band) with those determined before the administration of penicillin. The smallest reproducibility of mutual positive links was observed in beta-1 and delta bands (both reproduced only one link). In all bandwidths practically complete absence of negative type of links was observed – beta-2 band was an exception.

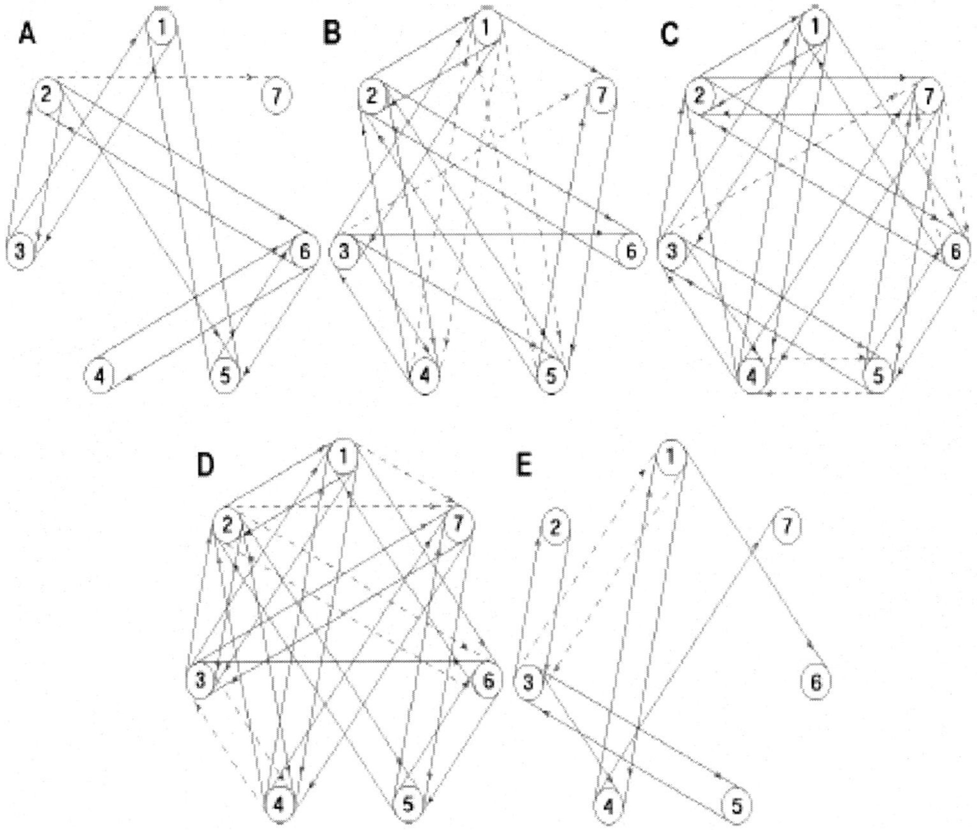


Figure 6. Polycycling multigraphs, which reflect the relationships between brain structures in WAG/rij rast in different bandwidths of EcoG during the period of penicillin- induced bursts of SWD activation. Notes: the same as on Figure 2.

The mutual interhemispheric links were not identified in beta-2 and delta band, while their number was maximal in beta-1 and alpha bands (both displayed two links). There were no links between cerebellum and hemispheres in delta and beta-1 bands, while other bands maintained the involvement of cerebellar structures into epileptogenesis at this stage of epileptogenesis development. Hence, the prevalent role of alpha-along with theta-activity in creation of interstructural “links” was pertinent for WAG/Rij rats at the stage of substitution of SWD with spikes in the course of penicillin-induced generalized epileptogenesis precipitation. It is also worth noting that delta, as well as high-frequency bands were markedly reduced in comparison with alpha and theta bands. The almost complete absence of negative type of links was also quite characteristic for this stage of epileptic activity development.

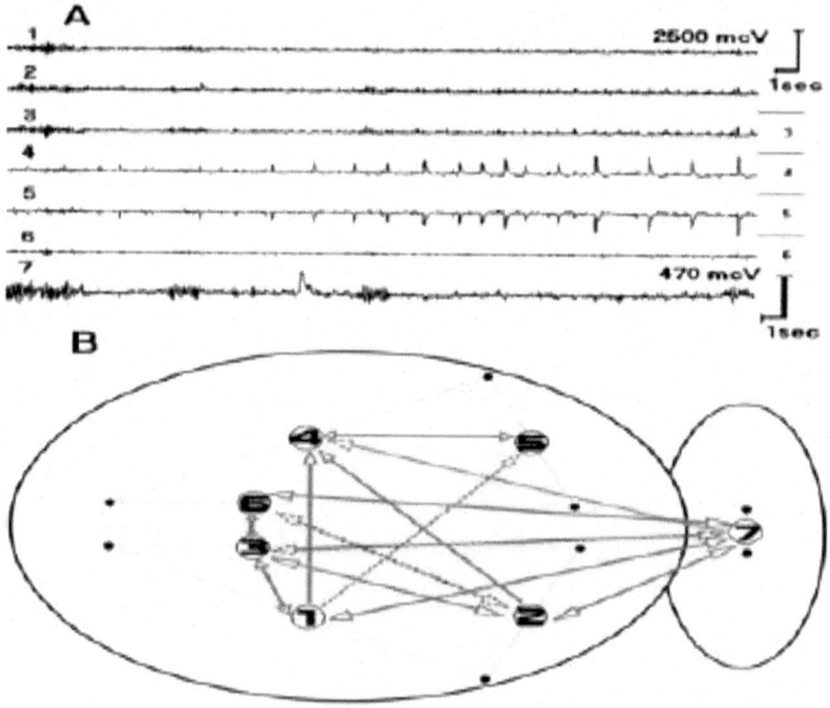


Figure 7. The appearance of spikes in brain structures and simultaneous suppression of bursts of SWD under the influence of sodium benzilpenicillin action, which was noted in 12 min from the moment of i.p. epileptogen administration (300.000 IU/ 100 g of body weight). Notes: on “A” and “B” are the same as on correspondent fragments on Figure 1.

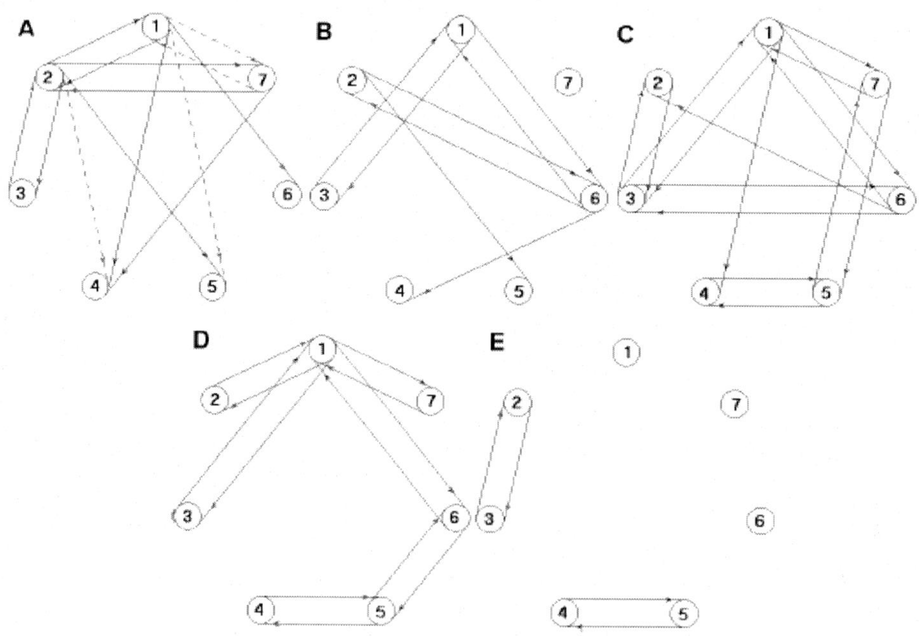


Figure 8. Polycycling multigraphs, which reflect relationships between WAG/rij brain structures in certain bandwidths of ECoG at the stage of substitution of SWD bursts with spike discharges (transition of absence epilepsy into seizure one). Notes are the same as at Figure 2.

## DISCUSSION

Obtained data revealed that ECoG manifestations of generalized absence and clonic seizures might be characterized from the point of view of the analysis of the ratio between different signals simultaneously registered via MLR method.

The comparative analysis of the whole frequency spectrum ECoG activity in Wistar and WAG/Rij rats revealed that the differences might be confined to more pronounced expression of mutual positive interhemispheric interactions in rats suffered from absence epilepsy. Besides, a more active involvement of cerebellar structures in functional links with cortical structures was also evident in WAG/Rij rats.

Most relations between structures were found in the theta-band in Wistar rats, while less pronounced they also were equally evident in high-frequency (beta-1 and beta-2) and alpha bands. At the same time functional links in rats with absence epilepsy (WAG/Rij) were most pronounced in theta-and delta, and to a less extent-in high frequency bands.

Hence, obtained data are in favor for the idea that spontaneous generation of SWD in WAG/Rij is going on in parallel with the reduction of high-frequency activity. As far as fast ECoG rhythms corresponds to arousal and activation of antiepileptic brain mechanisms (3, 10, 17), the net reduction of antiepileptic brain defense could be suspected. The marked synchronization is most pronounced in the delta band as a result.

Intensification of SWD bursts generation in WAG/Rij rats was shown as initial stage of penicillin action upon brain activity. The increase of total number of mutual positive (from 8 up to 10) as well as negative (from 2 up to 3) links was characteristic for this stage. Thus, the involvement of all structures of left hemisphere in the mutual positive interaction and the increase of the number of links between paleocerebellar cortex and hemispheres were seen during this period of epileptic activity development. Almost all mutually positive links (9 out from 10) were preserved in the structure of multigraph created in alpha band. Besides, a pronounced decrease of mutual negative links in the delta band was also found. Along with these mentioned peculiarities, a relative resistance to penicillin action of the mechanisms of rhythms generation in theta, beta-1, and beta-2 bands was observed.

At the background of precipitation of the generalized type of activity (substitution of SWD with spikes synchronized in prolonged periods) the relatively small reduction of total number of links between structures was combined with the suppression of interhemispheric functional relations. Also a high level of paleocerebellar cortex interstructural interaction has been seen. These changes were determined mainly by interaction of structures in the alpha band. Also a marked reduction of links in theta and delta as well as high-frequency bands was also seen.

Hence, obtained data demonstrates a pronounced susceptibility of mechanisms, which underlie delta-activity generation, to the action of penicillin. The reduction of links in the delta band coincided with the reduction of links in alpha band. This fact rejects the notion of the primary role played by mechanisms of desynchronization, as responsible for delta-activity suppression. The mechanisms of SWD generation, as far as it represents the antagonism between SWD and delta-waves, might be worth studying. Previously it was established that deep slow wave sleep and SWD in WAG/Rij are not compatible (18, 19). In this respect it is worth mentioning that the incompatibility of alpha and delta waves was noted with regard to so-called "rhythmical delta activity" (RDA) (5, 20). This rhythm is determined by low excitability of main neuronal cortical populations along with the almost complete absence (inactivation) of backward both positive and negative influences (5, 20). Hence, it might be assumed that under penicillin action prevalent RDA is provoked. That is why it is quite possible that greater level of "isolation" of brain structures, which was noted in form of reduction of links in delta-band is originated from RDA mechanisms, namely, from the reduction of backward negative influences. Such effects are characteristic for the penicillin action (2, 15).

It should be stressed that high number of links, which were registered in background activity of WAG/Rij rats in the delta band, might support another source of origin. Thus, its is possible that this kind of delta activity, represents non-regular delta activity (FIRDA) (20). This type of delta activity is determined by the high level of backward positive influences (20), which might be sooner connected with the facilitation of epileptogenesis.

Taking into consideration the functional antagonism between cerebellar and neocortical structures observed in the course of epileptic syndrome development (3, 10), it is possible to analyze the present data on the basis of this paradigm of interaction. Hence, while in Wistar rats links from cerebellar cortex are not directed to cortex, in the course of SWD generation in WAG/Rij rats the two-sides influences are precipitated. A further increase of the number of mutually positive links was found at early stage of penicillin induced epileptogenesis development in WAG/Rij rats. This result might be in favor that epileptogenic excitation originated from telencephalon caused the active involvement of cerebellar structures into the processes of excitability control.

It should be stressed that greater involvement of cerebellar structures into SWD bursts generation assumes some form of involvement of cerebellar structures into manifestations of absence epilepsy. For example, such manifestations as tremor (vibrisses), eye-ball movements (nystagmus-like), "starings," timely disturbances of autonomic system are also known for cerebellar hyperexcitable state and might be induced by electrical or chemical stimulations (21, 22). Moreover, there are some neurophysiologic data, namely, greater threshold of locomotor reactions induced via n.dentatus electrical stimulations in those rats prone for absence-like manifestations in the course of pentylenetetrazol-induced kindling (3), strongly suspect certain role of cerebellar – thalamo-cortical chains in the precipitation of absence like-manifestations. Hence, cerebellum might contribute substantially to thalamo-cortical loops activity engendered in the course of the generation of epileptiform manifestations.

When the involvement of frequency-specific aspects of paleocerebellar structures into more intensive interaction with brain cortex is concerned, it should be noted that the reduction of links in high-frequency bandwidth as well as delta bandwidth were the characteristic features for WAG/Rij rats in comparison with Wistar rats. That was the case both for WAG/Rij background activity and for penicillin-induced seizure syndrome. The heightening of the interaction in the alpha-band along with the relatively stable links in the theta-band was also seen in WAG/Rij rats. It might be assumed that the precipitation of generalized seizure activity is connected with a certain critical decrease of the high-frequency activity. This assumption is supported by the well known role of desynchronization in the development of cerebellar structures antiepileptic effects (3, 10).

It might be assumed that pacemakers of corresponding rhythmogenesis are in charge for the functional links between neocortical structures and paleocerebellar cortex in animals with genetic predisposition to absence epilepsy.

The increase of the links in alpha band is in favor for the involvement by the alpha-activity pacemaker (presumably thalamic nuclei) of telencephalic and cerebellar structures. The synchronous character of SWD bursts generation in mentioned structures is in favor of this possibility (13, 18, 19, 23, 24).

Hence, the obtained data suggest a principal possibility of application of MLR method for the analyses of ECoG. Proposed method of the presentation of the data serves for the better interpretation of functional relationships between brain structures.

## REFERENCES

[1] Coenen AML, Drinkenburg WHIM, Inoue M, van Luijtelaar ELJM. Genetic models of absence epilepsy, with emphasis on the WAG/rij strain of rats. Epilepsy Res 1992;12:75–86.

[2] Gloor P. Generalized epilepsy with spike and wave discharge: reinterpretation of its electrographic and clinical manifestations. Epilepsia 1990;20:571-88.

[3] Kryzhanovsky GN. Central nervous system pathology: A new approach. New York: Raven Press, 1986.

[4] Kostopoulos GK. Spike-and-wave discharges of absence seizures as a transformation of sleep spindles: the continuing development of a hypothesis. Clin Neurophys 2000;111:S27-S38.

[5] van Luijtelaar G, Coenen A. Two types of electrocortical paroxysms in an inbred strain of rats. Neurosci Lett 1986;70:393–7.

[6] Azen R, Budescu DV. The dominance analysis approach for comparing predictors in multiple regression. Psychol Methods 2003;8:129-48.

[7] Lobasyuk BA. Mapping of relationships between amplitudes and frequencies in electrocorticogram of different cortical regions in rats. Odessa Med J 2005;1:10-5 (Russian)

[8] Lvovsky EN. Statistical methods of building up of empirical equations. Moscow: High School, 1982 (Russian)

[9] Lueders H, Bustamante L, Zablow I, Krinsky A., Goldensohn EG. Quantitative studies of spike foci induced by minimal concentrations of penicillin. Electroencephalogr Clin Neurophysiol 1980;48:80-9.

[10] Godlevsky LS, van Luijtelaar ELJM, Shandra AA, Coenen AML. Cause and effect relations in disease; lessons from epileptic syndromes in animals. Med Hypothesis 2002;58:237-43.

[11] Karceski S, Mullin P. Expanding therapeutic options: devices and the treatment of refractory epilepsy. Curr Neurol ZNeurosci Rep 2004;4:321-8.

[12] Kandel A, Buzsaki G. Cerebellar neuronal activity correlates with spike and wave EEG patterns in the rat. Epilepsy Res 1993;16:1-9.

[13] Drinkenburg WH, Coenen AM, Vossen JM, van Luijtelaar ELJM. Spike-wave discharges and sleep-wake states in rats with absence epilepsy. Epilepsy Res 1991;9:218-24.

[14] Mrangoz C, Bagrici F. Effects of L-arginine on penicillin-induced epileptiform activity in rats. Jpn J Pharmacol 2001;86:297-301.

[15] Woodburry DM. Convulsant drug: mechanisms of action. In: Penry JK, Woodburry DM, eds. Antiepileptic drugs: Mechanism of action. New York: Raven Press, 1980:249-303.

[16] Paxinos G, Watson C. The rat brain in stereotaxic coordinates. New York: Academic Press, 1982.

[17] Buzsaki G, Laszlovszky I, Lajtha A, Vadasz C. Spike and wave neocortical patterns in rats: genetic and aminergic control. Neurosci 1990; 38: 323-33.

[18] Sitnikova E, van Luijtelaar G. Electroencephalographic precursors of spike-wave discharges in a genetic rat model of absence epilepsy: Power spectrum and coherence EEG analyses. Epilepsy Res 2009;84:159-71.

[19] Sitnikova E. Thalamo-cortical mechanisms of sleep spindles and spike-wave discharges in rat model of absence epilepsy: A review. Epilepsy Res 2010;89:17-26.

[20] Stam CJ, Pritchard WS. Dynamics underlying rhythmic and non-rhythmic variants of abnormal, waking delta activity. Int J Psychophysiol 1999;34:5-20.
[21] Heinen SJ, Oh DK, Keller EL. Characteristics of nystagmus evoked by electrical stimulation of the uvular/nodular lobules of the cerebellum in monkey. J. Vestib Res 1992;2:235-45.
[22] Kim JM, Jeon BS. Survivors from beta-fluoroethyl acetate poisoning show a selective cerebellar syndrome. J Neurol Neurosurg Psychiatry 2009;80: 528-32.
[23] Meeren H, van Luijtelaar G, Lopes de Silva FH, Berdiev RK, Chepurnova NE, Chepurnov SA, Coenen A. The cotico-thalamic theory for generalized spike-wave discharges. Uspehi Fiziologicheskih Nauk 2004;35:3-19 (Russian)
[24] Żygierewicz J, Blinowska KJ, Durka PJ, Szelenberger W, Niemcewicz SZ, Androsiuk W. High resolution study of sleep spindles. Clin Neurophysiol 1999;110:2136-47.

In: Considering Consciousness Clinically
Editors: Gerry Leisman and Joav Merrick

ISBN: 978-1-63484-260-0


*Chapter 18*

# DISCUSSION OF A MODEL ON HUMAN CONSCIOUSNESS

***Steven L Strauss****
Neurologist, Private Practice, Baltimore, Maryland,
United States of America

## ABSTRACT

The study of human consciousness has historically sought to align prevailing models of psychology and neuroanatomy. Behaviorism rejected mentalistic constructs and sought explanation in stimulus-response networks, the latter rooted in neuroanatomic reflex arcs. It therefore denied the existence of consciousness altogether. Information processing cognitive psychology sees mental life as the serial transformation of sensory inputs into conceptual outputs, regulated and controlled by thalamocortical pathways and increasingly abstract cortico-cortical pathways. It characterizes the content of human consciousness as the product of such neuroanatomically driven information processing. Eye movement studies of reading support constructivist psychology as uniquely capable of explaining the complex psychological phenomenon of predicting. The material basis for this psychology is the emerging neuroanatomic understanding of the primacy of feed-forward, cortico-thalamic connections. The contents of human consciousness therefore reflect not merely inputs through the sense organs, but also the outputs of subconscious mechanisms that generate predictions about the world, and seek evidence in the world for or against these predictions. Information processing therefore does not express the highest mechanisms of consciousness generation, since it is subordinate to the even deeper, purposeful efforts of the mind to make sense of the world.

## INTRODUCTION

The study of human consciousness has, quite properly, captured the attention of philosophers, psychologists, and neuroscientists. I say "quite properly" because the profundity of the subject matter demands that we not confuse distinctions in academic disciplines for real

* Correspondence: Steven L Strauss, MD, PhD, 6830 Hospital Drive, Suite 104, Baltimore, MD 21237, United States. E-mail: strauss.md@hotmail.com

epistemological boundaries. Consciousness is an achievement of evolution whose apprehension and explanation will demand broad and deep integration of knowledge.

Having said that, I want to address the topic of human consciousness from what may at first glance seem like an overly narrow angle, but which in fact opens a wide lens on how the human mind works and what it means to be a conscious human. I want to discuss the scientific study of reading. I will consider some essential aspects of the reading process. I will then consider the kinds of psychological processes that must exist in order for reading to occur as it does. I will then turn to implications that these psychological processes have for our understanding of human consciousness. Finally, I will discuss recent and emerging concepts in neuroanatomy that support this psychology of consciousness.

Everyone is familiar with optical illusions, such as the Müller-Lyer illusion, in which two bidirectional arrows of the same length appear to be unequal in length (see Figure 1a), or the one in which a straight stick placed in a glass of water appears to be bent (see Figure 1b):

I want to discuss another illusion, and what it entails for a theory of human consciousness. My example is well-known, though its implications have not been fully elucidated. It is a type of cognitive illusion, in which the source of the erroneous conclusion lies in the workings of cognitive processes.

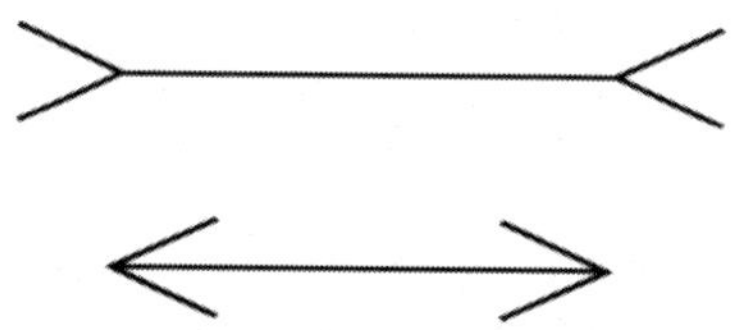

Figure 1a. Two lines of equal length appear to be of unequal length.

Consider what you believe is occurring as you read a page from a book or magazine, or, better yet, what you believe is occurring as you read a page aloud. The subjective impression most people have is that they look at each word, interpreting them individually as they proceed through the text, from left to right, top to bottom. How else could they have read the page aloud with all the right words, no wrong words, and all in the right sequence?

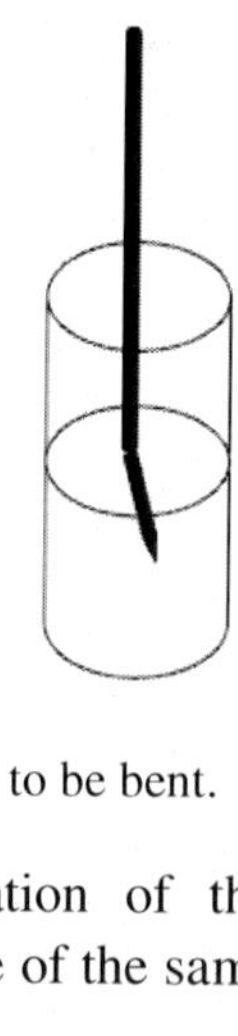

Figure 1b. A stick immersed in water appears to be bent.

What does an empirical investigation of the matter tell us? If we measure the bidirectional arrows, we find out they are of the same length. If we remove the stick from the water, we find out it is really straight. What happens if we use a piece of technology that can tell us which words the reader is really looking at, really fixating on?

Such machines, called eye-tracking machines, have been used for decades. Studies that employ them are called "eye movement studies." A virtual treasury of eye movement studies has established what the eyes do when we read. And what the eyes do is not what we subjectively sense they are doing.

The eyes do not look at each word. In fact, they only look at about two thirds of the words on the page. The eyes do not move uniformly from left to right and from top to bottom. They dart around the page, usually proceeding in the same direction as the text, but often turning around and going back. Here is an example showing the eye movements seen in typical, proficient reading (1).

The dots on the page are the places where the reader fixated, as revealed by the eye tracker. The lines show the quick, saccadic transitions from one fixation to the next. As is well-known, the eyes only transmit visual information to the brain during periods of fixation, and no information is transmitted during saccades.

In this quite typical scenario, the reader reads each word aloud, even though it is empirically clear that he or she did not fixate on each and every word, nor did the sequence of saccades and fixations proceed linearly through the text. Yet the common subjective impression of a reader is that each word was looked at, one at a time, from left to right and then top to bottom.

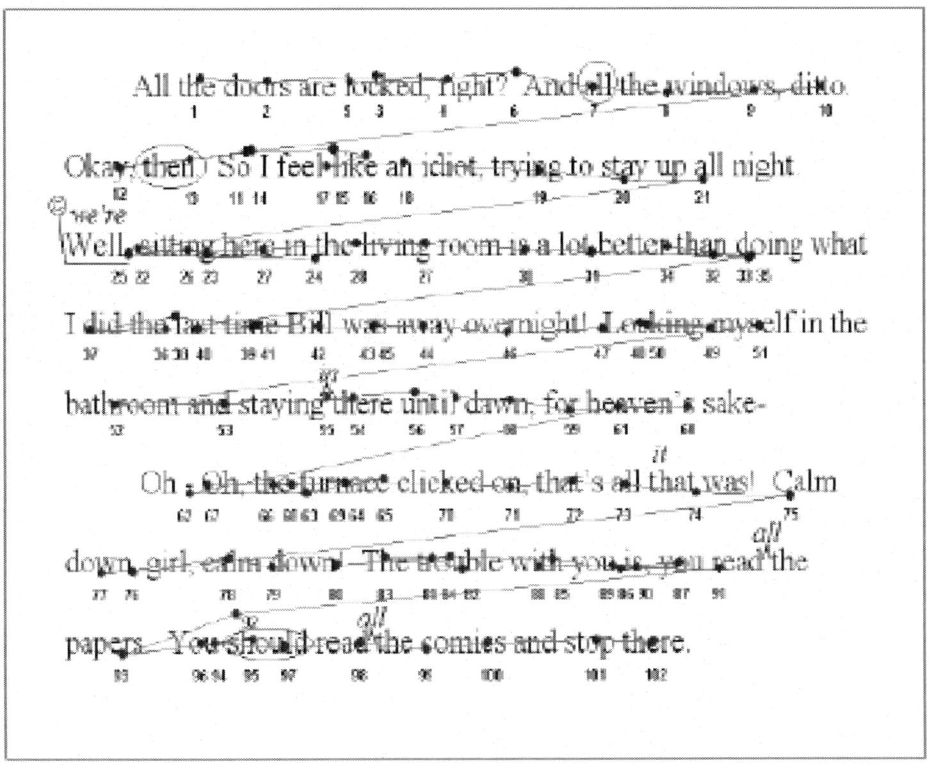

Figure 2. Eye movement sequence of a typical proficient reader (© 2003 by Eric J. Paulson and Ann E. Freeman. From Insight from the Eyes: The Science of Effective Reading Instruction. Portsmouth, NH:Heinemann).

This is the illusion of reading, which, despite having been identified by many researchers, has only achieved a full and adequate explanation via the transactional socio-psycholinguistic model of reading developed by Kenneth Goodman (2), combined with the empirical investigations of readers' eye movements carried out by Eric Paulson (3) and others. I will therefore call it the Goodman-Paulson illusion.

## EXPLAINING THE GOODMAN-PAULSON ILLUSION

How do we explain the Goodman-Paulson illusion? At the outset, we can note that it is not possible to say that individual fixations create visual fields that include large chunks of text, thereby allowing the reader to in fact look at all the words. A typical fixation has a foveal field, that is, a field of sharp focus, which spans only three to six letter spaces. A typical parafoveal field, with reduced focus, adds about fifteen additional letter spaces.

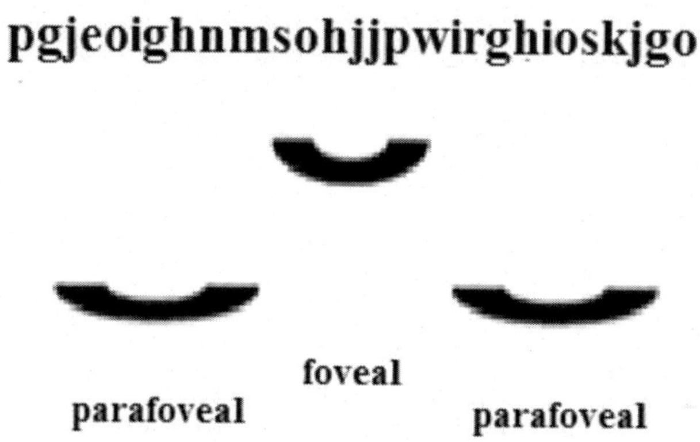


Figure 3. The fovea (area of maximum visual acuity) subsumes three to six letter spaces. Each parafovea space subsumes up to seven additional letter spaces.

If we add together all of the reader's actually fixated foveal and parafoveal territories, they do not summate to include the full size of the text.

In other words, not all the words are looked at. Analyses carried out by Goodman, Paulson, and others clearly show that many of the words that the proficient reader does not look at are "small" words. But they are not just any small words. They are the grammatically functioning class of words, the prepositions, determiners, particles, grammatical suffixes, and so on. In fact these function words and morphemes are twice as likely as content words to not get a fixation. What is interesting about this class of words from a linguistic point of view is that, in the use of language, their appearance is relatively, sometimes entirely, quite predictable. There are two reasons for this. First, grammatical words, unlike nouns, verbs, and adjectives, are a closed class of words, that is to say, they are finite in number. There is only a small inventory to choose from. New words that enter the language are "content" words, usually nouns, which are limitless. The neologistic creations of receptive aphasics typically occupy only the noun, verb, and adjective slots in sentences.

Second, the choice of a grammatical word is tightly constrained by syntax. You can say "I climbed the mountain," or "I climbed a mountain," but not "I climbed walked mountain."

Small, grammatically functioning words must occupy certain positions to render the syntax well-formed: "I climbed *and* walked *the* mountain." Syntax constrains the choices of grammatically functioning terms, and makes them relatively predictable to a language user. Therefore, the words that are not fixated by a proficient reader are often linguistically predictable.

This tells us that the proficient reader, the one who left out a full third of the words on the page when reading aloud, looked at the less predictable words and did not look at the predictable words, but merely filled them in based on predictions. The predictions themselves were based on evolving syntactic constructions and meaning. Therefore, *the illusion that we look at each word as we read is really the phenomenon whereby what we think we looked at has in fact only been predicted.*

The illusion is even deeper. Some content words are also predicted. These are the ones whose likelihood of appearing is dramatically increased by preceding text and surrounding context, and by the meanings and syntax the reader has already apprehended. If the right hand page of a book ends with the line, "*The boy kissed the ...*," and continues on the next, still unseen page, the proficient reader will say aloud the word *girl*. Or, if the story is about a boy and his dog, the good reader will say *dog*. Both syntactic information, which prompts the likely appearance of a noun, and semantic information, derived from the text meaning already carried along by the reader, aid in the correct prediction of the upcoming word. In the case of a word not even on the page, it goes without saying that it must have been "read" without having been looked at.

With the understanding that reading involves the mental construction of predictions, it is now possible to explain why the eyes sometimes regress to earlier portions of the text. If a reader predicts, then it follows that the reader must also test the predictions against incoming text. That is, the predictions must be either confirmed or disconfirmed, so the reader may return to earlier text for such confirmation or disconfirmation.

These processes can be seen in the passage discussed earlier (see Figure 2). The markings in this passage show where this reader has inserted words (*and staying <in> there until dawn*), omitted words (*And <all> the windows*), and substituted words (*That's all <that → it> was*). The reader has also corrected certain orally read words *(<we're → well> sitting here in the living room*). Except where the reader self-corrects, the oral renditions retain syntactic and semantic acceptability. There is no evidence, in other words, that the construction of meaning has gone awry. However, the self-correction occurs in a reading that renders the phrase syntactically and semantically unacceptable.

This finding is entirely what we would expect on the view that reading is, as Goodman described it, "a psycholinguistic guessing game" (2), a process by which the reader samples text cues in order to predict meanings. Meaning is *constructed* by the reader during the course of reading. Each chunk of meaning is really a tentative hypothesis, to be confirmed or disconfirmed. If confirmed, it becomes incorporated into the semantic quilt being constructed by the reader. If disconfirmed, it is discarded.

This view also explains why a proficient reader often reads aloud a word or phrase that is not on the page. As long as the produced word or phrase coheres semantically with surrounding text, the proficient reader generally does not go back and correct. As long as the meaning makes sense in the context of the passage, the reader has no reason to consider that a prediction was incorrect. Constructing coherent meaning is what counts.

But notice that, on this understanding of reading, the proficient reader is reading for meaning. The proficient reader is not reading for accurate word or letter identification. The *purposeful* nature of the event is the defining element in reading. Reading for meaning is reading. Reading to identify letters and words is not reading. Poor reading generates words that do not make sense, yet still remain uncorrected by the reader. In other words, poor reading is such because it is not reading for meaning. Compare the following good and poor readings:

In Figure 4a, the reader produces miscues, that is, words and other linguistic material that are not what is on the printed page. But these miscues are syntactically and semantically acceptable. This reader produces his or her own meaningful text, alongside or parallel to the author's text, thereby demonstrating the purposeful act of making sense of print.

The reader of 4b, on the other hand, treats reading as a word and letter identification process. The miscues are syntactically and semantically unacceptable, in the sense that the reader's own text does not express coherent meaning. The construction of meaning is sacrificed to the extent that the reader's purpose in reading is letter and word identification.

In many cases, perhaps the majority of cases, such poor reading is an artifact of instruction, and is therefore an artifact of instruction based on a scientifically incorrect view of the reading process, one which sees it as the serial identification of letters and words. As a corollary, reading is considered proficient only if it is accurate.

*front* *mailman* *dad*

- **Kay was waiting by the ^ door for the postman. Her father**
- **had promised to write her a letter. He told Kay the letter**
- **would have a blue stamp on it. Kay saw the**

*mailman* *road* *house*

- **postman walking up the street toward her home. The man was carrying a**
- **big bag. The man reached into his bag and gave Kay some letters. One of the**
- **letters**

*dad* *dad*

- **had Kay's name on it. The letter was from her father. In the letter Father told**
- **Kay he was coming home soon.**

(A)

*clis* *fare stuction* *faremin*

- **Ann's class went to visit a fire station. One of the firemen**

*clis*

- **was at the door. He said he was happy to see the class. He**

*fare trick* *trick* *lidder*

- **showed the class a big fire truck. The truck had a long ladder**

*faremin*

- **on it. The fireman let them see many things. Then the**

*clis*

- **class went back to school. They were very happy. They told**

*tieder*

- **their teacher they wanted to go again.**

(B)

Figure 4. (A) Syntactically and semantically acceptable miscues, demonstrating the purposeful act of making sense of print. (B) The miscues are syntactically and semantically unacceptable (4).

But it should now be clear that this view of reading is analogous to a scientific theory which seeks to discover the laws of physics that force a stick to bend as it enters water. In other words, it is based on an illusion. The scientific study of reading is no different from any other scientific endeavor. It seeks to differentiate that which *appears* to happen from that which *actually* happens.

The letter and word identification paradigm is, in fact, the favored view of federally funded research and federally promoted models of reading in the United States. Leading architects of this view have expressed the principles in a variety of ways. For example, according to a prominent pediatric reading researcher from Yale University, and a major architect of federal policy on reading research and instruction:

> "The task of the reader is to transform the visual percepts of alphabetic script into linguistic ones—that is, to recode graphemes (letters) into their corresponding phonemes. To accomplish this, the beginning reader must first come to a conscious awareness of the internal phonological structure of spoken words. Then he or she must realize that the orthography— the sequence of letters on the page—represents this phonology. That is precisely what happens when a child learns to read" (5).

The former director of reading research at the National Institute of Child Health and Human Development rejects the notion of guessing, i.e., predicting, in reading:

> "Scientific research, however, simply does not support the claim that context and authentic text are a proxy for decoding skills. To guess the pronunciation of words from context, the context must predict the words. But content words—the most important words for text comprehension—can be predicted from surrounding context only 10 to 20 percent of the time .... Instead, the choice strategy for beginning readers is to decode letters to sounds in an increasingly complete and accurate manner" (6).

In general, advocates of this paradigm have insisted on word-based models of reading, stating that "Unless the processes involved in individual word recognition operate properly, nothing else in the system can either" (7). But it is precisely the *empirical evidence* itself which leads to a fundamentally different understanding of reading. Reading is the process by which a reader attempts to make sense of print. Making sense is an active process of meaning construction. Each piece of meaning constructed by the reader is really a tentative hypothesis, a prediction or guess, to be confirmed or disconfirmed.

## Communication Between Mutually Impenetrable Minds

We have seen that an adequate theory of reading must explain the Goodman-Paulson illusion, in which the reader does not look at fully one-third of the words on the page despite a firm belief in having looked at all of them, and at having looked at them in a left-to-right and top-to-bottom fashion. The scientific study of reading instead informs us that words which appear in the reader's oral recitation may have been placed there by a process of predicting, and not by word identification.

This underlying phenomenon of good guessing can appear to the conscious mind as a phenomenon of accurate identification precisely because the contents of conscious awareness are generated by subconscious mechanisms.

Despite being strictly subconscious, these mechanisms can be discovered by scientific analysis. But because they are not immediately accessible to the conscious mind, the contents of that conscious mind appear to have a reality independent of the subconscious mechanisms which generated them. They appear to "already be there," waiting to be grasped by just so many acts of direct identification.

But if the scientific study of reading informs us that predicting, confirming, and disconfirming are the fundamental processes of meaning construction, then the visual material on the page is not the direct reflection of the author's intended meaning. Rather, it is the author's presentation of *clues* to meaning, selected by the author to convey his or her intended meaning.

Both the reader and the writer participate in this psycholinguistic guessing game. This is precisely how two private minds, each unable to directly access the other, communicate and exchange meanings. Minds that are not mutually interpenetrable achieve the illusion of such by exchanging *material clues* to meaning.

## TRADITIONAL ALIGNMENTS OF READING, PSYCHOLOGY, AND NEUROSCIENCE

There is a psychology that goes along with the view that readers visually fixate on each word, just as there is a psychology that goes along with the view that readers fixate selectively, building mental perceptions in the process of constructing meaning. The former, generally speaking, is called information processing cognitive psychology. The latter is called constructivist psychology.

There is a neuroscience that goes along with each of these psychologies. And there is a philosophy of consciousness that also goes along with each of these psychologies. Of course, neuroscience studies more than the human brain, psychology studies more than reading, and reading has a cultural, social, and historical dimension that propels it beyond the reach of mere psychological reductionism. As a result, neuroscience, psychology, and reading have their own logical and methodological traditions. Not all of the results of one can be easily nestled inside the paradigms of the others. Even more, each has its own set of competing models.

But because the sites of intersection of the three disciplines are certainly neither accidental nor arbitrary, they can be thought of as together constituting another well-demarcated reality -- *the neuropsychology of reading*. Attempts to align neuroscience, psychology, and reading have been part of the modern history of these fields.

Behaviorism, for example, invoked the neuroscientist's reflex arc to lend plausibility to its stimulus-response explanation of human behavior. In a typical reflex arc, a stimulus to the body evokes an observable response via the connection that exists between the sensory neuron (nerve cell) that is sensitive to the stimulus and the motor neuron that converts this energy to movement. Touching the cornea of the eye evokes contraction of the muscle that closes the eyelid. Touching the pharynx evokes a gag response.

The appeal of such a neuroscientific basis for stimulus-response psychology lay not only in providing an organic mechanism connecting the body to behavior, but in doing so without appeal to any allegedly unobservable mental categories. The latter would include notions like intentionality, purpose, and goal. This satisfied behaviorist strictures on scientific methodology, in which no reality was ascribed to any unobservable categories of an alleged mind.

Nearly a century ago, stimulus-response psychology, in turn, influenced the way linguists understood certain aspects of language. For example, Leonard Bloomfield wrote in the 1930s that the meaning of an utterance was just the set of stimuli that produced that utterance and the set of responses to it (8). One can certainly wonder how this would be observable or measureable, but at least the concept seemed consistent with the larger principles of the enterprise.

As a special case of language use, Bloomfield characterized a proficient reader as one who "has an overpracticed and ingrained habit of uttering one phoneme of the English language when he sees the letter *p*, another when he sees the letter *i*, another when he sees the letter *n*, still another when he sees the letter *m*, still another when he sees the letter *d*, and so on."(9) Bloomfield's thinking was influenced by the belief that writing was an artificial, cultural invention, unlike speech, that it was a mere "notation for speech," and therefore needed to be converted to speech before it could be interpreted. This conversion process was to proceed by applying phonics patterns to the letters. Bloomfield was a leading figure in the development of the field of phonics.

This is one example of an alignment among neuroscience, psychology, and reading. Its unifying principle is a pairing together of categories according to the formula: *A brings about B*. In neuroscience, this is the essence of the reflex arc, in which touch, pain, light, stretch, or some other physical event acting on a neuron (*A*) leads automatically, without the imposition of thought, to another neuron producing an observable movement or other physical change (*B*). In psychology, this is the essence of the stimulus (*A*)-response (*B*) formula. In reading, this is the essence of phonics, in which the visual identification of a letter (*A*) brings about the oral production of a sound (*B*).

Cognitive psychology has also sought an alignment with neuroscience. This is particularly evident in the information processing branch of the field, certainly the most influential. While information processing also turns *A* into *B*, neither *A* nor *B*, nor the mechanisms that turn *A* into *B*, have to derive, ultimately, from directly measureable phenomena residing outside the human mind. The obvious advantage of this paradigm over behaviorism is its capacity to explain problem-solving, language use, and other psychological events that require logics that go beyond associative links.

Information processing finds expression in the field of reading through what its advocates call "phonological processing" (10). The reader of an alphabetic language must process the letters on the page in order to convert them, by phonics rules, to their corresponding sounds. The sounds are then processed into words, and these, ultimately, into meaningful phrases and meaning itself.

Information processing likewise finds expression in the field of neuroscience by means of two complementary mechanisms of information flow. In the first, primary sensory information is transferred from sense receptors in the periphery to the thalamus, a structure deep in the brain which has been considered the "relay station" for sensory processing. Visual information from the eyes goes to the lateral geniculate nucleus of the thalamus. Auditory information from the ears goes to the medial geniculate nucleus of the thalamus. Tactile information from the skin goes to the dorsolateral nucleus of the thalamus. (Only the sense of smell bypasses the thalamus and goes directly to the limbic system of the brain).

This first order relay is connected to a second set of nerve fibers that now send the sensory information to the cortical surface of the brain, where they are further processed. As A.R. Luria described it more than fifty years ago, the cortical surface is itself arranged in a pattern of primary, secondary, and tertiary regions for each sensory modality (11). Thus, visual information goes to the occipital region of the brain, where the primary neurons identify color, shape, movement, and other raw visual characteristics. The secondary and tertiary neurons take the primary characteristics and assemble them into perceptual and conceptual structures – recognizable objects, scenes, and so on. Similar trains of information processing occur in the auditory cortex of the temporal region of the brain and in the tactile cortex of the parietal region. Heteromodal regions can now combine these distinct cortical sensory outputs into even more abstract mental representations.

This neuroanatomic schema for information processing has been widely described. Thalamus experts Sherman and Guillery, for example, point out that, on the "classical" view, the thalamus is "the *major relay to the cerebral cortex*" and "*the gateway to the cortex.*" According to this view, *"almost everything we can know about the outside world or about ourselves is based on messages that have had to pass through the thalamus*" (12).

In a similarly philosophical interpretation of the neuroanatomic facts, Mesulam writes:

> "Sensory information undergoes extensive associative elaboration and attentional modulation as it becomes incorporated into the texture of cognition.... The resultant synaptic organization ... allows each sensory event to initiate multiple cognitive and behavioural outcomes. Upstream sectors of unimodal association areas encode basic features of sensation such as colour, motion, form and pitch. More complex contents of sensory experience such as objects, faces, word-forms, spatial locations and sound sequences become encoded ... by groups of coarsely tuned neurons. The highest synaptic levels .... bind multiple unimodal and other transmodal areas into distributed but integrated multimodal representations. Transmodal areas in the midtemporal cortex, Wernicke's area, the hippocampal–entorhinal complex and the posterior parietal cortex provide critical gateways for transforming perception into recognition, word-forms into meaning, scenes and events into experiences, and spatial locations into targets for exploration. All cognitive processes arise from analogous associative transformations of similar sets of sensory inputs" (13).

Again, the three areas of neuroscience, psychology, and reading have achieved a mutual alignment. The neuroscience describes sequential synaptic connections and electrical transmission from the periphery to the center, psychology describes the mechanisms of information processing, and reading emphasizes the more specific notion of phonological processing.

## THE ALIGNMENT OF CONSTRUCTIVISM AND NEUROSCIENCE

Until recently, an alignment has existed between yet another psychological paradigm and its corresponding view of reading, though without a neuroanatomic correlate. Coexisting with behaviorism and information processing, constructivist psychology has sought to explain the mechanisms by which mental structures create meanings and other cognitive representations that go "beyond the information given" (14). Qualitatively different from behaviorism, it acknowledges the existence of mental structures that exist independently of associative links of experience. Qualitatively different from information processing, it projects its own representations of reality prior to the presentation of information.

Thus, constructivism has figured significantly in models of how humans make sense of their world. Crucial notions include purposefulness and goal-directed behavior. A typical expression of constructivist psychology can be seen in the now widely accepted view of speaking as an intentional act, in which purpose and goal initiate and drive the event:

> "In planning an utterance, there is an initial phase in which the speaker decides on a purpose for his next move. This decision will depend on a variety of factors, and not in the last place on the speaker's needs, beliefs, and obligations" (1).

In reading, constructivist psychology relies on the notion that the act itself is a purposeful, non-automatic effort to make sense of print. The reader makes a decision to attend to this goal. It is a deliberate, purposeful decision. Therefore, making sense of print can be thought of as the purposeful, goal-directed intention of the reader that is analogous to the speaker's intention of conveying a message.

The constructivist model of reading derives from this crucial insight, that reading, a receptive language process, is as much a purposeful act as speaking, a productive language process. More generally, both receptive language processes (listening, reading, sign interpretation) and productive language processes (speaking, writing, signing) are purposeful acts. The purpose that drives receptive language is making sense. Making sense is not an automatic, passive response to sensory input, but rather the active interplay between the subject and the interlocutor, intimately driven by the subject's own mental representation of purpose, itself derived from background knowledge and prior experience. Fundamentally, every newly constructed representation of meaning is tentative, subject to adjustment according to incoming linguistic material. Thus, meaning is simultaneously a prediction of what will come next, what counts as making sense. Incoming linguistic material provides evidence for or against the language user's predictions. Tentative meanings are revised accordingly.

Emerging insights in neuroanatomy are beginning to clarify the mechanisms by which the human brain constructs predictions and then finds evidence for or against them, that is, confirms or disconfirms them. Thus, we are beginning to understand the neuroanatomic bases of constructivist psychology.

This emerging understanding turns on a new interpretation of the relationship between the cortex of the brain and the thalamus, and, more generally, between the cortex and deeper structures. Though traditionally understood as a relay station that passes peripheral incoming sensory data to the cortex, the thalamus is an organ that also receives input from the cortex. This is well-known, and is traditionally viewed as representing *cortical feedback*, that is to say, the means by which the cortex puts the breaks on the thalamus, or otherwise modifies thalamic activity. The very term *feedback* connotes the idea that the thalamocortical projection is primary and fundamental, whereas the corticothalamic projection is secondary and subordinate.

But it has been pointed out by a number of neuroscientists that the ratio of corticothalamic nerve fibers to thalamocortical nerve fibers is 10:1. How can this strictly quantitative fact be accommodated within a framework that regards corticothalamic fibers as subordinate to thalamocortical ones? One might use the metaphor of brakes on an automobile that have to be more powerful than the car's accelerator in order to create deceleration. But there is no electrical evidence that so many more corticothalamic nerve fibers than thalamocortical ones are needed to decelerate the thalamocortical impulses.

Other neuroanatomic facts challenge the traditional notion that the primary processes utilize thalamocortical tracts. For example, distinct thalamic components emit electrical discharges unconnected to one another in decorticated preparations (the cortex has been experimentally removed), whereas the electrical discharges are synchronized when the cortex and the thalamus remain intact. Thus, the cortex organizes the thalamic electrical activity, raising the idea that perhaps the corticothalamic pathways are primary, feed-forward neural tracts and the thalamocortical ones operate in a subordinate, feedback fashion (16).

This indeed would be a quite plausible explanation of the 10:1 pattern. The cortical activity is primary in the sense that it operates independently of thalamic input, but sends its products to the thalamus for further processing. Whereas information processing conceives of the thalamus as a relay station for sensory input, directing this input to the cortex, where more refined and elaborate processing now takes place, a different psychology is needed to rationalize a system in which cortical representations precede the arrival of sensory information. A number of neuroscientists have noted that this is precisely the psychology of predicting (16, 17).

The cortical surface creates visual, auditory, and tactile representations of the world. It creates semantic representations associated with language and other semiotic systems. If an auditory-visual scene is projected by the cortex, and if such a scene is regarded as a prediction, then the role of the thalamus is to search for sensory information that will confirm or disconfirm the cortex's representation.

Thus, when the cortex creates a mental representation that includes purpose (I am looking for my car in the parking lot), memory (my car is red, I parked it in the last row), and a variety of other social and physical knowledge and beliefs (I parked legally so it won't be towed), the thalamus is directed to seek out a car shape, a red color, and a location. Checking one's license plate number, or looking for the tell-tale scratch on the front bumper, is not routinely necessary. Relatively few thalamically-sensitive sensory findings will suffice to tell the cortex that the car has been correctly identified.

Thus, the cortex and corticothalamic tracts, along with cortical connections to other subcortical structures, constitute the organ of prediction (16, 17). The thalamocortical tracts constitute the organ of confirmation and disconfirmation.

Now we can more easily appreciate that there is no neuroanatomic obstacle to constructivist psychology. To the contrary, constructivist psychology can claim, as behaviorism and information processing have, that it has a strong, empirically-supported neural underpinning.

It goes without saying that the mere existence of a neuroanatomic basis for constructivist psychology is, in itself, no argument for a constructivist model of the reading process. An empirically based model of reading must be based on a detailed study of the phenomenon of reading. It is not given in advance what level of psychological complexity will be needed to explain how readers interact with print to arrive at meaning.

But the converse is also true. The absence of a neuroanatomic basis for constructivist psychology is no argument against constructivist psychology or a constructivist model of reading. There is an accepted system of formal logic, without which much scientific research cannot proceed. But no neuroscientist has a clue how the brain accomplishes syllogistic reasoning.

It is therefore a simple matter to dismiss the silly claims of some neuroscientists that constructivist models of reading "*ascribe children's reading problems entirely to sociological or educational factors and totally deny the biology*" (9). Even before the most recent elucidations of cortical and subcortical connections, reading scholars were quite aware that the brain is the organ that enables and instantiates reading. Until a neuroanatomic basis for constructivism is discovered, constructivist models of reading anticipate what neuroscientists will one day discover.

## CONSTRUCTIVISM AND CONSCIOUSNESS

The neuroanatomic basis of constructivism is now emerging in broad outline. The cortex initiates mental events. It generates mental representations of reality, guided and influenced by one's immediate purposes and goals. It feeds its representations forward to subcortical structures, like the thalamus, directing these to obtain sensory evidence that will fill in any blanks, or confirm and disconfirm any representations that are tentative and predictive in character. These pieces of evidence revise and reshape the cortex's mental representations, leading to another feed forward transmission to the subcortical structures.

It is likely that billions of such cortex-subcortex-cortex loops operate simultaneously. It is likely that this is the constant, non-stop living activity of the whole brain. It is likely that the neuroanatomic manifestation of psychological purpose is the identification and recruitment of specific regions of the cortex likely to solve the problem at hand. It is likely that these loops are solving many problems at once, though conscious awareness allows us to see the end result of just one problem at a time. Subconscious problem solving can assert itself into conscious awareness, however, such as when a conversation is suddenly arrested by the emergence of the answer to a question one had been considering for the past week.

This type of experience feels like what happens when one's conversation is interrupted by the thalamic transmission of an immediately noxious stimulus, like the pin you may have just sat down on. A conscious visual representation of the pin, provoked by a tactile experience that does not involve actually seeing the pin itself, demonstrates recruitment of the cortex. One gets up from the chair and reaches for the offending object. This can only be a cortically-based predictive behavior. Visual identification of the pin, tactile identification of it with one's fingers, provides the confirmatory feedback.

The difference between the two events is that the latter is immediate and driven by an immediate sensory stimulus. The bottom-up part of the loop asserts itself over the top-down part. Both are ways in which a loop that is both active and in conscious awareness can be displaced by a different loop, as the working space for conscious awareness permits only one loop at a time.

The conception of the brain as an organized assembly of integrated loops of cortical-subcortical tracts still provides no explanation for how cortical activity is driven, that is, how plans, goals, thoughts, and so on are generated in the first place. It is likely that they emerge in a most rudimentary form, a general notion for example of what one's behavioral or ideational goal is. This is revised and refined by the loops themselves, in a process that adds texture and detail to the emerging cortical representation. This is the same problem implicit in Noam Chomsky's notion of "stimulus free" thought:

> "... the normal use of language is not only innovative and potentially infinite in scope, but also free from the control of detectable stimuli, either external or internal. It is because of this freedom from stimulus control that language can serve as an instrument of thought and self-expression, as it does not only for the exceptionally gifted and talented, but also, in fact, for every normal human being" (18).

While it is no doubt true that our conscious reflection on language use may fail to identify internal or external "stimuli" that prompt the construction of thought, we do not wish to conclude that specific instances of language use arise from a vacuum. The source of answers to this problem must be the subconscious mind, from which only one representation can enter into and occupy the space of conscious awareness. But the panoply of neural loops remains fully active whether in subconscious thought or held before us in conscious awareness.

Psychologies and their neuroanatomical correlates have generated broad views on the nature of human consciousness. Obviously, the conception of consciousness aligns neatly with its presumed neuroanatomic and psychological substrate.

Before Burrhus F Skinner (1904-1990) purged consciousness from the study of human behavior, John B Watson (1878-1958) wrote that "the time has come for psychology to discard all reference to consciousness," because it is as non-provable as the soul, and because "*the Behaviorist must discard from his scientific vocabulary all subjective terms*" (19).

Information processing psychologists, though acknowledging consciousness, characterize it as "the *capacity to integrate information*."(20) Tononi further describes the neuroanatomic substrate of this capacity in the claim that "*consciousness is generated by a distributed thalamocortical network that is at once specialized and integrated....*" According to Tononi, "*a well-functioning thalamocortical system is essential for consciousness.*" Indeed, "*the fact that consciousness as we know it is generated by the thalamocortical system fits well with the information integration theory, since what we know about its organization appears ideally suited to the integration of information.*"

This notion of consciousness has nothing to say about the purposeful element in human mental life, since this lies outside the mechanisms of automatic information processing. Yet, as we have seen, purpose is a defining criterion in understanding how the conscious mind makes sense of the world. Making sense of written language in particular is purposeful for both the author and the reader.

And it has nothing to say about the primacy of cortico-thalamic tracts over thalamocortical tracts, since it regards the former as informationally subordinate to the latter, providing only a feedback influence. Yet we have seen how a new understanding of corticothalamic connections is emerging within neuroscience to explain otherwise recalcitrant and theoretically embarrassing facts, like the 10:1 ratio discussed earlier.

## CONCLUSION

The emerging understanding of the relationship between the cortex and the thalamus and its associated constructivist psychology demands a different view of consciousness. It demands, in fact, that we recognize the tentative, inexact nature of the relationship between the conscious brain and the world. It demands that the purposeful non-automaticity of this relationship be incorporated into an adequate explanatory model of the conscious human brain. It identifies the active pursuit of sense and meaningfulness as the fundamental non-automatic purpose in conscious behavior. And, finally, it identifies predicting and the testing of prediction as the subconscious mechanisms which enable the conscious human mind to construct sense and meaningfulness.

Both behaviorism and information processing psychology see an organism acted upon by the outside world. On the former view, the organism responds behaviorally to stimuli. On the latter view, the organism processes information. Neither sees the organism as the subjective agent in its own behavior and thinking. This is the fundamental limiting factor in these two psychologies, one rectified immediately by constructivism. If constructivism is the psychology that allows us to appreciate the subjective element in human action, then human consciousness, which is generated by that psychology, must express that subjective element as well.

## REFERENCES

[1] Paulson EJ Freeman AE. From insight from the eyes: the science of effective reading instruction. Portsmouth, NH: Heinemann, 2003.

[2] Goodman K S. Reading: a psycholinguistic guessing game. J. Read Specialist 1967;6:126-35.

[3] Paulson EJ. Are oral reading word omissions and substitutions caused by careless eye movements? Read Psychol 2002;23(1):45-66.

[4] Nichols, C.D., Literacy assessment: Theory and practice. URL: http:// clem.mscd.edu/~nicholsc/ literacy/modfied_miscue_analysis_assignm.htm.Accessed March 2, 2009.

[5] Shaywitz S. Dyslexia. Scientific American 1996;275(5):98-104.

[6] Lyons GR. Why reading is not a natural process. Educ Leadership 1998;55:14-8.

[7] Adams M. Beginning to read: thinking and learning about print. Cambridge, MA, MIT Press, 1990:1.

[8] Bloomfield L. Language. New Delhi, Motilal Banarsidas, 1994.

[9] Bloomfield L. Teaching children to read. In: Bloomfield L, Barnhart CL, eds, Let's read: a linguistic approach, Detroit, MI: Wayne State University Press, 1961:19-42.

[10] Shaywitz S. Overcoming dyslexia: A new and complete science-based program for reading problems at any level. New York: Alfred A Knopf, 2003.

[11] Luria A R. The working brain: an introduction to neuropsychology. New York, Basic Books, 1973.

[12] Sherman S M, R W Guillery. Exploring the thalamus and its role in cortical function, 2nd ed. Cambridge, MA: MIT Press, 2006.

[13] Mesulam M-K. From sensation to cognition. Brain 1998;121:1013-52.

[14] Bruner J. Beyond the information given: studies in the psychology of knowing, New York, Norton, 1973.

[15] Levelt W J M. Speaking: from intention to articulation. Cambridge, MA, MIT Press, 1989.
[16] Destexhe A. Modeling corticothalamic feedback and the gaiting of the thalamus by the cerebral cortex. J Physiol (Lond) 2000;94:394-410.
[17] Hawkins J. On intelligence, New York: Henry Holt, 2004.
[18] Chomsky N. Language and mind, New York, Harcourt Brace Jovanovich, 1972.
[19] Watson J B. Behaviorism, New York: People's Institute, 1925.
[20] Tononi G. An information integration theory of consciousness, BMC Neuroscience, 2004;5(42):1-22.

# SECTION TWO: ACKNOWLEDGMENTS

In: Considering Consciousness Clinically
Editors: Gerry Leisman and Joav Merrick
ISBN: 978-1-63484-260-0


*Chapter 19*

# ABOUT THE EDITORS

**Gerry Leisman, MD, PhD, BCFM** is an Israeli neuroscientist educated in the United Kingdom and the United States in medicine, neuroscience, and biomedical engineering at the University of Manchester, the City University of New York, and Union University. He holds the position of Director of the National Institute for Brain and Rehabilitation Sciences-Israel in Nazareth, Israel and Professor of Rehabilitation Sciences in the Department of Mechanical Engineering at O.R.T.-Braude College of Engineering in Karmiel, Israel. He is also Professor of Restorative Neurology at the Universidad de Ciencias Medicas de la Habana, Faculdad Manuel Fajardo, Institute for Neurology and Neurosurgery in Havana Cuba. He is also Editor-in-Chief of the journal Functional Neurology, Rehabilitation and Ergonomics.

He has been active since the early 1970s in the promotion of consciousness as a scientifically tractable problem, and has been particularly influential in arguing that consciousness can now be approached using the modern tools of neurobiology and understood by mechanisms of theoretical physics. He has also been influential in examining mechanisms of self-organizing systems in the brain and nervous system for cognitive function exemplified by his work in optimization, memory, kinesiology, consciousness, death, autism and dyslexia. It is in this context that he was one of the first to identify functional disconnectivities in the brain and nervous system.

Also, in his long work in rehabilitation sciences, he has been able to apply the tools of systems sciences in human rehabilitation and technology development to optimize human performance for those who have sustained traumatic brain injury and in those with developmental disabilities.

He has served as a consultant to the USA National Sciences Foundation. He was elected Fellow of the Association for Psychological Science in 1990, a Life Fellow of the American College of Forensic Examiners in 1994, Senior Member of the Institute for Electrical and Electronic Engineers Engineering in Medicine and Biology Society in 1988, a Life Fellow of the Institute for Functional Neurology and Rehabilitation and a recipient of its Lifetime Achievement Award in 2011. He is the author of over 500 papers, texts, chapters and holder of patents. He is the co-author of a text with Dr. Robert Melillo on "Neurobehavioral disorders of childhood from an evolutionary perspective." E-mail: gerry.leisman@staff.nazareth.ac.il

**Joav Merrick, MD, MMedSci, DMSc,** born and educated in Denmark is professor of pediatrics, child health and human development, Division of Pediatrics, Hadassah Hebrew University Medical Center, Mt Scopus Campus, Jerusalem, Israel and Kentucky Children's Hospital, University of Kentucky, Lexington, Kentucky United States and professor of public health at the Center for Healthy Development, School of Public Health, Georgia State University, Atlanta, United States, the medical director of the Health Services, Division for Intellectual and Developmental Disabilities, Ministry of Social Affairs and Social Services, Jerusalem, the founder and director of the National Institute of Child Health and Human Development in Israel. Numerous publications in the field of pediatrics, child health and human development, rehabilitation, intellectual disability, disability, health, welfare, abuse, advocacy, quality of life and prevention. Received the Peter Sabroe Child Award for outstanding work on behalf of Danish Children in 1985 and the International LEGO-Prize ("The Children's Nobel Prize") for an extraordinary contribution towards improvement in child welfare and well-being in 1987. E-mail: jmerrick@zahav.net.il

In: Considering Consciousness Clinically
Editors: Gerry Leisman and Joav Merrick
ISBN: 978-1-63484-260-0


*Chapter 20*

# About the National Institute for Brain and Rehabilitation Sciences, Nazareth, Israel

The National Institute for Brain and Rehabilitation Sciences is a research center based in Nazareth Israel associated with that city's three hospitals. The Institute's purpose is to investigate solutions for all issues that impede the optimization of human performance. The ultimate aim is to get every individual from infancy to the fourth age, to contribute to himself, family and society at the highest level.

## Research agenda

As such, the Institute's research agenda includes the nature of stress, environmental toxins, and diet on pregnancy and on the development of the infant and child, neuroeducation, biomechanics cognitive motor interactions, autism and developmental disabilities, biological rhythms, ergonomics of classroom and workplace, functional and restorative neurology, aging, post-stroke and traumatic brain injury, and neurodegenerative conditions all from a management perspective. The institute is involved not in basic, but rather translational research, where the end result may be better programing or the development of patents and new technologies, but clearly the optimization of human potential.

## International and national collaborations

The Institute is formally affiliated with laboratories in the USA, the M.I.N.D. Institute at M.I.T. in Cambridge Massachusetts, The Institute for Neurology and Neurosurgery in Havana Cuba, s well as the Manuel Fajardo University of the Medical Sciences in Havana, and cooperative relationships with the School of Medicine of Bar-Ilan University in Safed, Israel and the National Institute of Child Health and Human Development, Jerusalem, Israel.

## Contact

Gerry Leisman
Director and Professor of Neuro- and Rehabilitation Sciences
O.R.T.-Braude College of Engineering
Karmiel, Israel
Professor of Restorative Neurology
Manuel Fajardo University of the Medical Sciences
Havana, Cuba
51 Snunit
POB 78 Kamiel, Israel
E-mail: gerry.leisman@staff.nazareth.ac.il

In: Considering Consciousness Clinically
Editors: Gerry Leisman and Joav Merrick

ISBN: 978-1-63484-260-0


*Chapter 21*

# About the National Institute of Child Health and Human Development in Israel

The National Institute of Child Health and Human Development (NICHD) in Israel was established in 1998 as a virtual institute under the auspices of the Medical Director, Ministry of Social Affairs and Social Services in order to function as the research arm for the Office of the Medical Director. In 1998 the National Council for Child Health and Pediatrics, Ministry of Health and in 1999 the Director General and Deputy Director General of the Ministry of Health endorsed the establishment of the NICHD.

## Mission

The mission of a National Institute for Child Health and Human Development in Israel is to provide an academic focal point for the scholarly interdisciplinary study of child life, health, public health, welfare, disability, rehabilitation, intellectual disability and related aspects of human development. This mission includes research, teaching, clinical work, information and public service activities in the field of child health and human development.

## Service and academic activities

Over the years many activities became focused in the south of Israel due to collaboration with various professionals at the Faculty of Health Sciences (FOHS) at the Ben Gurion University of the Negev (BGU). Since 2000 an affiliation with the Zusman Child Development Center at the Pediatric Division of Soroka University Medical Center has resulted in collaboration around the establishment of the Down Syndrome Clinic at that center. In 2002 a full course on "Disability" was established at the Recanati School for Allied Professions in the Community, FOHS, BGU and in 2005 collaboration was started with the Primary Care Unit of the faculty and disability became part of the master of public health course on "Children and society." In the academic year 2005-2006 a one semester course on "Aging with disability" was started as part of the master of science program in gerontology in our collaboration with the Center for Multidisciplinary Research in Aging. In 2010 collaborations with the Division of Pediatrics, Hadassah Hebrew University Medical Center, Jerusalem, Israel around the National Down Syndrome Center and teaching students and residents about intellectual and developmental disabilities as part of their training at this campus.

## Research activities

The affiliated staff have over the years published work from projects and research activities in this national and international collaboration. In the year 2000 the International Journal of Adolescent Medicine and Health and in 2005 the International Journal on Disability and Human Development of De Gruyter Publishing House (Berlin and New York) were affiliated with the National Institute of Child Health and Human Development. From 2008 also the International Journal of Child Health and Human Development (Nova Science, New York), the International Journal of Child and Adolescent Health (Nova Science) and the Journal of Pain Management (Nova Science) affiliated and from 2009 the International Public Health Journal (Nova Science) and Journal of Alternative Medicine Research (Nova Science). All peer-reviewed international journals.

## National collaborations

Nationally the NICHD works in collaboration with the Faculty of Health Sciences, Ben Gurion University of the Negev; Department of Physical Therapy, Sackler School of Medicine, Tel Aviv University; Autism Center, Assaf HaRofeh Medical Center; National Rett and PKU Centers at Chaim Sheba Medical Center, Tel HaShomer; Department of Physiotherapy, Haifa University; Department of Education, Bar Ilan University, Ramat Gan, Faculty of Social Sciences and Health Sciences; College of Judea and Samaria in Ariel and in 2011 affiliation with Center for Pediatric Chronic Diseases and National Center for Down Syndrome, Department of Pediatrics, Hadassah Hebrew University Medical Center, Mount Scopus Campus, Jerusalem.

## International collaborations

Internationally with the Department of Disability and Human Development, College of Applied Health Sciences, University of Illinois at Chicago; Strong Center for Developmental Disabilities, Golisano Children's Hospital at Strong, University of Rochester School of Medicine and Dentistry, New York; Centre on Intellectual Disabilities, University of Albany, New York; Centre for Chronic Disease Prevention and Control, Health Canada, Ottawa; Chandler Medical Center and Children's Hospital, Kentucky Children's Hospital, Section of Adolescent Medicine, University of Kentucky, Lexington; Chronic Disease Prevention and Control Research Center, Baylor College of Medicine, Houston, Texas; Division of Neuroscience, Department of Psychiatry, Columbia University, New York; Institute for the Study of Disadvantage and Disability, Atlanta; Center for Autism and Related Disorders, Department Psychiatry, Children's Hospital Boston, Boston; Department of Pediatric and Adolescent Medicine, Western Michigan University Homer Stryker MD School of Medicine,

Kalamazoo, Michigan, United States; Department of Paediatrics, Child Health and Adolescent Medicine, Children's Hospital at Westmead, Westmead, Australia; International Centre for the Study of Occupational and Mental Health, Düsseldorf, Germany; Centre for Advanced Studies in Nursing, Department of General Practice and Primary Care, University of Aberdeen, Aberdeen, United Kingdom; Quality of Life Research Center, Copenhagen, Denmark; Nordic School of Public Health, Gottenburg, Sweden, Scandinavian Institute of Quality of Working Life, Oslo, Norway; The Department of Applied Social Sciences (APSS) of The Hong Kong Polytechnic University Hong Kong.

## Targets

Our focus is on research, international collaborations, clinical work, teaching and policy in health, disability and human development and to establish the NICHD as a permanent institute at one of the residential care centers for persons with intellectual disability in Israel in order to conduct model research and together with the four university schools of public health/medicine in Israel establish a national master and doctoral program in disability and human development at the institute to secure the next generation of professionals working in this often non-prestigious/low-status field of work.

## Contact

Joav Merrick, MD, MMedSci, DMSc
Professor of Pediatrics, Child Health and Human Development
Medical Director, Health Services, Division for Intellectual and Developmental Disabilities, Ministry of Social Affairs and Social Services, POB 1260, IL-91012 Jerusalem, Israel.
E-mail: jmerrick@zahav.net.il

In: Considering Consciousness Clinically
Editors: Gerry Leisman and Joav Merrick
ISBN: 978-1-63484-260-0


*Chapter 22*

# About the Book Series "Functional Neurology"

**Functional neurology** is a book series with publications from a multidisciplinary group of researchers, practitioners and clinicians for an international professional forum interested in the broad spectrum of neurology and human development.

- Vojdani A. Neuroimmunity and the brain-gut connection. New York: Nova Science, 2015.
- Leisman G, Merrick J, eds. Neuroplasticity in learning and rehabilitation. New York: Nova Science, 2015.
- Leisman G, Merrick J, eds. Considering consciousness clinically. New York: Nova Science, 2015.

## Contact the editors

Professor Gerry Leisman, MD, PhD
Director, The National Institute for Brain and Rehabilitation Sciences Biomechanics Laboratory, Department of Mechanical Engineering
ORT-Braude College of Engineering
Snunit 51 Street
POBox 78, IL-21982 Karmiel, Israel
E-mail: gerry.leisman@staff.nazareth.ac.il

Professor Joav Merrick, MD, MMedSci, DMSc
Medical Director, Medical Services
Division for Intellectual and Developmental Disabilities
Ministry of Social Affairs and Social Services
POBox 1260, IL-91012 Jerusalem, Israel
E-mail: jmerrick@zahav.net.il

# SECTION THREE: INDEX

# INDEX

## A

## B

## C

## D

## E

## F



## G

## H



## I

## J



## K



## L

## M

## N

## O



## P

## Q



## R

## S

## T

## U



## V



## W



## Y